Neurology and Neurobiology

EDITORS

Victoria Chan-Palay
University Hospital, Zurich

Sanford L. Palay
The Harvard Medical School

ADVISORY BOARD

Albert J. Aguayo
McGill University

Günter Baumgartner
University Hospital, Zurich

Masao Ito
Tokyo University

Tong H. Joh
Cornell University Medical
College, New York

Gösta Jonsson
Karolinska Institute

Bruce McEwen
Rockefeller University

William D. Willis, Jr.
The University of Texas, Galveston

NEUROPLASTICITY, LEARNING, AND MEMORY

NEUROPLASTICITY, LEARNING, AND MEMORY

Proceedings of a Symposium held at the University of Toronto,
Scarborough, Ontario, March 25, 1986

Editors

N.W. Milgram
Colin M. MacLeod
Ted L. Petit
Department of Psychology
Division of Life Sciences
University of Toronto
Scarborough, Ontario, Canada

ALAN R. LISS, INC., NEW YORK

Address all Inquiries to the Publisher
Alan R. Liss, Inc., 41 East 11th Street, New York, NY 10003

Copyright © 1987 Alan R. Liss, Inc.

Printed in the United States of America

Library of Congress Cataloging-in-Publication Data
Neuroplasticity, learning, and memory.

    (Neurology and neurobiology; v. 29)
    1. Memory—Physiological aspects—Congresses.
2. Learning—Physiological aspects—Congresses.
3. Neuroplasticity—Congresses. I. Milgram, N.W.
(Norton William) II. MacLeod, Colin M. III. Petit,
Ted L. IV. Series. [DNLM: 1. Learning—physiology—
congresses. 2. Memory—physiology—congresses.
3. Neuronal Plasticity—congresses. W1 NE337B v.29 /
WL 102 N4995 1986]
QP406.N53   1987   153.1   87-3932
ISBN 0-8451-2731-4

Contents

Contributors

D.L. Alkon, Section on Neural Systems, Laboratory of Biophysics, IRP, NINCDA-NIH, Marine Biological Laboratory, Woods Hole, MA 02543 **[17]**

B. Bank, Section on Neural Systems, Laboratory of Biophysics, IRP, NINCDA-NIH, Marine Biological Laboratory, Woods Hole, MA 02543 **[17]**

D.A. Coulter, Section on Neural Systems, Laboratory of Biophysics, IRP, NINCDA-NIH, Marine Biological Laboratory, Woods Hole, MA 02543 **[17]**

J.F. Disterhoft, Department of Cell Biology and Anatomy, Northwestern University Medical School, Chicago, IL 60611 **[17]**

B.J. Farnell, Departments of Physiology and Medicine, Faculty of Medicine, University of Toronto, Toronto, Ontario M5S 1A8, Canada **[45]**

Eva Fifkova, Department of Psychology, University of Colorado, Boulder, CO 80309 **[61]**

Peter Graf, Department of Psychology, University of Toronto, Toronto, Ontario M5S 1A1, Canada **[279]**

Gwen O. Ivy, Division of Life Sciences, University of Toronto, Scarborough, Ontario M1C 1A4, Canada **[125]**

Edward W. Kairiss, Department of Psychology, University of Otago, Dunedin, New Zealand **[173]**

Colin M. MacLeod, Division of Life Sciences, University of Toronto, Scarborough, Ontario M1C 1A4, Canada **[xi,1]**

Etan J. Markus, Division of Life Sciences, University of Toronto, Scarborough, Ontario M1C 1A4, Canada **[87]**

Donald R. Crapper McLachlan, Departments of Physiology and Medicine, Faculty of Medicine, University of Toronto, Toronto, Ontario M5S 1A8, Canada **[45]**

N.W. Milgram, Division of Life Sciences, University of Toronto, Scarborough, Ontario M1C 1A4, Canada **[xi,1]**

Ted L. Petit, Division of Life Sciences, University of Toronto, Scarborough, Ontario M1C 1A4, Canada **[xi,1,87]**

Ronald J. Racine, Department of Psychology, McMaster University, Hamilton, Ontario, Canada **[173]**

The numbers in brackets are the opening page numbers of the contributors' articles.

Menahem Segal, Center for Neurosciences, The Weizmann Insitute of Science, Rehovot, Israel [265]

P.H. St. George-Hyslop, Departments of Physiology and Medicine, Faculty of Medicine, University of Toronto, Toronto, Ontario M5S 1A8, Canada [45]

Earl Thomas, Department of Psychology, Bryn Mawr College, Bryn Mawr, PA 19010 [199]

Richard F. Thompson, Department of Psychology, Stanford University, Stanford, CA 94305 [151]

Robert Thompson, Department of Physical Medicine and Rehabilitation, University of California Irvine, College of Medicine, Orange, CA 92668 [231]

Wayne A. Wickelgren, Department of Psychology, University of Oregon, Eugene, OR 97403 [301]

Elna Yadin, Department of Psychology, Bryn Mawr College, Bryn Mawr, PA 19010 [199]

Jen Yu, Department of Physical Medicine and Rehabilitation, University of California Irvine, College of Medicine, Orange, CA 92668 [231]

Preface

This volume grew out of a symposium held at the Scarborough Campus of the University of Toronto in March of 1986. The symposium brought together scientists of diverse backgrounds in psychology and neurobiology who share a primary interest in understanding learning and memory. The researchers invited to take part represented the current range of perspectives on the problem, from the study of the physiology of neurons to work on amnesia in adult humans. It was our hope that a mutually beneficial cross-fertilization of ideas would result; happily, both the participants and the audience indicated that the symposium succeeded in this goal.

This book is intended to capture the diversity of approaches and the excitement of the research, as well as to foster further interdisciplinary contact. We believe such communication to be essential to the complete understanding of the operation of learning and memory that we all seek. In addition to the participants in the symposium, we recruited a number of other investigators in the field to contribute chapters to the book. In this way, we hoped to display the breadth and the depth of the research on learning and memory mechanisms. As we will discuss in our introductory chapter, there have been important new advances on a number of fronts, and an examination of these under a common umbrella is certainly timely.

As with any enterprise of this sort, we have a number of people to thank for their assistance. To begin, we wish to acknowledge the major contribution of our students to the symposium. The student body as a whole, via the Student Council, helped with funding and mechanics. We are especially grateful, though, to the students in the Neuroscience Programme, who not only assisted with funding but also contributed much time and effort to making sure the conference was successful. We could not have done it without them, and we are particularly grateful for the yeoman service of George Thorne and Surrinder Toor.

We of course thank the Division of Life Sciences and the Scarborough Campus for their support, financial and otherwise. One of the advantages of working in a smaller campus environment is the fluid interaction it permits. And we should not forget the participants, who came from all over North America and gave interesting (and even inspiring) talks. We truly enjoyed their participation.

Finally, in preparing this book, we appreciated the advice and encouragement of the staff of Alan R. Liss, Inc. As well, we are grateful to Lucy Willard and most especially to Brenda Brown for putting so much effort and care into making the manuscripts look good in final form. We trust that you, the reader, will find these chapters interesting and informative, and we hope that you will share with us the fascination of uncovering the operation of learning and memory.

N. W. Milgram
Colin M. MacLeod
Ted L. Petit
Scarborough, Ontario
December 1986

Neuroplasticity, Learning, and Memory, pages 1–16
© 1987 Alan R. Liss, Inc.

NEUROPLASTICITY, LEARNING AND MEMORY

N. W. Milgram, Colin M. MacLeod, and Ted L. Petit

Division of Life Sciences, University of
Toronto, Scarborough Campus, Scarborough,
Ontario M1C 1A4   CANADA

This is an exciting time to be involved in the
study of learning and memory. Regardless of perspective,
it is fair to say that advances in our understanding are
accruing at an ever accelerating pace. We are closing in
on the mechanisms that underlie the most remarkable feature
of the nervous system -- its ability to change and, in so
changing, to represent experience in a lasting way. From
uncovering the cellular basis of memory to determining the
nature of amnesic disorders, great strides are being made.
The purpose of this book, and of the symposium out of which
it grew, is to bring together researchers in the many areas
that make up the study of learning and memory. The purpose
of this chapter is to set out the basic issues and to
provide an introduction to the chapters that follow.

The symposium which provided the impetus for this
volume arose from our interest in the modifiability of the
nervous system, a collection of different kinds of changes
that have come to be called neuroplasticity. We know that
both the structure and the physiology of neurons can be
modified by providing specific experiences. As the
succeeding chapters will show, we also know a good deal
about the mechanisms. We even possess the tools to allow
us to graft embryonic neurons into adult brains where they
will establish functional synaptic connections with host
tissue. Such discoveries have established that plasticity
is an inherent property of the nervous system, as
biologists and psychologists have long assumed. It is no
longer far-fetched to suggest that we will be able to
identify how the nervous system is modified during learning

and how stable memories are formed.

These developments in neurobiology are paralleled by revolutionary changes in the conceptual framework of experimental psychology. In the past quarter century, the cognitive approach has largely replaced the long entrenched and sterile behaviorism which dominated psychological thought for much of this century. A major contribution of this cognitive approach has been to emphasize that learning and memory are dynamic processes which create and use central representations of specific events and relations. Moreover, in an information processing framework, it has been possible to set out specific (and testable) models of how events are encoded, stored, and retrieved. These models necessarily constrain neurobiological thinking about learning and memory, and vice versa. Just as we do not want to build conceptual models of cognitive functioning which are incompatible with our understanding of nervous system function, we do not want to propose neurobiological models that cannot accommodate cognitive abilities as we understand them. The strong implication is that we must work together if we are to gain a full appreciation of the nature of learning and memory.

The first goal of this chapter is to survey the progress that has been made in understanding learning and memory. We also will take this as an opportunity to define terms with an aim toward providing a bridge between experimental psychologists and neurobiologists. Because this chapter will present an overview of recent developments in both disciplines, at points it will seem elementary to one group of researchers or the other. We believe, nevertheless, that this somewhat tutorial level is worthwhile, and we hope this will allow each group to gain an increased appreciation for what the other group is doing.

SOME BASIC DEFINITIONS OF LEARNING AND MEMORY

What do we mean by terms like learning, memory, and plasticity? Before beginning to discuss them in detail, we think it valuable to provide some working definitions, although we are aware of the risks involved in such an undertaking. One strategy is to resort to dictionary definitions, so that (according to Webster) "learning" becomes "gaining or acquiring knowledge of or skill in" and "memory" means "the power, capacity or faculty of the mind by which it retains the knowledge of past events or ideas." "Plasticity" would then be "the capability of change or modification." In fact, these are fair definitions at a global level, but scientists demand more precise definitions. Let us consider each of these terms in turn.

To an experimental psychologist, learning is any relatively long-lasting change in behavior that is contingent upon the occurrence of a specific event or events. An important addition of this definition to that of the dictionary is its emphasis on behavior, an observable entity. Of course, this definition has its ambiguities, too. Psychologists are keenly aware of the learning-performance distinction. We cannot be certain whether something has been learned without appropriate demonstration. On the other hand, a demonstration of an apparently learned response does not guarantee that learning has occurred, just as the absence of such a response does not preclude learning having occurred. For example, amnesics had been thought to be unable to form new memories, yet we now can establish that learning often does occur, but that it may be inaccessible to conscious recollection.

A neurobiologist might attempt to refine this definition further by insisting that there must also be a corresponding change in neuronal responsiveness that does not stem from incidental factors such as changes in metabolism, biochemical deficiencies, or organic damage. This definition would not obviate the learning-performance distinction; one need only substitute "performance" for "neuronal responsiveness". Still, these definitions are becoming increasingly precise, despite continuing to cover a broad range of phenomena. Thus, one need grapple no longer with the issue of learning in one-celled organisms, or other complex organisms which still lack true nervous systems.

Learning can be subdivided further into types of learning, a major distinction being that of associative versus nonassociative learning. Associative learning requires that a connection be established between two or more events due to their contiguity in time, space, or some other dimension of experience. Classical conditioning of a cue to a situation, so that the previously neutral cue comes to signal the situation, is the most frequently studied example. The antithesis of this type of learning, nonassociative learning, involves only a single stimulus. Habituation, a waning in responsiveness to repeated stimulation, is the most often studied example here.

Each of these types of learning must have some impact on the nervous system -- the contingency must be stored and the repetition must be represented. The distinction may be critical, however, since much of the work on human learning and memory involves associative learning (see, e.g., Anderson & Bower, 1973), while some of the most prominent work with animal models has used the nonassociative paradigm (see, e.g., Kandel, 1979). Thus, Kandel's elegant studies elucidating the mechanisms underlying sensitization and habituation in aplysia, a marine snail, take a very different route than do Anderson's (1983) studies of language processing. We might reasonably expect that the rules governing the two types of behavioral changes will turn out to be considerably different. How generalizable are these diverse studies that all go under the heading of learning? This is a fundamental question.

There are some grounds for suggesting that the degree of overlap depends on the learning paradigm employed. The work described by Coulter et al. in this volume indicates a surprising resemblance in mechanisms underlying classical conditioning in hermissenda, an invertebrate, and in the rabbit. The critical cellular change appears to be the same in both species: It relates to a modification of a specific ion channel. Cross-species comparisons on the same or similar tasks can be very useful in understanding the continuity of learning.

Now we will turn our attention to memory. The first thing to realize is that it is extremely difficult to disentangle learning and memory. Memory is a reflection of the retention, durability and specificity of learning; put more simply, memory is a consequence of learning. To complicate matters, learning is itself often dramatically affected by what is already held in memory. We can measure memory in general by behavior and neuron responsiveness, but there are many subprocesses to memory. As with learning, a failure to remember does not imply that the representation no longer exists. There must also be neural processes that permit the retrieval of what has been learned previously. When retrieval succeeds, we remember; when it fails, we sometimes spontaneously remember at a later time, or sometimes not at all. We simply do not know whether memories can ever be completely lost, or whether they are permanent but become irretrievable. Still, we do have some useful ideas about how memory might work.

Every introductory psychology text makes the distinction between short-term memory (STM) and long-term memory (LTM). Although in recent years this distinction is associated primarily with the model set forth by Atkinson and Shiffrin (1968), it can be traced back through William James (1890) and on to Aristotle (Sorabji, 1972). Basically, STM is a state wherein some representation of the outside world is held in a labile form, subject to many potential sources of disruption. STM has a small capacity and is of brief duration, and can be thought of as a kind of "working memory", the part of which we are conscious. It appears to be intact even in many deeply amnesic patients who seem unable to acquire long-lasting memories. LTM, then, is the more permanent memory on which the dictionary definition focused.

Experimental psychologists have been particularly interested in the possibility that there exist more than one kind of memory. The STM-LTM distinction is one of several such dichotomies. Thus, we distinguish within LTM a semantic memory that holds general knowledge and an episodic memory that is autobiographical in content (Tulving, 1972, 1983). Or, we separate procedural knowledge -- knowledge of skills, or how to perform some action -- from declarative knowledge -- knowledge of facts (Squire, 1986). In this volume, for example, Graf distinguishes between implicit and explicit memory. If a person is asked to remember a specific event, then reliance is placed on explicit memory. If, however, something from the past influences present behavior without the intention to remember, then this is an instance of implicit remembering. The theoretical importance of such distinctions is indicated by the finding that amnesic patients often show extreme deficits in explicit memory while appearing to have normal implicit memory.

The evidence from experimental psychology of

different memory systems strongly suggests that there are
also different underlying neural substrates. The brain
lesion literature in animals provides compelling support
for this assumption. For example the research described in
this volume by Thompson and Yu indicates that the effects
of brain damamge on memory depend upon the task. On the
one hand, the visual cortex appears essential for visual
discrimination learning, but not for a nonvisual
discrimination (e.g., inclined plane). Conversely, the
mediodorsal thalamus is critical for the nonvisual but not
for the visual discrimination. On the other hand, Thompson
and Yu have also discovered a collection of structures
which are critical for all sorts of memory tasks, which
they have labeled a "general memory system." These
structures appear to mediate processes such as attention
and motivation, which are necessary for learning and for
performance although it has not been established that they
are involved in the actual storage of information.

Clearly, there is more to defining learning and
memory than would be realized on the basis of consulting a
dictionary. While we have been trying to tie together the
experimental psychology and the neurobiology as we go, our
focus has been on the former. Still, it was the
neurobiological work that led to this compilation, and our
point has been to emphasize that different kinds of
learning and memory may well involve different processes
and potentially rely on different neurological substrates.
It is here that the plasticity of the system comes into
play, the issue to which we turn now.

NEUROPLASTICITY

Like the STM-LTM distinction, introduced by James
(1890) and not really of major influence until the 1960s,
plasticity has a long past but a short history.
Interestingly, James attempted to explain habit formation
(or learning) using this concept. For him, plasticity was
"the possession of a structure weak enough to yield to an
influence, but strong enough not to yield all at once" (p.
105). He went on to write that "organic matter, especially
nervous tissue, seems endowed with a very extraordinary
degree of plasticity of this sort" (p. 105). His clear
intention here was to hinge modifiability of behavior on a
corresponding modifiability of the nervous system. He also

recognized, however, that plasticity subserved other functions as well.

Over the years, plasticity has continued to be thought of as the quality of the nervous system that underlies long-lasting behavioral change. However, the term also has been used more and more in a generalized sense to refer to any kind of experience-dependent modification in neural structure or function. Thus, all of the following (and others) have been considered as instances of neuroplasticity: growth and death of cells during development; structural modifications induced in intact neurons by brain damage; changes in transmission characteristics following neural activation; changes in density of receptors; and development of grafted embryonic tissue in host nervous systems. These examples certainly indicate that plasticity can refer to many, diverse phenomena. Yet it also seems clear that at least some kinds of plastic changes are not relevant to learning and memory processes. Axonal regeneration, for example, is an adaptive response to injury, yet it is difficult to see any relevance to learning. Of course, it may turn out to be the case that they share the same underlying cellular mechanisms.

There are three general categories of neural events which have been referred to as examples of plastic neural events. The first -- developmental plasticity -- applies to changes which occur early in an organism's development. Early on, cellular potentiality is remarkable. It becomes more restricted as neurons grow (and discard) processes. These plastic processes are mediated largely by internal events such as the chemical environment and growth patterns occurring in other cells. Environmental factors, such as those related to level of general stimulation, also can produce profound effects on neural growth (Rosenzweig, 1984). There is also considerable plasticity in the establishment of synaptic connectivity. Not only is the size of synapses subject to external influence, but the number of synapses is variable as well. Petit and Markus raise the intriguing suggestion that the same kinds of changes occur during normal learning. It is widely accepted that synaptogenesis continues until adulthood and that the molecular composition of the synapses in adult animals is similar to that of developing animals. This makes more likely the possibility that the cellular

mechanisms producing synaptic modifications are the same
during development and learning.

In considering development, it is appropriate to
discuss changes at both ends of the continuum. Aging is
characterized by a progressive decrease in behavioral
modifiability. We know surprisingly little about the
cellular mechanisms underlying the aging process, but we
would expect that they would incorporate a decline in
plasticity. The work described in this volume by Ivy
suggests that there is a specific group of enzymes
(thiol-proteinases) that becomes progressively inactive
during aging and produces a disruption of the machinery
involved in normal cellular maintenance. Ivy's work
demonstrates that interfering with these enzymes produces
anatomical changes in the cells of young rats which are
strikingly similar to those seen in aged rats. This class
of enzymes has also been proposed to control the changes in
synaptic responsiveness which underlie learning (Lynch &
Baudry, 1984). Thus, the cellular changes and the decrease
in behavioral modifiability may both result from changes in
the activity of common enzymes. Alternatively, the changes
in plasticity may be a result of secondary cellular
modifications: It is possible that aging causes changes in
plasticity rather than the reverse.

A second general category of plasticity is provided
by anatomical plasticity, which refers to distinct changes
in cellular structure that are experientially induced.
These events occur after normal developmental growth and
differentiation have ceased. Hebb (1949) generally is
credited with providing the impetus for a renewed search
for growth processes which occur during learning, although
the basic idea is not at all new. In fact, James (1890)
again suggested this and also proposed a mechanism. In
discussing habits as being due to brain plasticity, he
wrote: "The only impressions that can be made upon them are
through the blood, on the one hand, and through the
sensory-nerve roots, on the other; and it is to the
infinitely attentuated currents that pour in through these
latter channels that the hemispherical cortex shows itself
to be so peculiarly susceptible. The currents, once in,
must find a way out. In getting out they leave their
traces in the paths which they take. The only thing they
can do, in short, is to deepen old paths or to make new
ones."

We now know that both James and Hebb were at least partially right. A variety of studies have shown that such prominent changes in structure can be induced by neural activation produced with chemical, electrical or environmental stimulation. Some of these changes are reviewed in the chapters by Petit and Markus and by Fifkova, including dendrites, dendritic spines, and also synaptic terminals. Indeed, there is evidence that entirely new synapses can be formed under certain conditions, a point also taken up by Segal in his chapter on the grafting of neural tissue between organisms. These kinds of findings have become so firmly established that the capacity of additional neuronal growth now is taken for granted. It is worthwhile to point out that as recently as 1949 the dogma was that, after birth, the only thing nerve cells could do was die.

Having established that such changes can occur, considerable effort is being devoted to understanding the mechanisms that promote them. There is a surprising degree of consensus to the suggestion that a critical first step is an inflow of calcium (see the chapters by Coulter et al., Fifkova, McLachlan & George-Hyslop, and Petit & Markus). The next step -- the actual induction of a physical change -- is still problematic. The work described by Fifkova introduces a novel possibility. Neurons contain the same kinds of proteins which are responsible for muscular contraction: Perhaps the activation of these proteins (by calcium) can induce changes in neuronal shape leading to an increase in synapse size and connectivity. Naturally, calcium can also influence other aspects of cellular function. An alternative is suggested by very recent evidence that calcium influx due to neural activation can initiate gene expression (Greenberg, Ziff & Greene, 1986). This result raises the possibility of a biochemical coding for excitation-induced structural changes.

Certainly, we need more research to determine the functional significance of these structural changes. Like so much of the research on learning and memory, this work has been largely correlational. Two areas of study which might assist in clarifying the role of these changes are (1) comparative studies focusing on several different regions of the nervous system, and (2) studies establishing a functional (i.e., causal) link between synaptic change and learning. We need to answer questions such as whether there are uniquely modifiable areas of the nervous system (most work has focused on limbic and neocortical structures thus far), and whether preventing the formation of structural changes would predictably influence learning and memory processes.

The third category of neuroplasticity is physiological plasticity. This can be thought of as a change in level of responsiveness, threshold of firing, or pattern of activation which can be related to experienced events. For example, Thomas's work shows that behavioral conditioning can produce consistent changes in firing pattern. Whether the change is an increase or a decrease depends both on the nature of the conditioned stimulus and on which anatomical structure is sampled. An unusual example is provided in the findings described by Segal: It appears that grafting of embryonic tissue can restore the pattern of slow-wave electroencephalographic activity (theta) after that activity has been disrupted by brain damage. However, the restored activity occurred only when the animals were inactive, while theta normally occurs during activity.

Although it seems reasonable to suggest that plastic physiological changes have underlying structural correlates, this may not always be the case. First, there may be short-term changes which have no structural basis other than a change in ionic concentration. Thus, repeated activation could lead to an accumulation of intracellular calcium, which in turn could produce a short-term change in transmitter release. Such short-term potentiation effects may relate to transient memory processes (Racine, Milgram, & Hatner, 1983). As well, the region of interest may be remote from -- but synaptically connected to -- the locus of change. This may be the case for many of the types of cells discussed by Thomas. Further, the plastic change could be at the subcellular level, and thus not evidenced in a change in synaptic size or number. The articles by Coulter et al. and by McLachlan and George-Hyslop propose this kind of change.

Possibly the most important example of physiological plasticity is the phenomenon of long-term potentiation (LTP) which is dealt with in the chapter by Racine and Kairiss. There appears to be a specific set of

pathways which become modified when they are activated
above some threshold level. Since this modification can
last for several days (or longer), LTP has been suggested
as a possible basis for memory. This conception receives
support from the work described by McLachlan and
George-Hyslop, who report a suppression of LTP in brain
tissue taken from animals treated with aluminum salts, a
treatment which also produces memory deficits.

On the other hand, there are some problems relating
LTP to other work on memory. LTP does decay, but far more
rapidly than does normal memory. As well, the hippocampus,
the structure most responsive to LTP, is not critical for
storing memories (see the chapter by Thompson and Yu). It
seems more likely that LTP assists in the storage of memory
but does not provide the only substrate. As Racine and
Kairiss stressed, all of this underlines the importance of
distinguishing the plasticity at the cellular level from
the plasticity involved in normal learning. An entirely
different set of rules may be involved.

THE MODEL SYSTEM APPROACH

The study of normal learning has proved to be
extraordinarily difficult and even frustrating. For much
of this century, a disproportionate amount of attention was
paid to understanding learning in the laboratory rat. A
major outcome was acceptance of the Harvard law of animal
behavior which asserted that "In the end, the rat will end
up doing what it damn well pleases." One of the problems
was the difficulty in making clear to the uncooperative rat
what, exactly, it was supposed to learn. Inevitably, far
more learning went on than was desired or intended, and it
was difficult to know what the measures really told us.

This difficulty from a behavioral perspective has
parallels in the complexity of neural organization. For
example, Thompson and Yu provide evidence in their chapter
that there are multiple, quasi-independent systems which
participate in the learning and remembering involved in any
task. In addition, as we have already discussed,
investigators of human memory recognize that there are many
different ways to retain experience and to use it at a
later time. Wickelgren's chapter, for example, illustrates
the degree of complexity required to model such processes

using (as he would be the first to admit) an oversimplified nervous system.

The model system approach is one way to deal with the complexities of the problem. If we can understand certain specific principles in the context of a simpler system, be it mathematical or invertebrate, perhaps we can relate these to more complex systems. This approach has considerable appeal, as evidenced in the chapters by Richard Thompson, Racine and Kairiss, and Coulter et al. Numerous insights have been gleaned from this approach. However, the inevitable tradeoff arises; one danger is that this approach tends to distract one from the "big picture". Thus, although LTP is a manifestation of the kind of plasticity which could play a role in learning, as we have pointed out previously, there are some problems with this model. Moreover, most people working in this field have tended to ignore or avoid the difficulties, focusing instead on the features which are common to LTP and normal learning.

A related drawback of this approach is the danger of overgeneralization. A number of nontrivial leaps may be required to move from invertebrate to vertebrate, from one kind of learning to another, and from the cellular level to the intact organism. Such generalizations often are open to question on evolutionary grounds, given their basis in species from markedly divergent lines. Of course, there are also potential logical problems when it comes to generalizing from single cells to intact systems, which may involve many diverse cell types and a variety of nonlinear interactions among them.

We do not mean to challenge the value of model system approaches. To the contrary, they have opened avenues that were previously unreachable. However, the complexity of normal mammalian learning should not provide an excuse to avoid studying the problem. The discoveries based on analysis of model systems should be scrutinized carefully to determine their utility in furthering our understanding of more complex learning. While some model systems have provided specific predictions about human or mammalian learning, others may have a more restricted range of generality.

LOCUS OF THE ENGRAM

The final issue which warrants discussion here is that of the locus of memory in the nervous system. There are at least four quite different theoretical perspectives. The first is that memories are discretely localized. Intuitively, most people find this conception to be the easiest to understand because it corresponds with our perception of the organization of the external world: Objects are located (stored) in specific places. This sort of intuitive approach also works in designing machines, in that computers store information at specific addresses. However, there is evidence that the brain may work differently. Thus, Lashley (1929) showed that memory for maze learning could survive extensive damage to the neocortex. He then devoted most of the rest of his scientific career to an unsuccessful attempt to discover the locus of memory.

It now appears probable that we will be able to identify a discrete locus for some memories. Memories in the invertebrate, hermissenda, apparently can be stored in an identifiable cell. The research summarized by Thompson shows that a relatively simple classically conditioned response can be localized to a discrete region within the cerebellum. Such work raises the intriguing possibility that the cerebellum may serve as a site of storage for relatively simple kinds of motor learning. Eventually, it may be possible to relate this notion to the arguments for different kinds of memories put forward by experimental psychologists.

The second alternative is that memory is organized in a distributed neural assembly, as proposed by Hebb (1949). Such circuitry would probably involve both cortical and subcortical structures, as well as their interconnections. As a consequence, it is also likely that there would be considerable built-in redundancy. Such a theoretical formulation is consistent with the fact that memories show a surprising resistance to brain damage. It would also be suitable for handling multisensory problems like maze learning. Here, animals use visual and olfactory cues, but cognitive and emotional elements are also involved. While such a conception is intuitively appealing (and consistent with a large body of literature), it is difficult to demonstrate experimentally. To our knowledge, no instance of the location of such circuitry has been reported.

The third alternative does not focus on the site of synaptic change at all, but emphasizes more molar properties of organization. Gestalt psychology's field theory, Lashley's (1929) concept of mass action, and Pribram's (1971) holographic theory can be considered within this framework. This kind of approach generally has been advocated to account for perceptual learning, but it also relates to the evidence that memories can survive extensive brain damage.

The work reported by Thompson and Yu provides a fourth alternative. Apparently, certain kinds of complex memories can be seriously disrupted by lesions in any one of several distinct subcortical structures. On this basis, Thompson and Yu suggest that there is a general memory system in which these structures are involved. Of course, the problem of distinguishing storage from retrieval deficits makes strong conclusions difficult here, just as it does in the cognitive literature on human memory. Still, their work does serve to underline the pervasive problems in trying to locate memory. Like learning, memory is probably complexly organized, involving participation of a number of diverse neural systems.

Not surprisingly, these issues remain unresolved despite the rapid overall progress that has been made in the field. There may be no resolution other than to point out that the question concerning where memory is located is not necessarily the right question upon which to focus. Once we recognize that neither learning nor memory represent unitary processes, it becomes clear that the storage of memories will depend upon what has been learned. Thus, the multisensory maze learning tasks preferred by Lashley probably required that rats store visual, olfactory and auditory cues. Each of these sensory systems has projections to various subcortical regions as well as to the neocortex. It is not so difficult to see that such learning might survive extensive removal of cerebral cortex, while highly discrete learning such as eyelid conditioning might depend on a highly localized neuronal circuit. After all, these are different kinds of learning.

CONCLUDING COMMENTS

The issues which we have discussed in this chapter have been discussed elsewhere in the past. What is new is that the clarification or resolution of them is now much more than a remote possibility. The most impressive achievements in neurobiology have been the advancements in knowledge at the cellular and subcellular levels. Future work should seek to establish not only what initiates these molecular changes but also which molecules can serve as a memory substrate, how the memory system is organized in the brain, and how all this ties in with gene expression. For experimental psychologists, the major advancements have been in characterizing normal and amnesic memory, and in describing different categories of performance that suggest different types of memory. Too often, these achievements have been completely divorced one from the other, no doubt to the detriment of both. Our hope is that this will not continue, and that we will find ways to build the necessary bridges between our disciplines on the way to a complete understanding of the marvels of learning and memory.

ACKNOWLEDGEMENTS

Preparation of this chapter was facilitated by grants from the Natural Sciences and Engineering Research Council of Canada to each of the three authors.

REFERENCES

Anderson, JR (1983). "The Architecture of Cognition." Cambridge, MA: Harvard University Press.
Anderson, JR, Bower, GH (1973). "Human Associative Memory." New York: Wiley.
Atkinson RC, Shiffrin, RM (1968). Human memory: A proposed system and its control processes. In Spence, KW, Spence, JT (eds): "The Psychology of Learning and Motivation, Vol 2." New York: Academic Press.
Greenberg, ME, Ziff, EB, Greene, LA (1986). Stimulation of neuronal acetylcholine receptors induces rapid gene transcription. Science, 243: 80–83.
Hebb, DO (1949). "The Organization of Behavior." New York: Wiley.

James, W (1890). "Principles of Psychology." New York: Holt.

Kandel, ER (1979). Cellular aspects of learning. In Brazier, MAB (ed): "Brain Mechanisms in Memory and Learning: From the Single Neuron to Man." [International Brain Research Organization Monograph Series, Vol 4.] New York: Raven Press.

Lashley, KS (1929). "Brain Mechanisms and Intelligence." Chicago: University of Chicago Press.

Lynch, G, Baudry, M (1984). The biochemistry of memory: A new and specific hypothesis. Science, 224: 1057-1063.

Pribram, KH (1971). "Languages of the Brain." Englewood Cliffs, NJ: Prentice-Hall.

Racine, RJ, Milgram, NW, Hafner, S (1983). Short-term potentiation phenomena in the rat limbic forebrain. Brain Res, 260: 217-231.

Rosenzweig, MR (1984). Experience, memory and the brain. Amer Psychol, 39: 365-376.

Sorabji, R (1972). "Aristotle on Memory." Providence, RI: Brown University Press.

Squire, LR (1986). Mechanisms of memory. Science, 232: 1612-1619.

Tulving, E (1972). Episodic and semantic memory. In Tulving, E, Donaldson, W (eds): "Organization of Memory." New York: Academic Press.

Tulving, E (1983). "Elements of Episodic Memory." Oxford: Oxford University Press.

Neuroplasticity, Learning, and Memory, pages 17–43
© 1987 Alan R. Liss, Inc.

PERSISTENT CONDITIONING-SPECIFIC CHANGES OF POST-SYNAPTIC
MEMBRANE CURRENTS IN HERMISSENDA AND HIPPOCAMPUS

D.A. Coulter, J.F. Disterhoft, B. Bank,
and D.L. Alkon
Laboratory of Biophysics, IRP, NINCDA-NIH
at The Marine Biological Laboratory
Woods Hole, MA 02543

Many possibilities have been proposed as cellular
storage mechanisms of learning and memory. These include
changes in synaptic morphology (Fifkova and Van Harreveld,
1977; Greenough, 1984; Lee et al., 1980; Tsukahara, 1984),
alterations in synaptic efficacy (Lynch and Baudry, 1984;
Mamounas et al., 1984), and/or use-dependent modifications
of channel properties in existing neurons or neuronal
processes (Alkon, 1980; Alkon, 1984; Alkon et al., 1985;
Disterhoft et al., 1986; Hawkins et al., 1983; Walters and
Byrne, 1983; Woody et al., 1986; Woollacott and Hoyle, 1977;
Hoyle, 1982). Recent work in our laboratory has revealed a
remarkable similarity in the mechanism of conditioning-
induced increases in neuronal excitability between
Hermissenda, a nudibranch mollusc, (Alkon, 1984; Alkon et
al., 1985) and rabbits (Disterhoft et al., 1986; Coulter et
al., 1985, 1986) following Pavlovian classical conditioning.
These changes in two disparate phyla involve channel
property alterations, specifically persistent reductions of
potassium and calcium currents. Transient alteration in
potassium and/or calcium currents has been shown to occur
in many systems in response to neuromodulator exposure.
Substances acting in this way include noradrenaline (Dunlap
and Fischback, 1981; Galvan and Adams, 1982; Madison and
Nicoll, 1982), acetylcholine (Cole and Nicoll, 1984;
Halliwell and Adams, 1982; Benardo and Prince, 1982)
histamine (Pellmar, 1986; Haas and Konnerth, 1983) and
serotonin (Segal, 1980). This conservation of mechanism
between neuromodulation and the cellular storage of
experience across phyla may reflect activation of common
second messenger systems, i.e., similar cellular machinery

may be activated initially during both storage of learned associations and neurohumoral modulation across phyla.

In this chapter, we describe and compare the changes in conductances occurring in Hermissenda photoreceptor and rabbit hippocampal pyramidal cells at least one day after Pavlovian conditioning of intact animals, and discuss the possible biochemical mechanisms which may underlie these alterations.

HERMISSENDA: BEHAVIORAL MODIFICATIONS WITH CONDITIONING

Hermissenda's normally positive phototaxic response is reduced for weeks (Harrigan and Alkon, 1985) following repeated pairings of light with rotations (Figure 1a). Randomized presentations of light and rotation do not produce this decrease in positive phototaxis, nor do repeated presentations of either stimuli alone (graph in Figure 1a, Crow and Alkon, 1978). This provides evidence against either habituation or sensitization contributing to the behavioral change. The data indicate that a temporal association between the two stimuli (light and rotation) is important in generating the behavioral change. Training with brief light and rotation stimuli (<3.0 sec) shows a remarkably specific requirement for a precise temporal interval (1.0 sec) between the onset of the conditioned stimulus (CS-light) and the onset of the unconditioned stimulus (UCS-rotation). No significant training results when the UCS onset precedes the CS onset or when the UCS follows the CS by 1.5 seconds or more (Lederhendler and Alkon, 1986). Further support for the strictly associative nature of the learned behavior was provided by recent work demonstrating the necessity for a predictive relationship between the two stimuli. Degrading this predictability by interspersing either additional light or rotational stimuli during training with paired stimuli reduces the normal conditioned response (Farley, 1984). Other work has demonstrated an associative transfer between the CS and UCS: Following training, light elicits a new muscular response from the foot of Hermissenda, causing it to contract, a response normally elicited only by the aversive rotational stimulus. Thus, training causes the animal's response to the CS to acquire aspects of its response to the UCS (Lederhendler et al., 1986). Finally, although Hermissenda can "remember" its training for days or weeks (Harrigan and

Alkon, 1985), it will "forget" the experience with time.
If the animal is re-exposed to training, it will relearn the
pairing-specific behavior in fewer trials, i.e., it shows
"savings" as has been demonstrated in vertebrate Pavlovian
conditioning (Crow and Alkon, 1978). Extinction due to
unpaired presentations of the CS during retention has also
been demonstrated (Richards et al., 1984).

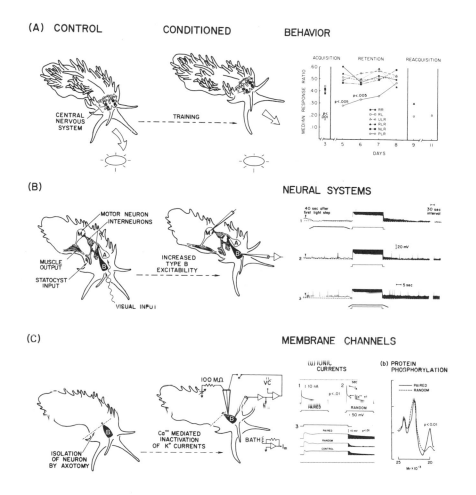

Figure 1: Cellular analysis of Hermissenda associative
learning (a) Behavior. Reduction of positive phototaxic
response in Hermissenda as a result of conditioning
procedure. The plot on the right represents data on the

(Continued on next page)

Fig. 1. (*continued*)

median response ratios for acquisition, retention and
reacquisition of a long-term behavioral change after a light
stimulus [random rotation (●), random light (◨), unpaired
light and rotation (▲), random light and rotation (▲),
nothing (◖), and paired light and rotation (○)]. (b) Neural
systems. Critical input and output neurons, a few of many
that mediate learning the association of light and rotation.
Type B and Type A photoreceptors are indicated by B and A;
M indicates the pedal ganglion motor neuron whose activity
regulates turning movements. Intracellular recordings from
intact Type B cells during and after light and rotation
stimuli. (Trace 1) Responses to the second of two
succeeding 30 second light steps (with a 90-second interval
intervening) each preceded by rotation. (Trace 2) Responses
to the second of two light steps without rotation. (Trace 3)
As in Traces 1 and 2 with the onset of each light step
followed by onset after 1 second of maximal rotation.
(c) Membrane channels. Type B cells are isolated by axotomy
subsequent to behavioral measurements made before and after
training. The circuit for the voltage clamp experiment
with two microelectrodes is shown in the center. The
ionic currents were measured from holding potential of -60
mV. (Trace 1) Paired I_A (early peak outward K^+ current)
and $I_{Ca^{2+}-K^+}$ (late current, maximum at 300 msec after onset
of command) are smaller than random (Trace 2) or control
values (not shown). (Trace 3) Paired steady state
depolarization during and after (shaded areas) a light step
(monitored by top trace) are larger than random and control.

The data on protein phosphorylation are represented
by densitometric scans of autoradiograms of samples of eye
proteins in the molecular weight range of 20,000 to 25,000
obtained 1 to 2 hours after animals received the third
training session of paired or random light and rotation.
For references, see text; reprinted from Alkon, 1984.

HERMISSENDA: NEURAL CORRELATES OF CONDITIONING

Intracellular recording from Type B photoreceptors of
Hermissenda on days following conditioning reveals a
conditioning-specific increase of input resistance and
excitability. These changes are reflected in an increased
light response of conditioned Type B photoreceptors compared
to random and naive controls (Figure 1b, Alkon, 1980).
Type B photoreceptors inhibit Type A photoreceptors, which

excite, via interneurons, motorneurons responsible for turning of the foot (Alkon, 1983, 1984). Thus, these changes can be directly responsible for decreased phototaxis in trained animals (Figure 1b). These excitability differences are intrinsic to the Type B soma, and can be measured in cells isolated via axotomy. Learning could be simulated in intact Hermissenda nervous systems by exposing them to repeated pairings of light and rotation, or current injection simulating statocyst stimulation, while recording intracellularly responses of the Type B photoreceptors. These pairings in the intact nervous system caused gradual cumulative depolarization (Alkon, 1980) and prolonged elevation of internal calcium concentration (Connor and Alkon, 1984) in the Type B photoreceptors, resulting in excitability differences identical to those seen in trained animals. Impalement and stimulation mimicing training of Type B photoreceptors in living animals demonstrated a predictability between excitability changes elicited by the training stimuli, and subsequent behavior of the animal, a very strong argument for the excitability differences in photoreceptors measured with training causally underlying the conditioning-induced decrease in phototaxis (Farley et al., 1983).

Voltage-clamp recording in isolated Type B photoreceptor somata has revealed reductions in specific ionic conductances which can account for the input resistance and excitability changes seen in the Type B photoreceptor under current-clamp recording conditions. The fast, transient potassium current, I_A, the calcium-dependent potassium current, I_C, (Alkon, 1984; Alkon et al., 1985; Figure 1c, Figures 2 and 3), and the voltage-dependent calcium current I_{Ca++} (Collin et al., 1986) are all significantly reduced in conditioned animals on days following training. The delayed rectifier potassium current, a slowly activating and non-inactivating outward current, is apparently unaffected by training.

RABBIT: BEHAVIORAL MODIFICATION AND EXTRACELLULAR RECORDING

The nictitating membrane/eyeblink conditioning paradigm in rabbit is one of the best studied examples of simple Pavlovian conditioning of striated muscle response (see Gormezano et al., 1983 for review). Animals exposed to repeated pairings of tone (CS) overlapping and coterminating with either periorbital shock or airpuff to the cornea (UCS) rapidly learn to blink to the tone before the onset of the UCS. Once learned, this conditioned response (CR) is retained for many weeks. Extracellular recording throughout the brain in animals during training has demonstrated that many areas are activated and involved in conditioning.

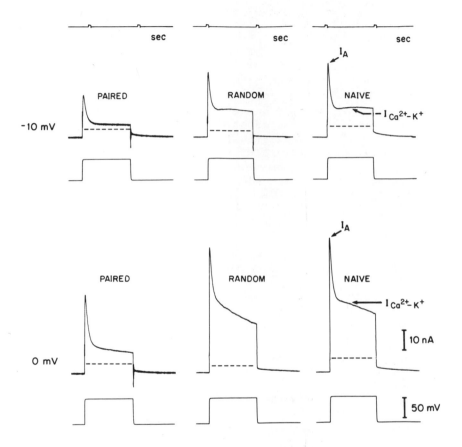

Figure 2: Comparison of voltage-dependent K^+ currents measured in Type B somata isolated from paired, random, and naive animals. The records were chosen to illustrate the reduction of I_A and $I_{Ca^{2+}-K^+}$ for paired as compared to random and naive animals (see Tables 2 and 3). Reprinted from Alkon et al., 1985.

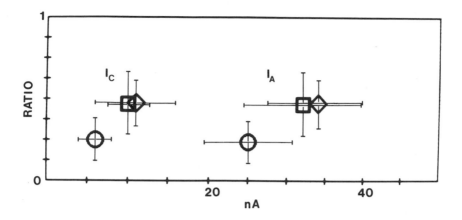

Figure 3: Mean phototaxis suppression ratios in relation to
ionic current magnitude. For individual animals of each
group (Paired, ● ; Random ◻ ; and Naive, ◇) a suppression ratio
(in the form B/A + B where A = post-treatment latency and
B = pretreatment latency) was obtained and the magnitude of
$I_{Ca^{2+}-K^+}$ (on the left) and I_A was measured at - 10 mV
(absolute) across the isolated soma membrane of the medial
Type B cell. The values presented ($\pm$ SD) are the mean ionic
currents ($I_{Ca^{2+}-K^+}$ and I_A) measured in relation to the mean
suppression ratio for each group. The Paired mean ratios
and ionic currents are all clearly lower than for the Random
and Naive groups. Reprinted from Alkon et al., 1985.

These areas include many cerebral cortical areas (Disterhoft
and Stuart, 1976; Disterhoft et al., 1982), brainstem (lesion
work--Desmond and Moore, 1982, recording--Desmond and Moore,
1985), cerebellum and associated deep nuclei (recording--
McCormick and Thompson, 1984; lesion studies--Yeo et al.,
1985a,b; McCormick et al., 1981, 1982) as well as the
hippocampus (Berger and Thompson, 1978a,b; Berger et al.,
1983). Multiple-unit activity in pyramidal cell layers of
the hippocampus has shown massive activation of these cells
during the CS and UCS period. This activation precedes and
predicts the onset of the behavioral response in training,
and precedes the onset of a CR within a given trial (Berger
and Thompson, 1978a,b). Peristimulus-time histograms of
neural activity correlate significantly with the shape of
the behavioral response in these cells. Single-unit

recording in the hippocampus demonstrated that more than 50%
of identified pyramidal cells show increases in firing rate
during either the CS or UCS period during conditioning
(Berger et al., 1983). No direct afferent to the pyramidal
cells of the hippocampus recorded to date has shown similar
degrees of modification with conditioning, suggesting that
the change in behavior of these pyramidal cells may be due
to intrinsic changes, and not be a reflection of neural
activity increases "upstream" (Berger and Weisz, 1985). The
actual role of the hippocampus in storage or generation of
the behavioral conditioning is not known. Complete lesions
of hippocampus and neocortex do not abolish conditioning of
the eylid/NM response (Oakley and Russell, 1972; Solomon and
Moore, 1975). Hippocampal lesions have been reported to
disrupt trace conditioning of the NM response (conditioning
with a time interval separating the CS stimulus termination
and onset of the UCS) (Weisz et al., 1980) and to disrupt
reversal learning of the NM response (Berger and Orr, 1982).
The hippocampus may be involved in encoding other aspects of
the training, such as temporal, contextual and/or associative
information (Olton et al., 1979; Solomon, 1980).

HIPPOCAMPUS: INTRACELLULAR NEURAL CORRELATES OF CONDITIONING

Intracellular recording in CA1 pyramidal neurons one day
following training has revealed conditioning--specific
alterations in membrane properties measured blind in the
isolated in vitro hippocampal slices (Disterhoft et al.,
1986; Coulter et al., 1985, 1986). These changes may explain
the increased excitability seen in hippocampal extracellular
recording in vivo (Berger and Thompson, 1978a,b).
Conditioning significantly reduces the amplitude of the
afterhyperpolarization (AHP) which occurs following current-
injection evoked spike activity in these cells (Figure 4)
(Coulter et al., 1985; Disterhoft et al., 1986). This
reduction occurs without any significant differences in
membrane potential, input resistance or spike height between
groups. The AHP reduction with conditioning occurs at all
stimulus amplitudes that elicit spikes. This AHP difference
gets larger between conditioned and control cells as the
stimulus eliciting the AHP increases from 1-4 spikes (Figure
5). Thus, conditioning does not just shift AHP amplitudes
by subtracting a constant amount of hyperpolarization, as
might occur with either a shift in membrane potential, input
resistance, or the potassium equilibrium potential. Rather,

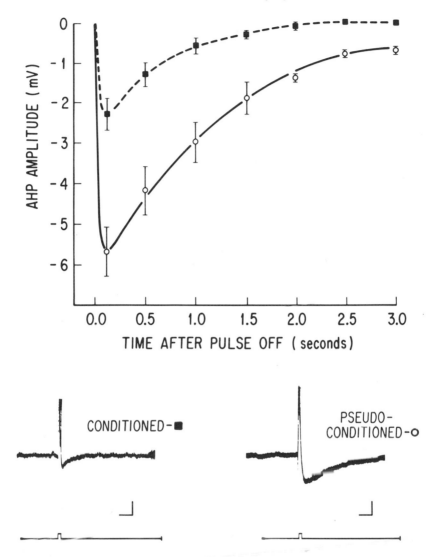

Figure 4: AHP amplitude and duration is reduced by
conditioning. Top: Plot of means + 1 SE of AHP amplitude
at isochronal times after stimulus offset for 18
pseudoconditioned cells (open circles) and 19 conditioned
cells (filled squares). Bottom: Typical AHP traces for
conditioned and pseudoconditioned cells following a 100 msec
depolarizing current pulse eliciting 4 spikes. Calibration
5 mV, 0.5 sec. Modified from Coulter et al., 1985.

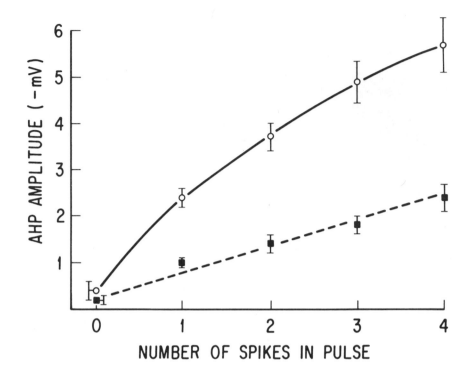

Figure 5: AHP differences with conditioning increase with increasing stimulus strength. Plot of mean + SE of AHP amplitude for pulses eliciting 0-4 spikes for 22 pseudoconditioned cells (open circles), and 20 conditioned cells (filled squares). Lines fit by eye. Modified from Coulter et al., 1985).

conditioning affects the dynamic properties of AHP generation, the effect varying with the strength of the stimulus eliciting the AHP (Coulter et al., 1986). The duration and time course of the AHP are also shortened by conditioning, compared to pseudoconditioned and naive controls. Conditioned animals, in addition to having smaller amplitude AHPs, have significantly shorter duration AHPs following a 4 spike stimulus (1.32 second + 0.85, mean + SD) which decay much more swiftly (time constant of average decay, 0.61 seconds, Figure 6) compared to pseudoconditioned (duration 2.70 + 0.56 sec, time constant

= 1.31 sec) and naive controls (duration 2.74 + 0.76 sec, time constant = 1.01 sec). These conditioning-correlated reductions in AHP are entirely intrinsic to the CA1 pyramidal cells. In 0.5 um TTX and 5mM TEA medium, synaptic transmission is abolished in the hippocampal slice, but AHP reductions with conditioning still persist following a current-injection evoked calcium spike (Figure 7c, Coulter et al., 1986). This AHP has been shown to be due to activation of a calcium-dependent potassium current (Hotson and Prince, 1980; Alger and Nicoll, 1980; Lancaster and Adams, 1986). It is thought to be important in shutting down repetitive firing in these cells, an intrinsic inhibitory current. Thus, reductions in amplitude and time course of the AHP should increase the excitability of a cell. We found conditioned cells to be significantly more

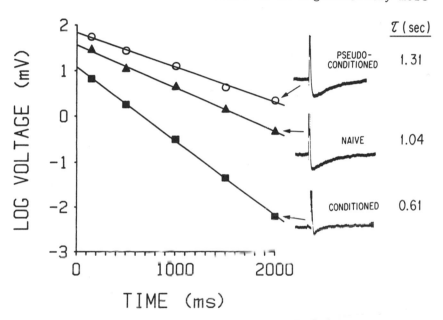

Figure 6: Time constant of average AHP decay is altered by conditioning. Mean AHP voltages at isochronal points were semilogarithmically plotted. Controls (pseudoconditioned, open circles; naives, filled triangles) had shallower slopes (and larger time constants) than did the mean of conditioned cells (filled squares). Lines fit by regression. Time constants calculated as reciprocal of negative slope of line. Modified from Coulter et al., 1985.

excitable to repetitive stimulation than pseudoconditioned
cells at all interstimulus intervals less than 4 seconds,
the first pulse adjusted to elicit 4 spikes (Coulter et al.,
1985).

To characterize the learning-induced AHP reduction,
recent work has focused on the interaction of calcium entry
and subsequent calcium-dependent potassium current
activation. In 0.5 um TTX and 5 mM TEA artificial
cerebrospinal fluid, CA1 pyramidal cells fire large, broad,
all-or-nothing calcium spikes, elicited by relatively large
current injections (Figure 7, Schwartzkroin and Slawsky,
1977). These spikes are followed by an AHP, again thought
to be due to activation of an underlying calcium-dependent
potassium current (this current in mammalian central neurons
has been found to be relatively resistant to TEA, cf.
Lancaster and Adams, 1986). Conditioned animals show a
much higher current threshold to elicit a calcium spike
(1.2 nA ± 0.78, mean ± SD, n = 11, 100 msec pulse) than do
pseudoconditioned or naive controls (0.62 nA ± 0.23, n = 12).

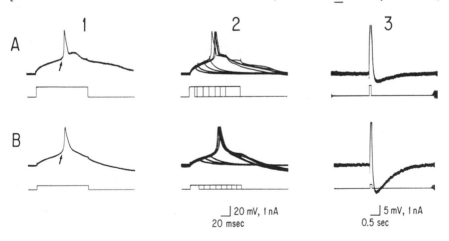

Figure 7: Calcium spike recordings in TTX/TEA medium. Row
A: Representative records of conditioned cell. Row B:
Representative records of pseudoconditioned cell. Columns 1
and 2: Current threshold to elicit calcium spike (arrows in
Column 1--voltage threshold). Note current threshold much
higher for conditioned cell. Column 3: Higher gain records
of AHP following calcium spike (top of spike clipped in
voltage traces) note reduced AHP in conditioned cell. From
Coulter et al., 1986.

This rise in current threshold does not reflect a dramatic increase in the voltage threshold between these cells (see arrows in Figure 7a). This suggests alterations in a subthreshold, depolarization-activated conductance, either a voltage-dependent decrease in an inward current with conditioning (probably a calcium current), or an increase in an outward current, responsible for shunting depolarizing current in conditioned cells. Once a calcium spike is elicited, however, there is no difference in either its amplitude or its duration between groups. Following the calcium spike, the AHP is still significantly reduced in conditioned vs. control groups (Coulter et al., 1986). Therefore, the AHP reduction is not secondary to a calcium current reduction, which may also occur with conditioning.

All of the above differences in AHP have been measured in animals one day following training to 80% or better CRS, i.e., in overtrained animals. Other work has focused on AHP amplitudes during acquisition of the learned response. Immediately following two days of training (compared to the three days of training, and one day of retention described above) animals were sacrificed and intracellular recordings made from CA1 pyramidal cells as above. Animals that showed higher percentage of CRs showed significantly smaller amplitude AHPs than did animals who did not learn as well (lower percentage CRs) (Figure 8). This is despite the fact that all animals in this experiment received identical numbers of paired trials, 80 per day for two days. This finding provides evidence that the conditioning-correlated AHP differences may be closely linked to the degree of learning (Disterhoft et al., 1986).

COMPARISON OF ELECTROPHYSIOLOGICAL CONDITIONING CHANGES IN HERMISSENDA AND RABBIT

Conditioning induces similar post-synaptic changes in both Hermissenda photoreceptors and the mammalian hippocampus. In both cases, training results in intrinsic increased excitability at the level of the neuronal soma and persists in synaptically isolated cells (via axotomy in Hermissenda, via TTX perfusion in the hippocampal slice). This increase in excitability is similarly achieved by reducing potassium currents, either directly, or possibly partially secondarily, through reducing calcium currents. In Hermissenda, the calcium current (Collin et al., 1986),

ACQUISITION

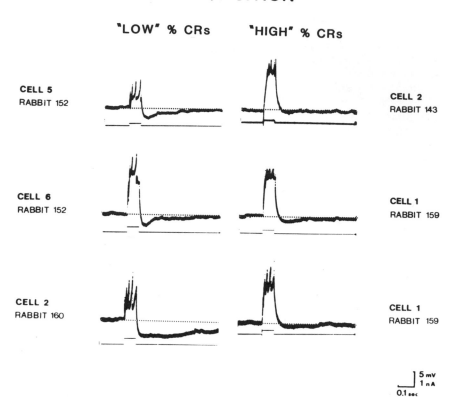

Figure 8: Acquisition of the reduced AHP. AHPs after 4 spikes are shown for three individual CA1 neurons in the "low CR" group as compared to CA1 neurons in the "high CR" group. All rabbits in this study received two 80 trial training sessions. Hippocampal neurons from those animals which had acquired the conditioned response tended to be reduced in amplitude and duration, as illustrated here. From Disterhoft et al., 1986.

the calcium-dependent potassium current, and the fast, transient potassium current (Alkon et al., 1982; Alkon et al., 1985) are reduced, while evidence only exists to date for reductions in the calcium-dependent potassium current, and possibly in both the subthreshold calcium current and the transient calcium current (responsible for the calcium spike) in the hippocampus (Coulter et al., 1985, 1986). The effect of conditioning on I_A in hippocampal CA1 cells is presently unknown, but experiments to address this question are planned.

The finding that Hermissenda and mammalian hippocampal neurons exhibit similar changes in membrane conductances, despite their being widely divergent phyla, is not totally unexpected, considering the membrane properties of individual neurons in both systems. At the biophysical level, the Hermissenda photoreceptor and the rabbit CA1 neuron are very similar. The Type B photoreceptor and the pyramidal cell of the mammalian hippocampus possess many similar voltage-dependent currents. Both have a slowly activating, non-activating potassium conductance, the delayed rectifier or I_K. Both are also endowed with a fast, transient potassium current, I_A. Both possess calcium-dependent potassium currents (the hippocampal pyramidal cell may contain several calcium-dependent potassium currents, one of which is fast enough to be responsible for spike repolarization). Both have voltage-dependent, non-activating calcium currents (the pyramidal cell may have more than one calcium current, with different kinetics and cellular distributions). Hermissenda photoreceptors and mammalian pyramidal cells also contain a similar voltage-dependent transmitter sensitive potassium current (Im in the hippocampus, sensitive to acetylcholine, and a similar current in the mollusc, sensitive to acetylcholine and α_2 agonists). Both types of cells also have a fast voltage-dependent sodium current. Thus, mollusc and mammal resemble one another at the cellular level (for reviews see Adams and Galvan, 1986; Alkon, 1980) and hence it is less surprising that, given similar challenges in terms of training protocols, both systems encode these experiences in similar ways.

POSSIBLE BIOCHEMICAL MECHANISMS UNDERLYING LEARNING

The biophysical changes which accompany associatively induced behavioral change must also have a corresponding underlying biochemical referent. To date the most widely studied biochemical cascade known to modulate ionic conductances is the second messenger activated protein kinase system. There are three well known protein kinase systems in nervous tissue which are activated by intracellular second messengers: cyclic nucleotide dependent protein kinases which are activated by cyclic AMP or cyclic GMP, calcium-calmodulin dependent protein kinases and the calcium/diacylglycerol activated phospholipid dependent protein kinase, protein kinase C (PKC) (see Nairn et al., 1985 for review). All three of these protein kinase systems have been shown to be present in both vertebrate (Nairn et al., 1985) and invertebrate (Neary et al., in press; DeRiemer et al., 1984; Castellucci et al., 1982) nervous systems.

The biophysical effect of protein kinase activation on vertebrate and invertebrate neurons is primarily on potassium and calcium conductances with no effect on sodium conductance (Levitan, 1985; Sakakibara et al., 1986; DeRiemer et al., 1985; Kubota et al., submitted). Protein kinases may alter ionic conductances via direct phosphorylation of ion channels as ion channels reconstituted into artificial phospholipid bilayers increase their open probability in the presence of activated protein kinase and ATP (Ewald et al., 1985).

In Hermissenda B photoreceptors, the two potassium currents and calcium current which are reduced after training (I_A, I_C and I_{Ca}) are also reduced by injection of type II calcium-calmodulin dependent protein kinase (Sakakibara et al., 1986). Activated protein kinase C reduces I_A and I_C only (Alkon et al., 1986; Kubota et al., submitted). Particularly interesting is the fact that calcium ion induced reduction of I_A and I_C can be prolonged by pairing kinase C activation with a calcium load (Figure 9) (Alkon et al., 1986). Therefore, the learning induced changes in potassium conductances may be mediated by a synergistic activation (via CS and US pathways) of calcium-calmodulin dependent protein kinase and protein kinase C.

Is there evidence that such a biochemical mechanism underlying learning exists in the vertebrate preparation? As mentioned, the most striking effect of learning on the behavior of CA1 pyramidal neurons is a reduction in the amplitude and duration of the AHP, which is mediated by a calcium-dependent potassium current. Recent studies have shown that phorbol ester activation of protein kinase C reduces the AHP in an identical manner to learning (Baraban et al., 1985; Nicoll et al., 1986). Therefore, in both Hermissenda and rabbit, identical biophysical substrates of

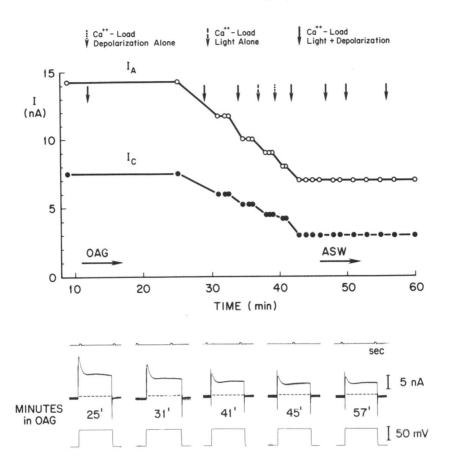

Figure 9: Effects of exposure to OAG on K+ currents across Type D soma membrane. Successive calcium loads (indicated by arrows) cause progressive persistent reduction of K+ currents, I_A and $I_{Ca^{2+}-K^+}(I_C)$, after OAG treatment. Conditions as described in Figure 1. Graphic representation of actual current values (after "leak" correction) is in upper panel. Cell was penetrated and voltage-clamped with two microelectrodes 9 min after exposure to OAG was begun. Lower records (for same cell) show actual currents elicited at times shown and after CA^{2+} loads indicated above. Note that Ca^{2+} loads were not followed by further persistent reduction of K+ currents after OAG was removed from the ASW (at 43 min) nor did the K+ currents recover their former amplitude in ASW. Reprinted from Alkon et al., 1986.

learning can be mimicked by activation of the same kinase systems.

Unlike Hermissenda, where it is difficult to isolate and biochemically analyze a single photoreceptor, the rabbit hippocampus affords such an opportunity due to the presence of homogenous cell populations (in our case the dorsal CA1 region). Therefore, we could directly analyze the effects of learning on kinase C activation.

Twenty-four hours after the last training session hippocampal slices were prepared from conditioned, pseudoconditioned and naive rabbits. The CA1 region was dissected out and membrane and cytosolic fractions prepared. The kinase C content of each fraction was determined after partial purification of the kinase and the extent to which it phosphorylated an exogenous substrate for this kinase. We found no difference in total kinase C levels between groups (membrane plus cytosol). However, when we analyzed the distribution of the kinase we found a significantly higher proportion of the kinase associated with the membrane fraction of conditioned animals versus pseudoconditioned and naive controls (Figure 9). This was paralleled by a concomitant decrease in cytosolic kinase C (Bank et al., 1986). This finding suggests that as a result of learning, kinase C is translocated (and hence activated) from a cytosolic to a membrane compartment. The biophysical consequences of this activation would be a lower threshold for modulation of ionic currents by subsequent extracellular signals. It is also possible that kinase C translocation is the mechanism whereby the AHP is reduced after training as suggested by the phorbol ester reduction of the AHP (Baraban et al., 1985; Nichol et al., 1986). Translocation of protein kinase C from cytosol to membrane has also been observed in hippocampus one hour after induction of long-term potentiation of synaptic transmission in the perforant path (Akers et al., 1986).

Although the B photoreceptor in Hermissenda is not amenable to direct biochemical study, the entire eye is. In vivo radiolabelling of Hermissenda eyes with organic orthophosphate revealed a conditioning-specific increase in the phosphorylation of a 20,000 Mr phosphoprotein (Neary et al., 1981) Figure 10). The phosphorylation of this protein was also found to be dependent on kinase C as judged by in vitro assays (Neary et al., in press). This finding is

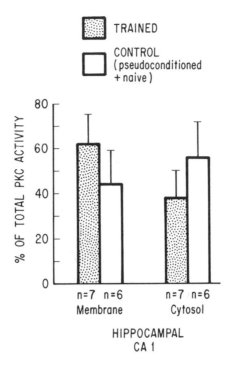

Figure 10: The effect of eyeblink/NM conditioning on the distribution of protein kinase C (PKC) in the CA1 region of rabbit hippocampus. Percent activity associated with each fraction is the specific PKC activity (pmols phosphate transferred/mg/min) of each fraction divided by the total specific activity (membrane and cytosol). From Bank et al., 1986.

compatible with the idea that kinase C is also activated during and after associative learning in Hermissenda. New techniques are currently being developed to test this hypothesis in individual B photoreceptors.

The reduction in I_{Ca++} found in Hermissenda after training may be mediated by an increase in calcium-calmodulin dependent protein kinase (Sakakibara et al., 1986). It is also possible that the calcium-calmodulin dependent protein kinase system mediates the increased threshold to fire a calcium spike found in rabbit hippocampal CA1 pyramidal neurons after learning (Coulter et al., 1986). In collaboration with Dr. Robert DeLorenzo and his colleagues at University of Virginia Medical School, we have recently found that learning decreases the in vitro auto-phosphorylation of calcium-calmodulin dependent protein kinase in CA1 cells. There was no effect of learning on dentate gyrus neurons (Bank, DeLorenzo and Alkon, work in progress). This change may mediate the biophysically observed increase in calcium spike threshold. Therefore, yet another parallel between biophysical and biochemical substrates of learning between invertebrates and vertebrates may emerge.

SUMMARY AND CONCLUSIONS

The results of our cellular neurophysiological and biochemical studies outlined above demonstrate remarkable similarities in the way Hermissenda photoreceptors and rabbit CA1 hippocampal pyramidal cells modify their membrane properties with conditioning. Both systems demonstrate conditioning-induced reductions in a calcium-dependent potassium conductance, and a calcium conductance (suggested but not proven for the rabbit). Hermissenda also exhibits reductions in a second potassium current, the fast, transient K^+ conductance I_A. Our experiments have also demonstrated possible similarities in biochemical mechanisms responsible for the conditioning-correlated conductance changes in both systems. Similar protein kinase systems (calmodulin kinase and kinase C) may mediate the observed biophysical changes in Hermissenda photoreceptors and rabbit hippocampus.

The power of these findings is increased by the nature of the approach. In both lines of investigation, intact, whole animal conditioning changes are measured 24 hours or more after training in isolated, whole or reduced nervous systems, precluding any possible involvement of hormonal or presynaptic modifications being responsible for the measured changes. The alterations described in both cases are unequivocally intrinsic to the cells in question, and can be measured in cells isolated from any synaptic stimulation, i.e., are entirely postsynaptic. This does not rule out the possibility that other changes in other parts of the brain or other changes within the same groups of cells may also be present, but not discovered as yet. This is undoubtedly true. Another advantage of measuring whole animal conditioning induced biophysical changes in isolated nervous tissue which we have begun to exploit is that further biochemical analysis of the same tissue used for the biophysical analyses is possible. Studies correlating biochemical changes with biophysical measurements allow interactive experimentation to explore possible cellular mechanisms underlying membrane property alterations. It may be possible with this kind of approach to determine the exact way a cell can recognize and store learned associations. A final advantage of our approach, which we hope to exploit in the future is that it may allow us to label (with antibodies, voltage-sensitive dyes, and/or metabolic or chemical markers) in vitro, possible sites within cell populations of conditioning-correlated change. With such labelling, it may be possible to analyze patterns of learned association storage at a systems level.

REFERENCES

Adams PR, Galvan M (1986). Voltage-dependent currents of vertebrate neurons and their role in membrane excitability. In Delgado-Escueta AV, Ward AA, Woodbury DM, Porter RJ (eds): "Advances in Neurology," New York: Raven Press.
Akers RF, Lovinger DM, Colley P, Linden D, Routtenberg A (1986). Translocation of protein kinase C activity may mediate hippocampal LTP. Science 231:587-589.
Alger BE, Nicholl RA (1980). Epileptiform burst afterhyperpolarization: Calcium-dependent potassium potential in hippocampal CA1 pyramidal cells. Science 210:1122-1124.
Alkon DL (1980). Cellular analysis of a gastropod (Hermissenda crassicornis) model of associative learning. Biol Bull 159:505-560.
Alkon DL (1980). Membrane depolarization accumulates during acquisition of an associative behavioral change. Science 210:1375-1376.
Alkon DL (1983). Learning in a marine snail. Sci Am 249: 70-84.
Alkon DL (1984). Calcium-mediated reduction of ionic currents: a biophysical memory trace. Science (Wash DC) 226:1037-1045.
Alkon DL, Kubota M, Neary JT, Naito S, Coulter D, Rasmussen H (1986). C-kinase activation prolongs Ca^{2+}-dependent inactivation of K^+ currents. Biochem Biophys Res Comm

134:1245-1253.

Alkon DL, Lederhendler I, Shoukimas JJ (1982). Primary changes of membrane currents during retention of associative learning. Science 215:693-695.

Alkon DL, Sakakibara M, Forman R, Harrigan J, Lederhendler I, Farley J (1985). Reduction of two voltage-dependent K^+ currents mediates retention of a learned association. Behav Neural Biol 44:278-300.

Bank B, Coulter DA, Rasmussen H, Chute DL, Alkon DL (1986). Effects of NMR conditioning on intracellular levels of protein kinase C. Soc Neurosci Abstr 12:182.

Baraban JM, Snyder SH, Alger BE (1985). Protein kinase C regulates ionic conductance in hippocampal pyramidal neurons: Electrophysiological effects of phorbol esters. Proc Nat Acad Sci USA 82:2538-2542.

Benardo LS, Prince DA (1982). Cholinergic excitation of mammalian hippocampal pyramidal cells. Brain Res 249: 315-331.

Berger TW, Orr WB (1982). Role of hippocampus in reversal learning of the rabbit nicitating membrane response. In Woody CD (ed): "Conditioning: Representation of Involved Neural Function," New York: Plenum.

Berger TW, Rinaldi PC, Weisz DJ, Thompson RF (1983). Single-unit analysis of different hippocampal cell types during classical conditioning of rabbit nicitating membrane response. J Neurophysiol 50:1197-1219.

Berger TW, Thompson RF (1978a). Neuronal plasticity in the limbic system during classical conditioning of the rabbit nictitating membrane response. I. The hippocampus. Brain Res 145:323-346.

Berger TW, Thompson RF (1978b). Identification of pyramidal cells as the critical elements in hippocampal neuronal plasticity during learning. Proc Nat Acad Sci USA 75: 1572-1576.

Berger TW, Weisz DJ (1985). Single unit analysis of hippocampal pyramidal and granule cells and their role in classical conditioning of the rabbit nictitating membrane response. In Gormezano I, Prokasy WF, Thompson RF (eds): "Classical Conditioning III: Behavioral, Neurophysiological and Neurochemical Studies in the Rabbit, I" Laurence Erlbaum.

Castellucci VF, Nairn A, Greengard P, Schwartz JH, Kandel ER (1982). Inhibitor of adenosine 3':5'-monophosphate-dependent protein kinase blocks presynaptic facilitation in Aplysia. J Neurosci 12:1673-1681.

Cole AE, Nicholl RA (1984). The pharmacology of cholinergic

excitatory responses in hippocampal pyramidal cells. Brain Res 305:283-290.

Collin C, Harrigan J, Alkon DL (1986). Differences between pharmacologic and conditioning-induced reduction of Hermissenda currents. Soc Neurosci Abstr 12:1153.

Connor JA, Alkon DL (1984). Light- and voltage-dependent increases of calcium ion concentration in molluscan photoreceptors. J Neurophysiol 51:745-752.

Coulter DA, Disterhoft J, Alkon DL (1986). Decreased Ca^{2+} entry and K^+ conductance contribute to AHP reductions with conditioning in rabbit hippocampus. Soc Neurosci Abstr 12:181.

Coulter DA, Kubota M, Moore JW, Disterhoft JF, Alkon DL (1985). Conditioning-specific reduction of CA1 afterhyperpolarization amplitude and duration in rabbit hippocampal slices. Soc Neurosci Abstr 11:891.

Crow TJ, Alkon DL (1978). Retention of an associative behavioral change in Hermissenda. Science 201:1239-1241.

Crow TJ, Alkon DL (1980). Associative behavioral modification in Hermissenda: cellular correlates. Science 209:412-414.

DeRiemer SA, Kaczmareck LK, Lai Y, McGuinness TL, Greengard P (1984). Calcium/calmodulin-dependent protein phosphorylation in the nervous system of Aplysia. J Neurosci 4:1618-1625.

Desmond JE, Moore JW (1982). A brain stem region essential for the classically conditioned but not unconditioned nictitating membrane response. Physiol Behav 28:1029-1033.

Desmond JE, Moore JW (1985). The classically conditioned rabbit nictitating response: excitatory and inhibitory conditioned activity from single units in the brain stem. Soc Neurosci Abstr 11:981.

Disterhoft JF, Coulter DA, Alkon DL (1986). Conditioning-specific membrane changes of rabbit hippocampal neurons measured in vitro. Proc Nat Acad Sci USA 83:2733-2737.

Disterhoft JF, Golden D, Read H, Coulter DA, Alkon DL (1986). AHP reductions in rabbit hippocampal neurons during conditioning require acquisition of the learned response. Soc Neurosci Abstr 12:180.

Disterhoft JF, Shipley MT, Kraus N (1982). Analyzing the rabbit NM conditioned reflex arc. In Woody CD (ed): "Conditioning: Representation of Involved Neural Function," New York: Plenum.

Disterhoft JF, Stuart DK (1976). The trial sequence of changed unit activity in auditory system of alert rat during conditioned response acquisition and extinction. J Neurophysiol 39:266-281.

Dunlap K, Fischbach GD (1981). Neurotransmitters decrease the calcium conductance activated by depolarization of embryonic chick sensory neurons. J Physiol 317:519-535.

Ewald DA, Williams A, Levitan IB (1985). Modulation of single Ca^{2+}-dependent K^+-channel activity by protein phosphorylation. Nature 315:503-506.

Farley J (1984). Cellular mechanisms for causal detection in a mollusc. In Alkon DL, Woody CD (eds): "Neural Mechanisms of Conditioning," New York: Plenum.

Farley J, Richards WG, Ling L, Liman E, Alkon DL (1983). Membrane changes in a single photoreceptor during acquisition cause associative learning in Hermissenda. Science 221:1201-1203.

Fifkova E, Van Harreveld A (1977). Long-lasting morphological changes in dendritic spines of dentate granular cells following stimulation of the entorhinal area. J Neurocytol 6:211-230.

Galvan M, Adams PR (1982). Control of calcium current in rat sympathetic neurons by norepinephrine. Brain Res 244: 135-144.

Gormezano I, Kehoe EJ, Marshall BS (1983). Twenty years of classical conditioning research with the rabbit. In Sprague JM, Epstein AN (eds): "Progress in Psychobiology and Physiological Psychology (10)," New York: Academic p 197-275.

Greenough WT (1984). Possible structural substrates of plastic neural phenomena. In Lynch G, McGaugh JL, Weinberger NM (eds), "Neurobiology of Learning and Memory," New York: Guilford Press.

Haas HL, Konnerth A (1983). Histamine and noradrenaline decrease calcium-activated potassium conductance in hippocampal pyramidal cells. Nature 302:432-434.

Halliwell JV, Adams PR (1982). Voltage-clamp analysis of muscarinic excitation in hippocampal neurons. Brain Res 250:71-92.

Harrigan JF, Alkon DL (1985). Individual variation in associative learning of the nudibranch mollusc Hermissenda crassicornis. Biol Bull 168:222-238.

Hawkins RD, Abrams TW, Carew TJ, Kandel ER (1983). A cellular mechanism of classical conditioning in Aplysia: Activity-dependent amplification of presynaptic facilitation. Science 219:400-405.

Hotson JR, Prince DA (1980). A calcium-activated hyperpolarization follows repetitive firing in hippocampal neurons. J Neurophysiol 43:409-419.

Hoyle G (1982). Cellular basis of operant-conditioning of leg position. In Woody CD (ed), "Conditioning," New York: River Press.

Kubota M, Alkon DL, Naito S, Smallwood J, Rasmussen H (submitted). C-Kinase: a molecular switch for K^+ channel regulation.

Lancaster B, Adams PR (1986). Calcium-dependent current generating the afterhyperpolarization of hippocampal neurons. J Neurophysiol 55:1268-1282.

Lederhendler I, Alkon DL (1986). Temporal specificity of the CS-UCS interval for Hermissenda Pavlovian conditioning. Soc Neurosci Abstr 12:40.

Lederhendler I, Gart S, Alkon DL (1986). Classical conditioning of Hermissenda: origin of a new response. J Neurosci 6:1325-1331.

Lee KS, Schottler F, Oliver M, Lynch G (1980). Brief bursts of high-frequency stimulation produce two types of structural change in rat hippocampus. J Neurophysiol 44: 247-258.

Levitan IB (1985). Phosphorylation of ion channels. J Membr Biol 87:177-190.

Lynch G, Baudry M (1984). The biochemistry of memory: A new and specific hypothesis. Science 224:1057-1063.

Madison DV, Nicholl RA (1982). Noradrenaline blocks accommodation of pyramidal cell discharge in the hippocampus. Nature 299:636-638.

Malenka RC, Madison DV, Andrade R, Nicholl RA (1986). Phorbol esters mimic some cholinergic actions in hippocampal pyramidal neurons. J Neurosci 6:475-480.

Mamounas LA, Thompson RF, Lynch G, Baudry M (1984). Classical conditioning of the rabbit eyelid response increases glutamate receptor binding in hippocampal synaptic membranes. Proc Natl Acad Sci USA 81:2548-2552.

McCormick DA, Guyer PE, Thompson RF (1982). Superior cerebellar lesions selectively abolish the ipsilateral classically conditioned nictitating membrane/eyelid response of the rabbit. Brain Res 244:347-350.

McCormick DA, Lavond DG, Clark GA, Kettner RE, Rising CE, Thompson RF (1981). The engram found? Role of the cerebellum in classical conditioning of the nictitating membrane and eyelid response. Bull Psychon Soc 18:103-105.

McCormick DA, Thompson RF (1984). Neuronal responses of the rabbit cerebellum during acquisition and performance of of a classically conditioned nictitating membrane-eyelid response. J Neurosci 4:2811-2822.

Nairn AC, Hemmings HC, Greengard P (1985). Protein kinases in the brain. Annu Rev Biochem 54:931-976.

Neary JT, Crow TJ, Alkon DL (1981). Change in a specific phosphoprotein band following associative learning in Hermissenda. Nature 293:658-660.

Neary JT, Naito S, DeWeer A, Alkon DL (in press). Ca^{2+}/diacylglycerol-activated, phospholipid-dependent protein kinase in the Hermissenda CNS. J Neurochem.

Oakley DA, Russell IS (1972). Neocortical lesions and Pavlovian conditioning. Physiol Behav 8:915-926.

Olton DS, Becker JT, Handelman GE (1979). Hippocampus, space, and memory. Behav Brain Sci 2:313-322.

Pellmar TC (1986). Histamine decreases calcium-mediated potassium current in guinea pig hippocampal CA1 pyramidal cells. J Neurophysiol 55:727-738.

Richards W, Farley J, Alkon DL (1984). Extinction of associative learning in Hermissenda: Behavior and neural correlates. Behav Brain Res 14:161-170.

Sakakibara M, Alkon DL, DeLorenzo R, Goldenring JR, Neary JT, Heldman E (1986). Modulation of calcium-mediated inactivation of ionic currents by Ca^{2+}/calmodulin-dependent protein kinase II. Biophys J 50:319-327.

Schwartzkroin PA, Slawsky M (1977). Probable calcium spikes in hippocampal neurons. Brain Res 135:157-161.

Segal M (1980). The action of serotonin in the rat hippocampal slice preparation. J Physiol 303:423-439.

Solomon PR (1980). A time and a place for everything? Temporal processing view of hippocampal function with special reference to attention. Physiol Psychol 8:254-261.

Solomon PR, Moore JW (1975). Latent inhibition and stimulus generalization of the classically conditioned nictitating membrane response in rabbits (Oryctolagus cuniculus) following dorsal hippocampal ablations. J Comp Physiol Psychol 89:1192-1203.

Tsukahara N (1984). Classical conditioning mediated by the red nucleus: An approach beginning at the cellular level. In Lynch G, McGaugh JL, Weinberger NM (eds), "Neurobiology of Learning and Memory," New York: Guilford Press.

Walters ET, Byrne JH (1983). Associative conditioning of single sensory neurons suggests a cellular mechanism for learning. Science 219:405-408.

Weisz DJ, Solomon PR, Thompson RF (1980). The hippocampus appears necessary for trace conditioning. Bull Psychon Soc Abstr 193:244.

Woody CD, Berthier NE, Kim EH-J (1986). Rapid conditioning of an eyeblink reflex in cats. In Alkon DL, Woody CD (eds): "Neural Mechanisms of Conditioning," Chapter 8, New York: Plenum.

Woollacott M, Hoyle G (1977). Neural events underlying learning: Changes in pacemaker. Proc R Soc London Ser B 195:395-415.

Yeo CH, Hardiman MJ, Glickstein M (1985a). Classical conditioning of the nictitating membrane response of the rabbit. I. Lesions of the cerebellar nuclei. Exp Brain Res 60:87-98.

Yeo CH, Hardiman MJ, Glickstein M (1985b). Classical conditioning of the nictitating membrane response of the rabbit. II. Lesions of the cerebellar cortex. Exp Brain Res 60:99-113.

Neuroplasticity, Learning, and Memory, pages 45–59
© 1987 Alan R. Liss, Inc.

MEMORY, ALUMINUM AND ALZHEIMER'S DISEASE

Donald R. Crapper McLachlan,
P.H. St. George-Hyslop and B.J. Farnell
Departments of Physiology and Medicine,
Faculty of Medicine, University of Toronto
Toronto, Ontario, M5S 1A8

The most common presenting feature of senile and presenile dementia of the Alzheimer type is an impairment in recent memory (McLachlan et al., 1984). Indeed, the memory deficit may precede by months or even years other symptoms and signs of this common, progressive and lethal disorder of the brain. The molecular mechanisms responsible for the failure in recent memory are unknown. Considerable experimental evidence indicates that failure in the cholinergic system is a contributing factor although the exact relation between the cholinergic failure and the onset and progression of memory impairment is uncertain (Bartus et al., 1982; Whitehouse et al., 1982). Choline acetyltransferase activity measured in brain biopsy material obtained from frontal cortex from 8 patients in the early stages of Alzheimer's disease, however, failed to reveal a significant correlation with performance of the Mini Mental Status task (Gauthier et al., 1986). The Mini Mental Status examination probably measures both memory and other cognitive functions. Interestingly, a significant correlation was observed between quantitative counts of neurons with neurofibrillary degeneration and the Mini Mental Status scores (r=-0.851). Cellular processes resulting in the formation of neurofibrillary degeneration may be more important overall determinants of altered brain function in Alzheimer's disease than deficits in a single neurotransmitter system.

Neurofibrillary degeneration is one of the principle histological markers for Alzheimer's disease. The change is characterized by shrinkage of affected neurons,

especially dendrites, and the intracytoplasmic accumulation
of dense argentophilic bundles of 10 nm paired helical
filaments (Kidd, 1963; Terry et al., 1964). Employing a mini-
sampling technique and atomic absorption spectrophotometry,
Crapper et al., (1973; 1976) reported that cerebral cortical
regions high in neurofibrillary degeneration in Alzheimer's
disease have elevated concentrations of aluminum. At least
9 independent laboratories employing 4 different techniques
have now reported elevated aluminum concentrations in brains
associated with Alzheimer's disease (see McLachlan, 1986 for
general review). Alzheimer affected brains with elevated
aluminum concentrations have been reported from several
geographic regions of North America, Britain, France,
Germany, Australia and Japan. Other neurodegenerative
diseases associated with Alzheimer type neurofibrillary
degeneration such as Down's syndrome with Alzheimer's
disease, Guam parkinsonism-dementia complex and Guam
amyotrophic lateral sclerosis have also been reported to
contain elevated aluminum concentrations.

Four principle loci within Alzheimer affected brain
tissues exhibit elevated concentrations of aluminum: DNA
containing nuclear structures, the insoluble residue of
neurofibrillary tangles, amyloid cores of the senile plaques
and ferritin (review: McLachlan, 1986). Despite the large
number of known neurotoxic properties of aluminum, the
precise contribution of aluminum to the pathogenesis of
Alzheimer's disease remains unknown. Furthermore, the stage
in the Alzheimer neurodegenerative process at which aluminum
begins to accumulate is also unknown. Nevertheless, aluminum
is a potent neurotoxic agent capable of inducing a progressive
encephalopathy of considerable scientific interest. The first
sign of the aluminum encephalopathy in cats and rabbits is a
progressive deficit in short term memory accompanied by the
histopathological change of neurofibrillary degeneration.
The ultrastructure of the aluminum induced neurofibrillary
degeneration differs from that found in Alzheimer's disease
because the argentiphilic material is composed of 10 nm
single filaments (Terry and Pena, 1965).

MEMORY AND THE ALUMINUM ENCEPHALOPATHY

The direct intracranial injection of soluble salts of
aluminum, in a sensitive species such as cat or rabbit,
induces a progressive and, if untreated with anticonvulsants

and fluid replacement, a lethal encephalopathy with unusual characteristics. Mean brain tissue aluminum concentrations only 4 to 6 times above the naturally occurring concentrations are sufficient to induce the encephalopathy. For several days following a single intracranial dose of aluminum the animals appear normal and able to perform several memory and motor tasks with unaltered scores. Between day 7 and 10 post-injection, cats exhibit impairment in precise motor control during jumping (Crapper, 1976) and alterations in the performance of learning and memory tasks (Crapper and Dalton, 1973a,b). Employing the Wisconsin test apparatus to measure delayed matching to sample performance, fully trained animals performing at 100% correct responses, initially demonstrate deficits at long delay intervals. The deficits in retention progress to involve shorter time intervals over the next several days. Impairment in the delayed matching to sample task was accompanied by a decreased rate of acquisition of a conditioned avoidance task. The behavioral deficits were selective in the early stages of the encephalopathy because no changes in performance of visual discrimination tasks were noted and the speed of motor response was not altered.

Rabbits also exhibit deficits in both acquisition of an active avoidance task 10 days post-aluminum and failed to retain the task when tested 3 days later (Petit et al., 1980). Infant rabbits injected intracerebral with 3.7 µM of aluminum demonstrated impaired learning in a water maze and this change in behavior was associated with aluminum induced neurofibrillary degeneration (Rabe et al., 1982). Repeated subcutaneous injections of aluminum in rabbits affected classical conditioning (Yokel, 1983). Clearly, one of the earliest manifestations of aluminum neurotoxicity is a disturbance in the cellular mechanisms responsible for short term memory.

To define more precisely the molecular events responsible for impairment in the performance of learning and memory tasks in the intact animal, electrophysiological studies were carried out on isolated hippocampal slices removed at various stages of the aluminum encephalopathy. These studies have revealed a number of molecular mechanisms which may contribute to the failure in performance of memory and learning tasks in the intact animal and are summarized as follows: During the asymptomatic stage of the encephalopathy there are a number of physiologically important changes. There is a progressive rise in total brain tissue calcium content and a decrease in the number of tissue slices demonstrating the electrophysiological phenomenon of long term potentiation (LTP). Furthermore, there is a decrease in calmodulin messenger RNA content and calmodulin becomes progressively less competent as an intracellular messenger in the links between membrane electrical and biochemical events. Since calcium flux and the resulting changes in conformation of the intracellular messenger, calmodulin, are thought to be one step in the molecular events responsible for conditioned responses in the invertebrate nervous system, the aluminum effect upon memory processes in the intact animal may operate upon this mechanism.

MOLECULAR MECHANISMS OF ALUMINUM TOXICITY

Total tissue calcium content rises progressively after a single intracanial dose of aluminum. Cerebral cortical and hippocampal tissue samples were dried to a constant weight and 100 mg ashed at 650 °C in platinum crucibles. The residue was taken up in 6% nitric acid and analysed by Inductively Coupled Plasma Emission Vacuum Spectroscopy. Control rabbit brain calcium content averages 263 + 15 SD µg/g dry weight of tissue (n=15). By twelve days post-injection, calcium content has risen to an average content of 294 µg/g (p<0.05) and by 20 days post-aluminum to 340 µg/g dry weight (Farnell et al., 1985). Thus, aluminum disturbs the mechanisms responsible for calcium homeostasis in brain.

A useful laboratory model of synaptic plasticity which has been considered important in studying total animal responses of learning and memory is long term potentiation (LTP). Following repetitive stimulation of synaptic inputs, the amplitude of the post synaptic response to a test stimulus is increased compared to pretetanus control evoked responses. Such potentiation can be produced by relatively low frequency stimulus trains of 10 to 20 Hz and may persist for hours in vitro or days in vivo (Bliss and Lomo, 1973; Schwartzkroin and Wester, 1978). During induction of hippocampal LTP there is uptake and redistribution of calcium. Several studies have demonstrated that calcium is an essential factor in LTP (Baimbridge et al., 1982). Furthermore, the hippocampus has been associated with learning and memory processes in both animals (Izquierdo, 1975; O'Keefe and Nadel, 1979; Olton et al., 1980) and humans (Milner, 1970).

Early in the aluminum encephalopathy, hippocampal slices taken from rabbits demonstrate a reduced ability to develop LTP (Farnell et al., 1985). Changes in LTP occur in both the apical and basilar orthodromic inputs to CA1 hippocampal neurons. By 10 days post-aluminum injection there is a significant decline in LTP, Figure 1. These electrophysiological changes correspond in time to the observed onset of behavioral changes in performance in learning and memory tasks in cats and rabbits. Interestingly, increasing the in vitro calcium concentration in the bath from the control value of 2.4 mM to 4.8 mM restored LTP in hippocampal slices taken from the early and middle stages of the encephalopathy to control values, Figure 1. This suggests that the aluminum effect upon LTP operates upon the component of the system influenced by calcium ion concentration. The mechanisms responsible for this calcium effect are largely unknown. However, a calcium conductance system is known to become active during membrane depolarizations ranging between -20 and 0 mv. These "high voltage" calcium conductance channels appear to be localized to the dendrites of hippocampal CA1 neurons and are completely blocked when intracellular ionic calcium is increased from the control concentration of 0.05 μM to 6 μM (Yaari et al., in press). Possibly, increasing the calcium concentration in the medium of the isolated hippocampal slices increased calcium uptake through partially inactivated "high voltage" calcium conductance channels resulting in restoration of the calcium mediated steps in LTP.

The principle mechanisms regulating intracellular calcium concentration are the Ca-Mg activated ATPase membrane pump and a Ca-Na counter-port. The Ca-Mg ATPase is activated by calcium bound to calmodulin and calcium is considered to regulate its own intracellular concentration. The Ca-Na counter-port may lead to increased intracellular calcium under conditions in which the chemical gradient for sodium is reduced secondary to an increase in intracellular sodium (Blaustein, 1974). Thus calmodulin has a central role in the overall regulation of intracellular calcium concentration and several other calcium mediated biochemical processes.

LONG-TERM POTENTIATION

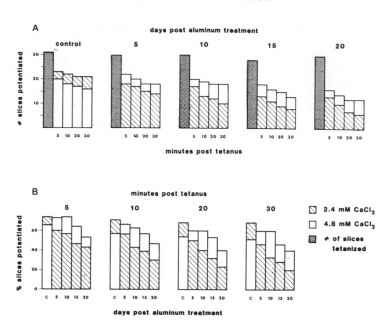

Figure 1. Long-term potentiation in rabbit hippocampi bathed in 2.4 and 4.8 mM $CaCl_2$, in vitro. A: days post-aluminum treatment and B: minutes post-tetanus. Experimental protocol as in Farnell et al., 1985.

ALUMINUM-CALMODULIN INTERACTIONS

Calcium bound to calmodulin exerts a pivotal role in several important cellular processes (Cheung, 1980; Wallaas et al., 1983). Recent experiments support the notion that aluminum interferes with calmodulin mediated messenger functions in the rabbit at two loci: aluminum alters the molecular conformation of calmodulin and prevents the molecule from activating receptor enzymes and aluminum reduces calmodulin messenger RNA content in brain. Several lines of evidence indicate that aluminum binds to calmodulin with approximately ten fold higher affinity than calcium (Siegel and Haug, 1983a,b) and induces a change in conformation in the molecule so that interaction with receptors is blocked. At aluminum to calmodulin ratios of 4:1 calcium-calmodulin dependent phosphodiesterase and Ca-Mg ATPase activity is completely inhibited. In preparations from rabbit hippocampus, the activity of calmodulin, as a calcium-calmodulin activator of the enzyme 3',5'-cyclic nucleotide phosphodiesterase, declined progressively as the aluminum encephalopathy progressed (Farnell et al., 1985). For hippocampal extracts, the Km for control tissue was 0.019 pM calmodulin, expressed in terms of calmodulin as measured by radioimmune assay, and 0.038 pM at 10 days post-aluminum. By 20 days post-aluminum, almost three times as much calmodulin was required to achieve the same rate of phosphorus release as calmodulin extracted from control rabbit hippocampus. This observation strongly supports the hypothesis that aluminum alters calcium homeostasis in rabbit hippocampus through an action upon calmodulin regulated calcium pumps.

Within 24 hours after intracranial injection of soluble aluminum salts, aluminum is found to be largely localized to DNA containing structures (DeBoni et al., 1974; Crapper et al., 1980). In rabbit brain, the yields of poly(A) RNA were significantly increased in the first 7 days post aluminum injection and then decreased as the encephalopathy progressed (VanBerkum et al., 1986). Importantly, the content of messenger RNA for calmodulin was significantly reduced by about 30% per gram of tissue compared to control mRNA calmodulin content. Furthermore, examination of the ratio of calmodulin mRNA to the ratio of mRNA content for each of the specific proteins actin, tubulin or neurofilament 68 kd revealed that calmodulin was selectively reduced during the first 10 days of the encephalopathy (VanBerkum and McLachlan, in preparation). Whether aluminum acts directly upon the calmodulin gene or upon degradation of the messenger RNA for calmodulin is unknown, however, the reduction could compound the effect of aluminum upon the cytoplasmic messenger functions of calmodulin by reducing the amount of available calmodulin peptide.

CALCIUM, CALMODULIN AND MODELS OF LEARNING

In each of the two invertebrate nervous systems in which associative conditioning has been studied in detail, calcium mediated steps are involved. Alkon et al., (1982) have studied conditioning of Hermissenda crassicornis to paired stimuli. In this organism, the presynaptic retinal neuron fires repetitive action potentials when exposed to the conditioning stimulus (light) paired about 1.5 seconds later with the unconditioned stimulus (rotation) (Coulter et al., this book). Intracellular recording from the photoreceptor after conditioning revealed a conditioning-specific increase in input resistance and excitability. Voltage-clamp recordings revealed reductions in specific ion conductances including the transient potassium current I_A, the calcium-dependent potassium current I_C and the voltage-dependent calcium current I_{Ca++}. In Hermissenda photoreceptors, the conditioning-specific potassium currents I_A, I_C and calcium current I_{Ca} are also reduced by intracellular injection of type II calcium-calmodulin dependent protein kinase (Sakakibara et al., 1986; Coulter et al., this book) and calcium-diacylglycerol activated phospholipid dependent protein kinase, protein kinase C (Alkon et al., 1986). Thus increased action potential activity results in an increase in intracellular Ca^{++} ion concentration in the presynaptic retinal neuron. Subsequent activation of Ca-calmodulin dependent protein phosphokinase, results in phosphorylation of voltage sensitive K^+ channels in the soma and axon of these retinal neurons (Alkon et al., 1982, 1983). The block in K^+ channels results in delayed repolarization which renders the presynaptic neuron more excitable. Since these alterations in presynaptic neuron excitability persist for several days, the consequent specific alterations in behavioral response of the intact animal to the conditioned stimulus is manifest as learning.

In another model of conditioning in an invertebrate, facilitation of the gill withdrawal reflex of Aplysia californica, Ca-calmodulin mediated changes are also involved (Hawkins et al., 1983; Walters and Byrne, 1983). In this model the conditioned stimulus was tactile stimulation of the gill and the unconditioned stimulus was electric shock to the tail. These workers demonstrated that the learned sensitization of the gill reflex results from presynaptic modulation of the gill sensory neuron. Specifically, serotonin or a serotonin-like substance, is released from a presynaptic facilitator interneuron and binds to the serotonin receptors on the presynaptic terminal of the gill sensory neuron resulting in stimulation of membrane bound adenylate cyclase. The resultant increase in intracellular cAMP in the presynaptic terminal of the gill sensory neuron promotes the cAMP dependent phosphorylation of presynaptic voltage dependent potassium channels. Phosphorylation of the voltage dependent potassium channels in turn results in decreased potassium conductance, thereby delaying repolarization and prolonging the inward calcium current. The net effect of these changes is to increase intracellular Ca-calmodulin complexes and enhanced neurotransmitter release. In both models Ca-calmodulin mediated messenger functions are steps in the formation of the long lasting change in excitability.

In mammals, the nictitating membrane-eyeblink conditioning in rabbit has been instructive. While many brain regions are involved, CA1 hippocampal neurons exhibit conditioning specific reductions in spike afterhyperpolarization. The reduction in hyperpolarization is intrinsic to mechanisms within CA1 neurons (Coulter et al., 1985). Afterhyperpolarization is due to activation of a calcium dependent potassium current. Biochemical analysis of the CA1 region of the hippocampus removed 24 hours after conditioning has demonstrated a translocation of protein kinase C from cytosol to membrane fractions compared to naive and pseudoconditioned rabbit hippocampal extracts. Thus, conditioning in the intact rabbit appears to utilize biophysical mechanisms similar to those found in invertebrates in the links between excitation and long-term changes in excitability. In each, calcium activated enzyme processes are important.

Calcium influx is also important for the rapid induction of gene transcription following stimulation of neuronal acetylcholine receptors (Greenberg et al., 1986). Cholinergic agonists rapidly and transiently induce transcription of the c-fos proto-oncogene and actin through a calcium influx mechanism. These recent observations suggest the possibility that gene induction could be related to long-term changes in excitability and offer future avenues of research into the biophysical mechanisms of long-term memory.

Consideration of the central role of calcium and calmodulin in the mediation of conditioning and the effect of aluminum upon both calcium homeostasis and calmodulin in the vertebrate experimental aluminum encephalopathy, suggests the hypothesis that the learning-memory deficit displayed by the intact animal operates through an

inhibition of calmodulin mediated biochemical changes. It
is further postulated that the biochemical sequence
responsible for these plastic changes represent "luxury"
functions of the neuron and operate in a range above that
necessary for the regulation of other "survival" or
"housekeeping" functions.

CALMODULIN IN ALZHEIMER'S DISEASE

      Unpublished work from this laboratory indicates that
calmodulin messenger RNA content, calmodulin measured by
radioimmune assay and calmodulin activation of 3'5' cyclic
nucleotide phosphodiesterase are all selectively depressed
in post mortem cerebral cortex from patients with end stage
Alzheimer's disease. Control brains were matched for age,
post mortem interval, drug ingestion, agonal process and
included non-Alzheimer dementia associated pathological
insults to the brain. Expressed as a percentage of non-
Alzheimer dementia control calmodulin messenger RNA per gram
of temporal lobe, Alzheimer calmodulin messenger RNA was
reduced to 36% ($p<0.02$) (McLachlan et al., in preparation).
Calmodulin measured by radioimmune assay was reduced from
an average control value of 635 µg/g soluble protein
extracted from cerebral cortex to an average value for
Alzheimer extracts of 446 µg/g ($p<0.001$) whereas the non-
Alzheimer cerebral cortex was not significantly different
from control: 691 µg/g soluble protein. Calmodulin
measurements were made on 17 control brains, 18 Alzheimer
affected brains and 15 non-Alzheimer affected brains.
Subcortical white matter also exhibited reduced calmodulin:
control=303 µg/g; Alzheimer=244 µg/g. Employing an enzymatic
assay for calmodulin-activity, Alzheimer extracts
demonstrated significantly reduced activity compared to
preparations from either the normal control or non-
Alzheimer affected extracts. Probably many molecular
mechanisms will be found disturbed in Alzheimer's disease
and no single molecular mechanism is likely to be solely
responsible for the observed alterations in behavior.
Nevertheless, the present observations suggest that a
disturbance in calmodulin at the level of gene expression,
synthesis or post-translational modification, occurring early
in the sequence of molecular events in Alzheimer's disease
could contribute to failure in memory, particularly if
"memory" processes represent a "luxury function" at
concentrations well above the amount required for cell

survival.

SUMMARY

Invertebrate models of conditioning and long term potentiation in hippocampal neurons are now known to involve a complex sequence of events linking membrane electrical excitability to calcium-calmodulin mediated enzymatic modification of electrical excitability. In intact animals, aluminum alters the performance of short term memory tasks and in isolated hippocampal neurons long term potentiation. At the molecular level, aluminum alters calmodulin gene expression and the competence of calmodulin to activate target enzymes. Both the molecular and behavioral toxic aluminum induced events are closely linked in time. A working hypothesis is that within neurons important in learning-memory performance, calmodulin content exceeds the content required for cell survival. In the early stage of the experimental encephalopathy, aluminum affects only a sufficient number of calmodulin molecules to affect the mechanisms responsible for memory functions but not cell survival. As more aluminum is released from intracellular stores, active calmodulin is reduced below the "luxury" level, and other vital cell functions are affected giving rise to the latter stages of the encephalopathy.

Alzheimer's disease is a complex metabolic disorder of brain in which aluminum accumulates in DNA containing structures of the neocortex and upon neurons with neurofibrillary degeneration. End stage Alzheimer affected neocortex has markedly reduced calmodulin messenger RNA and moderately reduced calmodulin. We speculate that if the disorder in calmodulin synthesis occurred at an early stage in the disease, the disorder in short term memory could be partially explained.

ACKNOWLEDGEMENTS

Supported by the Ontario Mental Health Foundation and the Scottish Rite Charitable Foundation.

REFERENCES

Alkon DL, Shoukimas JJ, Heldman E (1982). Calcium-mediated
decrease of a voltage-dependent potassium current.
Biophys J 40:245-250.
Alkon DL, Acosta-Urquidi J, Olds J, Kuzma G, Neary JT
(1983). Protein kinase injection reduces voltage-dependent
potassium currents. Science (Washington) 219:303-306.
Alkon DL, Kubota M, Neary JT, Naito S, Coulter D, Rasmussen
H (1986). C-kinase activation prolongs Ca^{2+}-dependent
inactivation of K^+ currents. Biochem Biophys Res Comm
134:1245-1253.
Baimbridge KG, Miller JJ, Parkes CD (1982). Calcium binding
protein distribution in the rat brain. Brain Res 239:519-
525.
Bartus RT, Dean RL, Beer B, Lippa AS (1982). The
cholinergic hypothesis of geriatric memory dysfunction.
Science (Washington) 217:408-417.
Blaustein MP (1974). The interrelationship between Na and
Ca flexes across cell membrane. Rev Physiol Biochem
Pharmacol 70:33-82.
Bliss TUP, Lomo T (1973). Long lasting potentiation of
synaptic transmission in the dentate area of the
unaesthetized rabbit following stimulation of the perforant
path. J Physiol London 232:331-356.
Cheung WY (1980). Calmodulin plays a pivotal role in
cellular regulation. Science (Washington) 207:19-27.
Coulter DA, Kubota M, Moore JW, Disterhoft JF, Alkon DC
(1985). Conditioning-specific reduction of CA1
afterhyperpolarization amplitude and duration in rabbit
hippocampal slices. Soc Neurosci Abst 11:891.
Coulter DA, Disterhoft JF, Bank B, Alkon DL (1986).
Persistent conditioning-specific changes of post-synaptic
membrane current in Hermissenda and hippocampus. This
book.
Crapper DR, Dalton AJ (1973a). Alteration and short-term
retention, conditioned avoidance response acquisition and
motivation following aluminum induced neurofibrillary
degeneration. Physiol and Behav 10:925-933.
Crapper DR, Dalton AJ (1973b). Aluminum induced
neurofibrillary degeneration, brain electrical activity
and alterations in acquisition and retention. Physiol
and Behav 10:935-945.
Crapper DR, Krishnan SS, Dalton AJ (1973). Brain aluminum
distribution in Alzheimer's disease and experimental
neurofibrillary degeneration. Science (Washington)

180:511-513.

Crapper DR, Tomko GS (1975). Neuronal correlates of an encephalopathy induced by aluminum neurofibrillary degeneration. Brain Res 97:253-264.

Crapper DR (1976). Functional consequences of neurofibrillary degeneration. In Terry RD, Gershon S (eds): "Neurobiology of Aging 3," Raven Press, New York, pp 405-432.

Crapper DR, Quittkat S, Krishnan SS, Dalton AJ, De Boni U (1980). Intranuclear aluminum content in Alzheimer's disease, dialysis encephalopathy and experimental aluminum encephalopathy. Acta Neuropath (Berlin) 50:19-24.

De Boni U, Scott JW, Crapper DR (1974). Intracellular aluminum binding: a histochemical study. Histochemistry 40:31-37.

Farnell BJ, Crapper McLachlan DR, Baimbridge K, De Boni U, Wong L, Wood PL (1985). Calcium metabolism in Aluminum encephalopathy. Exp Neurol 88:68-83.

Gauthier S, Leblanc R, Robitaille Y, Ouirion R, Carlsson G, Beaulieu M, Bouchard R, Dastoor D, Ervin F, Gauthier L, Gauvin M, Henry J, McLachlan DR, Palmour R (1986). Transmitter-replacement therapy in Alzheimer's disease using intracerebro-ventricular infusions of receptor agonists. Canadian J Neurol, in press.

Greenberg ME, Ziff EG, Greene LA (1986). Stimulation of neuronal acetylcholine receptors induces rapid gene transcription. Science (Washington) 234:80-83.

Hawkins RD, Abrams TW, Carew TJ, Kandel ER (1983). A cellular mechanism of classical conditioning in Aplysia's activity dependent amplification of presynaptic facilitation. Science (Washington) 219:400-404.

Isquierdo I (1975). The hippocampus and learning. Prog Neurobiol 5:37-75.

Kidd M (1963). Paired helical filaments in electron microscopy of Alzheimer's disease. Nature 197:192-193.

McLachlan DRC, Dalton AJ, Galin H, Schlotterer G, Daicar E (1984). Alzheimer's disease: clinical cause and cognitive disturbances. Acta Neurologica Scand 69:83-90.

McLachlan DRC (1986). Aluminum and Alzheimer's disease. Neurobiol. Aging 7, in press.

Milner B (1970). Memory and the medial temporal regions of the brain. In Pribram KH, Broadbent DE (eds): "Biology of Memory," Academic Press, New York, pp 29-50.

O'Keefe J, Nadel L (1979). The hippocampus as a cognitive map. Behav Brain Sci 2:487-533.

Olton DS, Becker JT, Handelmann GE (1980). Hippocampal

function: working memory or cognitive mapping? Physiol Psychol 8:239–246.

Petit TL, Biederman GB, McMullen PA (1980). Neurofibrillary degeneration, dendritic dying back and learning-memory deficits after aluminum administration, implications for brain aging. Exp Neurol 67:152–162.

Rabe A, Lei M, Shek J, Wisniewski H (1982). Learning deficit in immature rabbits with aluminum-induced neurofibrillary degeneration. Exp Neurol 76:441–446.

Sakakibara M, Alkon M, De Lorenzo DL, Goldenring JR, Neary JT, Heldman E (1986). Modulation of calcium-mediated inactivation of ionic currents by Ca^{2+}/calmodulin-dependent protein kinase II. Biophys J 50:319–327.

Schwartzkroin PA, Webster K (1978). Long lasting facilitation of a synaptic potential following tetanization in the in vitro hippocampal slice. Brain Res 89:107–119.

Seigle N, Haug A (1983a). Aluminum interactions with calmodulin. Evidence for altered structure and function from optical and enzymatic studies. Biochem Biophys Acta 744:36–45.

Seigle N, Haug A (1983b). Calmodulin-dependent formation of membrane potential in barley root plasma membrane vesicles: a biochemical model of aluminum toxicity in plants. Physiol Plant 59:285–291.

Terry RD, Gonatas NK, Weiss M (1964). Ultra structural studies in Alzheimer's presenile dementia. Amer J Path 44:269–297.

Terry RD, Pena C (1965). Experimental production of neurofibrillary degeneration. II. Electron microscopy, phosphatase histochemistry and electron probe analysis. J Neuropath Exp Neurol 24:200–210.

VanBerkum MFA, Wong YL, Lewis PN, Crapper McLachlan DR (1986). Total and poly(A) RNA yields during an aluminum encephalopathy in rabbit brains. Neurochem Res 11:1347–1359.

Walaas S, Nairn A, Greengard P (1983). Regional distribution of calcium- and cyclic adenosine 3':5'-mono-phosphate-regulated protein phosphorylation systems in mammalian brain. J Neuroscience 3:291–301.

Walters ET, Byrne JH (1983). Associative conditioning of single sensory neurons suggests a cellular mechanism for learning. Science (Washington) 219:405–408.

Whitehouse PJ, Price DL, Strumble RG, Clark AW, Coyle JT, De Long MR (1982). Alzheimer's disease and senile dementia: loss of neurons in the basal forebrain. Science

(Washington) 215:1237-1239.
Yaari Y, Hamon B, Lux HD (in press). Development of two
distinct types of calcium channels and cultured mammalian
hippocampal neurons. Science (Washington).
Yokel RA (1983). Repeated systemic aluminum exposure
effects on classical conditioning of the rabbit.
Neurobehav Toxicol Teratol 5:41-46.

Neuroplasticity, Learning, and Memory, pages 61–86
© **1987 Alan R. Liss, Inc.**

MECHANISMS OF SYNAPTIC PLASTICITY

Eva Fifkova

Department of Psychology,
University of Colorado
Boulder, Colorado 80309

The universal distribution of contractile proteins in
eukaryotic cells together with their involvement in a
number of critical cellular functions indicates that the
development of contractile proteins has been a crucial step
in the eukaryotic evolution (Fine and Blitz, 1976). The
role of the cytoplasm in neuronal functions has been so far
largely overlooked. The main emphasis has been on the
plasma membrane for fast electrical events and on
cytoplasmic organelles for the slower metabolic processes.
Studies of the cytoplasm were so far performed in non-
neural cells only, with the focus on the properties of
actin networks. These networks, because of their
capability of rapid phase (sol-gel) transitions (Stossel,
1982) may gain control over the state of the cytoplasm and
hence over important functions of the cell. In neurons,
such changes may affect among others, the geometry of
neuronal processes, in particular the geometry of dendritic
spines which may have an impact on their electrical
properties. In this way, actin networks may regulate
various plastic reactions in the CNS. Therefore, in this
review I shall discuss the behavior of actin networks and
their interactions with myosin and spectrin as they are
known in nonmuscle cells and speculate on their possible
function in neurons, in relation to neuronal plasticity
(Fifkova, 1985a).

ACTIN

In nonmuscle cells, actin occurs in the form of

monomers (G-actin) and filaments (F-actin). Since only
F-actin is physiologically active in the cell, the process
of filament assembly and its regulation is very important.
It is a self-sustaining process that is controlled by actin
associated proteins. Actin filaments may be cross-linked
into networks or bundles which are known as actin
superstructures that form the bases of actin gels. When
the gels are solated during the phase transitions of the
cytoplasm, the superstructures become disassembled; however,
the integrity of individual filaments remains intact. The
spatial organization of actin networks is highly variable
in nonmuscle cells. Actin-dependent activities are rather
flexible, because actin filaments are capable of continuous
reorganization which is based on an easy interconversion of
G- and F-actin. Actin networks may be transiently assembled
and disassembled in different domains of the cell. This
endows the cell with dynamic properties so that it can
speedily react to changing functional requirements (Stossel,
1982). However, such a property requires a strict control
over the assembly and organization of the network (Spudich
et al., 1982). The versatility necessary for such a control
is conferred on actin networks by actin associated proteins
(Isenberg et al., 1982; Stossel, 1982, Schliwa, 1981,
Schliwa et al., 1982a,b; Weeds, 1982). Since these
proteins are found in most of the cell types, it appears
that the actin regulatory complex is universally
distributed and forms an interactive system in the cell
(Pollard, 1986). The properties of actin networks are
determined by a number of factors, out of which actin
associated proteins and the concentration of free
cytoplasmic Ca^{2+} are the most important ones (Condeelis,
1983; Stossel, 1983). As to their function, they may be
divided into three groups (Pollard, 1981; Schliwa, 1981;
Weeds, 1982). 1) Actin filament cross-linking proteins
mediate lateral associations and branching polymerization
of actin filaments forming actin gels. These proteins in
general are either Ca^{2+} - insensitive or operate at
submicromolar Ca^{2+} concentrations. They make actin networks
stiffer, which has important consequences for the physical
properties of the cytoplasm. It will increase the
resistance of the cytoplasm affecting, e.g., the speed of
organelle movement and other processes related to such an
activity. This of course will change with the solation of
actin gels. 2) Actin modulators are Ca^{2+} sensitive, operate
at micromolar CA^{2+} levels, and regulate the rigidity of the
actin gels. They induce solation by breaking the links

formed by the actin cross-linkers. 3) <u>Actin depolymerizing</u>
<u>and polymerization inhibiting proteins</u> complex with actin
monomers (G-actin), so that they cannot enter the
polymerization cycle. These proteins are likely to account
for the large proportion (50%) of monomeric actin in nonmuscle cells and neurons (Flock et al., 1981), in spite of
the filament assembly-favoring conditions of the cytoplasm.
Profilin, e.g., suppresses spontaneous nucleation (the
first step in actin filament formation) while the brain
depolymerizing factor severs spontaneously formed actin
filaments. Thus, these two proteins allow the cell to
specify the time and place for actin assembly (Pollard,
1986). In the compartmentalized cytoplasm, it may be
easier to translocate complexed monomeric actin that is
readily polymerizable rather than to shift actin filaments
to places of demand (Schliwa, 1981). Since actin
polymerization is favored by the intracellular milieu
anyway, the primary concern of the cell may not be to
assemble actin into filaments but rather to keep a certain
proportion of actin non-polymerized.

The G- and F-actin conformations are suggesting a
possible dual role of actin in nonmuscle cells. The
polymerized actin may have a more static, skeletal function
while the non-polymerized but readily polymerizable actin
may subserve the dynamic properties of nonmuscle cells
(Pollard, 1981) and neuronal plasticity in the CNS (Fifkova,
1985a).

This overview indicates that actin is a protein
ubiquitous in eukaryotic cells that subserves diverse
cellular functions. This diversity is largely determined
by the concentration of free cytoplasmic CA^{2+} and by actin
associated proteins. These proteins, (including myosin
and brain spectrin [fodrin]), were recently isolated also
from the brain, and they were shown to have properties
similar to those of non-neural systems. Since free
cytoplasmic calcium fluctuates during neuronal activity,
it can be assumed that the properties and behavior of
neuronal actin will be similar to that of the non-neural
actin. Consequently, actin networks in neurons may undergo
transitions from gel to sol and may contract. Much of the
remodeling of the actin filament system is induced by
localized activation of myosin leading to a localized
contraction of the actin networks in the cell. The
organization of actin filaments can be understood at least

in part by the understanding of how myosin is activated at
specific locations and places in the cytoplasm (Pollard,
1986). Such types of changes may be involved in a variety
of plastic reactions observed in the nervous system (Fifkova
and Delay, 1982).

MYOSIN

The diversity of myosin molecules in nonmuscle tissues
and their involvement in a variety of functions may be
related to their evolutionary history. The specialized
contractile proteins in muscles may have actually evolved
from those more primitive ones of nonmuscle cells. The
colocalization of myosin with actin in various domains of
the nonmuscle cell argues for their contractile role (Karp,
1984); however, in some instances (not yet well defined)
myosin may merely cross-link actin filaments (Langer et
al., 1986). Nonmuscle actins from diverse sources have
preserved remarkably well their amino acid sequences during
evolution whereas myosins show more diversity. Actin is a
highly conserved molecule, ubiquitous within the cell while
myosin is less highly conserved with its specific location
in the cell unknown. Cytoplasmic consistency and
contractility are to a large extent determined by reversible
interactions among actin, myosin, and associated proteins
(Taylor and Condeelis, 1979). Although contractility and
movement are differentiated functions of nonmuscle cells,
nonmuscle motility is difficult to study. Actin and myosin
are less ordered and more labile in nonmuscle cells and
nonmuscle movements are far more discrete than muscle
contractions (Karp, 1984). According to the current view
of nonmuscle motive force production, myosin acts as a
mechanochemical transducer while actin is the major
structural protein in the contractile event (Pollard et al.,
1976).

Properties of Nonmuscle Myosin

The myosin molecule consists of two heavy and four
light chains. Each heavy chain (200,000 dalton) consists
of a head and a rod. The two rods are coiled in an α-helix
which represents the tail portion of the molecule. Two
light chains (20,000 and 16,000 dalton) are associated with
each head, and each head has an actin-binding site and a

catalytic site for ATP hydrolysis (Burridge, 1976; Pollard and Maupin, 1982). Individual myosin molecules tend to form tail-to-tail associated dimers which may aggregate into bipolar filaments. The nonmuscle myosin filaments are shorter and thinner than those from muscles and their varying size may be reflecting functional requirements of the respective cell types (Pollard and Maupin, 1982). All nonmuscle myosins are capable of interacting with actin filaments and all possess an actin-activated ATPase. The current hypothesis of the regulation of nonmuscle contraction is identical with that of the smooth muscle contraction, implicating phosphorylation of the 20,000 dalton myosin light chain as a crucial step in the cycle (Adelstein, 1982; Stossel, 1983). A stimulus that raises free cytosolic Ca^{2+} to micromolar levels causes CA^{2+} to bind to calmodulin, forming a complex that activates the myosin light-chain kinase which induces phosphorylation of the myosin light-chain. This facilitates activation of the myosin Mg^{2+}-ATPase, with a subsequent myosin ATP hydrolysis that provides energy for binding of myosin heads to actin filaments (F-actin), which then results in contraction (Stossel, 1983; Keller and Mooseker, 1982). The size of bipolar filaments (i.e., the number of aggregated myosin dimers) appears to be directly related to the amount of the motile force produced by the cell. In nonmuscle cells, myosin is present in a much lower concentration than actin (1:100) which may indicate a low power output requiring fewer force-generating units (Pollard et al., 1976). Also, its role in contraction may be the only myosin function, while actin is in addition also a major component of the cell microfilaments. The cytoskeletal function may require actin concentrations by far exceeding those necessary for motility (Taylor and Condeelis, 1979).

Conformation of Myosin

As to whether nonmuscle myosin is aggregated into bipolar filaments in vivo is a matter of a continuous debate since electron microscopy of nonmuscle cells has shown myosin filaments only infrequently. The myosin filaments (not dimers) are unstable and depend on ionic variations of their environment which may cause conformational changes. Recently two reports have suggested that myosin is always in the filamentous form which may be disrupted by the processing for electron microscopy (Trybus

and Lowey, 1984). However, even if the filament were not
disrupted, the sparseness of myosin filaments observed
under the electron microscope may be due not only to the
low myosin concentration, but also to the difficulty of
detecting an elongated myosin filament (300 nm long) which
is 5-6 times larger than the width of an ultrathin section
(50-60 nm). Given these problems some investigators have
concluded that nonmuscle myosin in vivo is not permanently
in the filamentous form (Pollard, 1982; Kuczmarski and
Rosenbaum, 1979a,b; Hirokawa et al., 1982) and that myosin
conformation reflects the functional state of the tissue
(Stossel, 1983; Hirokawa et al., 1982). In vitro isolated
brain myosin was shown to form very short filaments, much
shorter than those of smooth or skeletal muscles (Kuczmarski
and Rosenbaum, 1979a,b). In the noncontracted intestinal
brush border, myosin dimers were shown to be physically
associated with the cytoskeleton (probably with actin
filaments) by the tail end of the molecule. However,
phosphorylation of the myosin light chain releases the
dimers from the cytoskeleton and assembles them into bipolar
filaments. After contraction, when myosin is
dephosphorylated, the bipolar filaments are disassembled
and the myosin dimers are reattached to the cytoskeleton
(Hirokawa et al., 1982). While the question of myosin
conformation in nonmuscle cells in vivo remains so far
unresolved, the paucity of myosin in nonmuscle cells has
been unanimously acknowledged. In addition to all the
factors thus far mentioned, the paucity of myosin in
nonmuscle cells may be a form of "reciprocal" inhibition
at the cellular level, whereby myosin mobilization to one
compartment of the cell may temporarily paralyze the
function of another compartment (Berlin et al., 1978).
Thus, the availability of myosin may regulate the sequence
of individual cellular events (Stossel, 1983; Hirokawa et
al., 1982).

Conditions Affecting Myosin ATPase Activity

Filamentous conformation of myosin is essential for
binding to actin filaments and this can occur only in the
presence of myosin ATP and the actin-activated myosin Mg^{2+}-
ATPase (Kuznicki et al., 1985). The myosin ATPase activity
may be regulated by the length of actin filaments; the
maximal activity appears to be induced by actin filaments
that are 0.25-1.00 nm long (Coleman and Mooseker, 1985).

Given that the myosin ATPase activity is also enhanced by
actin-spectrin cross-linking, it is conceivable that actin
filaments cross-linked by spectrin are of the optimal length
that ensures the maximal ATPase activity (Coleman and
Mooseker, 1985). The actin-myosin interaction in nonmuscle
cells may be also modulated by cyclic AMP through cAMP-
dependent protein kinase which by phosphorylating the myosin
light chain kinase reduces its myosin phosphorylating
capacity. This will reduce the amount of myosin that can
interact with F-actin and consequently diminish the amount
of contraction (Hathaway et al., 1981, 1985).

Solation-Contraction Coupling Hypothesis

     Actin assumes different patterns of organization which
may or may not be amenable to contraction. Bundles of actin
filaments with a parallel orientation of individual
filaments (intestinal microvilli [Mooseker et al., 1984;
Herman and Pollard, 1981] or cilia of sensory hair cells
[Flock et al., 1981; Drenckhahn et al., 1982]) are not
capable of contraction. However, the respective structures
underlying the actin filament bundles (the terminal web or
the cuticular plate, respectively) may contract. While in
the latter regions actin colocalizes with myosin, no myosin
has been found in the microvilli or cilia (Mooseker et al.,
1984; Saunders et al., 1985). In general, actin regulatory
proteins that induce formation of actin bundles or networks
(actin gels) impede contraction by inhibiting the actin-
activated myosin ATPase, and thus prevent actin filaments
to interact with myosin (Condeelis, 1983). On the other
hand, actin regulatory proteins that cross-link actin
filaments into antiparallel arrays may be instrumental for
contraction (Condeelis, 1983). Although myosin colocalizes
only with actin patterns that are capable of contraction,
this colocalization per se is not sufficient to guarantee
contraction. Solation of the gelled actin must precede to
make the contraction possible. Cytosolic Ca^{2+} elevated by
physiological stimuli triggers solation of actin gels as
well as contraction (Taylor and Condeelis, 1979), since
Ca^{2+} differentially affects the respective polymerization
of actin and myosin. While submicromolar levels
($10^{-7}-10^{-8}$ M) of free cytoplasmic Ca^{2+} foster actin filament
assembly, micromolar Ca^{2+} levels (10^{-6} M) promote myosin
filament assembly (Stossel, 1983) and at the same time
induce solation of actin gels. The differential

distribution of myosin and free Ca^{2+} in various cell domains
may trigger regional contractions of the cytoplasm which
could result in directional movements (Stossel, 1983).
Because of the high volume to surface ratio in spines,
stimulation-induced elevated free Ca^{2+} may reach rather
quickly higher concentrations in spines than in dendrites.
Therefore, a movement of the spine could occur along the
concentration gradient between the respective domains of
high (spines) and low (dendrites) Ca^{2+} levels.

Cell Events Mediated by Contraction

     The available literature on myosin localization
suggests that myosin in resting conditions may be evenly
distributed through the cytoplasm and a stimulus may induce
its accumulation in regions that are related to the
physiological response of the cell. Another possibility
is that myosin may be located, even in resting conditions,
solely within the contractile domain. The following are
examples of both possibilities. Myosin in the mitotic
spindle could pull chromosomes to the pole during cell
division, and in the cleavage furrow of dividing cells it
could be involved in cytokinesis (Fujiwara and Pollard,
1976). It could also be involved in secretory activity of
platelets forming with actin a contractile ring, upon
stimulation, that exerts a pressure on secretory vacuoles
to fuse with the plasma membrane (Painter and Ginsberg,
1984). During capping, surface receptors are reorganized
by a contractile mechanism, whereby the receptors are
collected into the cap (Bourguignon et al., 1982).
Underneath the cap myosin together with actin, calmodulin
and myosin light chain kinase form a contractile, membrane-
associated complex (Kerrick and Bourguignon, 1984). The
terminal web of the intestinal brush border that is known
to contract, is the only region of the cell where myosin
and actin are colocalized (Mooseker et al., 1984).

Myosin in the Nervous System

     Since the pioneering work of Puzskin et al (1972) and
Berl et al. (1973), relatively little work has been done on
the localization of myosin in the nervous system. In most
of the studies on brain myosin, biochemical approaches have
been used for either myosin isolation or its identification

in individual fractions of brain homogenates. The molecule
of brain myosin is similar to that of other nonmuscle cells,
being composed of two globular heads and a 150 nm long tail
(Burridge, 1976; Burridge and Bray, 1975). In vitro, brain
myosin, phosphorylated with the chicken gizzard myosin
light chain kinase, has been shown to be capable to interact
with actin filaments (Barylko and Sobieszek, 1983). Several
proteins, like cofilin and caldesmon, known from non-neural
tissues to regulate myosin activity were also identified in
the brain. Thus, brain myosin seems to have properties
similar to those of other nonmuscle myosins. It has been
postulated that myosin together with actin is involved in
major neuronal functions like synaptic transmission, axonal
transport and growth, being localized in synaptosomes (Berl
et al., 1973; Blitz and Fine, 1974; Cotman and Kelly, 1980;
Drenckhahn and Kaiser, 1983; Drenckhahn et al., 1984) in
axons (Kuczmarski and Rosenbaum, 1979b; Lasek and Hofman,
1976), and axonal growth cones (Letourneau, 1981).
Systematic studies of myosin localization so far have not
been done, with the exception of the cuticular plate of
sensory hair cells (Drenckhahn et al., 1982), hippocampus
(Drenckhahn et al., 1984) and growth cones of cultured
neurons (Letourneau, 1981). All those studies employed the
light microscope techniques of immunofluorescent antimyosin
antibodies. However, this method does not permit us to draw
any conclusion as to the myosin function since the details
of myosin organization are beyond the resolving power of
light microscopy. There have been so far no attempts to
identify brain myosin in situ with immunoelectron
microscopy. The technical difficulties involved in
preserving and identifying unstable and infrequently
occurring structures like myosin filaments explains why
such a task has so far not been undertaken. However, it
is at present the only way how to approach the question of
myosin function.

In summary then, actin in conjunction with myosin is
likely to have a dual function: (1) as structural support
in the form of a microfilament cytoskeleton in which it is
aided by attached myosin dimers; (2) as a contractile
network when the phosphorylated myosin is released from
the microfilament cytoskeleton and aggregated in bipolar
filaments which bind to anti-parallel actin filaments and
induce contraction (Condeelis, 1983). The interplay between
phase transitions of actin networks and their contraction
and relaxation may underlie various forms of neuronal

plasticity (Fifkova, 1985a) as will be discussed in the last part of this article.

SPECTRIN

In close association with the cytoplasmic surface of the plasma membrane there is a two-dimensional network whose main component is spectrin, a long, fibrous tetrameric protein (composed of two head-to-head associated heterodimers, one heterodimer being composed of an α- and β-subunit) that, together with actin oligomers and 4.1 protein (=synapsin), forms a flexible membrane skeleton supporting the plasma membrane (for review see Goodman and Zagon, 1984). It associates with integral proteins of the plasma membrane via ankyrin and with cytoplasmic actin filaments via actin oligomers. Since spectrin was first identified in mammalian erythrocytes, the functional properties of the erythrocyte membrane skeleton were extrapolated to nonerythrocytes, when it was discovered that they too contain spectrin (Goodman and Zagon, 1984). However, while in erythrocytes spectrin plays an essential role in the membrane support and flexibility, in nonerythrocytes it has a high affinity for membrane receptors and links them through actin oligomers to cytoplasmic actin filaments (Painter et al., 1985a,b). Since brain spectrin is capable of binding calmodulin and activating myosin ATPase, it may form together with actin and myosin a force-generating complex associated with the plasma membrane. Such a network is uniquely suited to stabilize receptors in synaptic membranes and to mobilize and translocate them during a process that leads to an increased length of synaptic apposition after various experimental interventions (Connolly, 1984; Connolly and Graham, 1985; Peng and Phelan, 1984). If spectrin were also associated with the cytoplasmic aspects of individual organelles (Aunis and Perrin, 1984) in neurons, then, given the spectrin-actin affinity at resting Ca^{2+} levels, organelles like synaptic vesicles or the spine apparatus would be locked in time and space in the dense actin network of axon terminals and spines, respectively. Upon stimulation, the increased free Ca^{2+} would break the spectrin-actin filament bonds and cause solation of the actin network. Consequently, the organelles would be released during stimulation, for periods lasting as long as the cytoplasmic Ca^{2+} would be elevated to fulfill their respective functions.

In chromaffin cells, spectrin has been found on the cytoplasmic surfaces of chromaffin vesicles (Aunis and Perrin, 1984). In resting conditions, at low CA^{2+} concentractions ($10^{-8}M$), the vesicles positioned at the cell periphery are immobilized by the spectrin-actin filament bonds within the actin network. Upon stimulation, the surge of Ca^{2+} into the cell raises the free Ca^{2+} concentration, which breaks the actin filament - spectrin bonds causing solation of the actin network. Consequently, the vesicles are freed to undergo exocytosis (Aunis and Perrin, 1984). A system similar to this could also operate in axon terminals and regulate the transmitter release. The spine apparatus is another organelle whose function may be regulated by spectrin. Being positioned in the center of the spine, it represents an actin-anchoring site from which the actin filaments irradiate towards the plasma membrane and postsynaptic density (Fifkova, 1985a,b). Since the subplasmalemmal spectrin is instrumental in the association of actin filaments with the plasma membrane and probably also with the postsynaptic density, the same could apply to the membrane of the spine apparatus, if it were to contain (like the chromaffin vesicles) spectrin on its cytoplasmic surface. Although the function of the spine apparatus is not yet fully understood, there are indications that it could be involved in regulation of the levels of the free cytoplasmic Ca^{2+} in the spine (Fifkova et al., 1983). Spectrin might be expected to play an important role in this activity. In some spines, the spine apparatus is occupying most of the stalk cytoplasm (Fifkova, unpublished observations) which could increase considerably the resistance of the stalk. Since the spine contains a dense actin network, the spine apparatus could be locked in the resting state in one position within the spine stalk. However, during activity it might be released and change its position, which could affect the spine stalk resistance. Thus, spectrin on the cytoplasmic surface of the spine apparatus may play an important role in the dynamics of the stimulation-induced morphometric spine changes (Fifkova, 1985a,b).

Stimulation may also induce spectrin reorganization under the plasma membrane (Perrin and Aunis, 1985). In resting conditions, spectrin forms a continuous layer, which 10 min after stimulation that elicits a physiological

response (in chromaffin cell), becomes discontinuous for
about an hour before returning to the resting pattern.
Since this change is not accompanied by a discontinuity of
the plasma membrane, it is likely to be caused by spectrin
redistribution alone which indicates dynamic interactions
between activated membrane receptors and the submembrane
skeleton. Given that actin networks react to stimulation
within fractions of a second, it is likely that spectrin
reorganization actually reflects, with a delay, changes in
the actin network.

Brain spectrin (fodrin) has been so far examined only
at the light microscope level, mostly in the avian CNS
(Lazarides and Nelson, 1983a,b). Light microscope studies
of brain spectrin in mice with fluorescent antibodies have
revealed that heavy fluorescence is located in the perikarya
and large dendritic trunks and that attenuated fluorescence
in dendrites correlates with tapering of these processes
(Zagon et al., 1984). Little or no staining could be seen
in axons (Zagon et al., 1984), which contrasts with
observations describing spectrin as being axonally
transported (Levine and Willard, 1981). Such discrepancies
cannot be resolved at the light microscope level because
this method cannot reveal details as to the spectrin
localization and organization under the plasma and synaptic
membranes or within the postsynaptic density. It also
cannot show whether spectrin forms a submembrane skeleton
on the cytoplasmic face of neuronal organelles or whether
it occurs within the cytoplasm without any associations
with the membranes. Although fine structural details of
spectrin organization in small profiles like dendritic
spines and axon terminals are beyond the resolving power
of the light microscope, they could be studied with the
powerful technique of immunoelectron microscopy.

NEURONAL PLASTICITY, LONG-TERM POTENTIATION

From the present review on the properties of
contractile proteins in the brain it follows that myosin
and spectrin together with actin (Fifkova, 1985a,b,c).
actin-regulatory proteins, free cytoplasmic Ca^{2+} and
calmodulin may be involved in the molecular mechanism of
long-term plastic changes at the CNS synapses. Currently,
the best physiological model of synaptic plasticity is
long-term potentiation (LTP) which is elicited in the

dentate fascia by stimuli that may be generated in the
afferent perforant path by electrical stimulation that
matches physiological conditions (McNaughton, 1983). We
have shown distinct ultrastructural changes in dendritic
spines of the dentate fascia in preparations exhibiting
LTP. The organization of the perforant path in the dentate
fascia facilitates morphometric studies, since it terminates
solely on dendritic spines in a restricted zone of the
dentate molecular layer forming the majority of excitatory
synaptic contacts there (Fifkova, 1975; Matthews et al.,
1976; Nafstad, 1967). The stimulated spines show long-
lasting morphometric changes which include enlargement of
the spine head (cross section area and perimeter [Fifkova
and Van Harreveld, 1977; Fifkova et al., 1981], widening and
and shortening of the spine stalk [Fifkova and Anderson,
1981], and an increased length of synaptic appositions
[Fifkova, 1985c]). The relation between morphometric
changes and the increased synaptic activity may be as
follows: If the spine stalk were to widen, the longitudinal
resistance will decrease while the conductance will increase,
and the synaptic potentials will be enhanced (Rall, 1974;
1978). The increased length of the active synaptic zone
will contribute to this effect (Fifkova, 1985c). Since
1975 when we first reported these stimulation-induced
morphometric changes (Van Harreveld and Fifkova, 1975),
similar observations were done in dendritic spines of a
variety of species that were associated with a stimulation-
induced increase in synaptic activity (Bradley and Horn,
1979; Brown and Horn, 1979; Coss and Globus, 1978; Coss
et al., 1980; Brandon and Coss, 1982; Burgess and Coss, 1982;
1983; Desmond and Levy, 1983). Thus, the observed
morphometric changes in spines may represent a general
mechanism of synaptic plasticity. LTP in the dentate
fascia has all the characteristics expected for an
associative memory storage device. These may be summarized
in several points. The higher order sensory information
converges to the entorhinal cortex and is channeled through
the perforant path to the dentate fascia (Jones and Powell,
1970). This information may be modulated by the state of
the animal's consciousness (Winson, 1980). A conditioned
stimulus leads to a rapid, large increase in activity that
resembles LTP and is confined to the dentate fascia
leaving the activity of the entorhinal cortex unchanged
(Berger et al., 1976; Berger and Thompson, 1978; Patterson
et al., 1978). A parallel between LTP and spatial behavior
was shown in aged rats, which are dificient in both (Barnes,

1979). Since aged animals suffer from a loss of spines
that is not accompanied by a loss of the dentate granule
cells (Geinisman et al., 1977; 1978), spines may be
implicated not only in the mechanism of LTP but also in the
mechanism of memory. Therefore, clarification of the
molecular mechanism of morphometric changes in the spines
during increased activity may provide an extremely valuable
tool in studies leading towards understanding of higher
brain functions. The merit of these observations is that
they identify morphometric changes of the postsynaptic
spine as a possible factor modulating synaptic activity.

The type of morphometric changes in spines invited the
idea that contractile proteins might be involved in the
mechanism of these changes. While studying the actin
filaments with the S-1 fragment of myosin, it became
obvious that within the entire neuron the highest density
of actin filaments is in dendritic spines and that the
characteristic shape of the spine is determined by the
dense network in the bulbous head and by the lengthwise
oriented filaments in the slender stalk (Fig. 1). The
high density of the actin network, indicates a very low
cytoplasmic Ca^{2+} level (Fifkova, 1985a,b; Markham and
Fifkova, 1986; Fifkova et al., 1984), that may be
responsible for the absence of cytoplasmic organelles
from the spine. The only exception is the spine apparatus
which serves as one anchoring site for the actin filaments,
the other two being the plasma membrane and postsynaptic
density. The spine apparatus is likely to regulate Ca^{2+}
levels in the spine since it was shown to have an affinity
for, and capacity to sequester Ca^{2+}. The high surface to
volume ratio in spines may quickly raise the level of
intraspinous Ca^{2+} during synaptic activation. The influx
may be particularly dramatic during LTP when the synaptic
potentials are enhanced. The elevated Ca^{2+} could induce
solation of the actin network in the spine head and
contraction of filaments in the spine stalk resulting in
the observed changed configurations of the spine profile.
During LTP Ca^{2+} levels will be considerably higher in
spines than in dendrites, which will result in a
concentration gradient along which the spine stalk may
contract. The versatile nature of actin networks is going
to determine whether these changes will be short-lived
(Crick, 1982) or whether they will become stabilized by
Ca^{2+}-induced increase of protein synthesis in polyribosomes
at the base of the spine (Steward and Levy, 1982). The

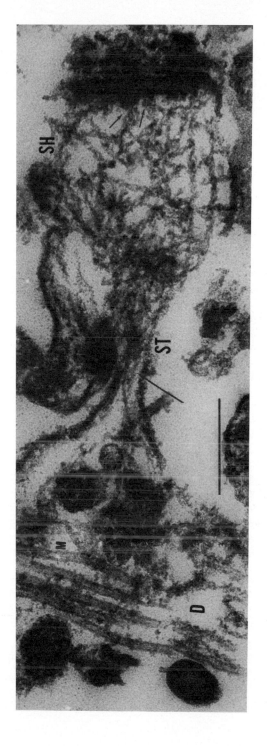

Fig. 1. Organization of actin filaments in a dendritic spine.
Dendritic spine head (SH) is attached with a stalk (ST) to a dendrite (D).
Note the actin filament network in the spine head and lengthwise oriented filaments
in the spine stalk (arrow). Actin filaments in the spine head are associated with
the postsynaptic density (small arrows). Within the dendrite there are microtubules
(M). The preparation was treated with S-1 fragment of myosin. Magnification
112,200 X; bar, 0.25 m. (Reprinted from Fifkova, 1985a).

merit of these observations is that they <u>identify</u>
<u>morphometric changes of the postsynaptic spine as a possible</u>
<u>factor modulating synaptic activity and single out</u>
<u>contractile proteins and Ca^{2+} as key factors in these</u>
<u>changes</u>.

The spine may be considered as a specific domain of the
neuron from the electrical as well as cytochemical aspect
(Steward and Levy, 1982). The absence of organelles from
the spine allows for a full use of the actin network, which
is regulated by the levels of free cytoplasmic Ca^{2+}. A
number of proteins known to be involved in actin-mediated
activities has been suggested (Drenckhahn and Kaiser, 1983)
or demonstrated (Carlin et al., 1980; Caceres et al., 1983;
Grab et al., 1979) in the spine. In addition, the
microtubule-associated protein MAP2 has also been observed
in spines (Caceres et al., 1984). This protein, in the
absence of microtubules, has an affinity to actin and
promotes a parallel organization of actin filaments
(Griffith and Pollard, 1982). Since such a pattern is
observed in the spine stalk, MAP2 could be responsible for
this organization (Fifkova and Delay, 1982; Fifkova et al.,
1984; Markham et al., 1984). In the spine head, however,
where actin forms a dense network, actin modulators and
cross-linking proteins may be involved. Free cytoplasmic
Ca^{2+} elevated by stimulation could activate the calmodulin
system of the spine and thus trigger a chain of events
leading to the formation of bipolar myosin filaments in the
spine stalk. These then would interact with actin filaments
and induce contraction of the stalk with a consequent
widening and shortening of its profile (Fifkova and Anderson,
1981). In the spine head, the increased Ca^{2+} levels may
induce solation of the actin network with a consequent
effect on the membrane cytoskeleton. The widened stalk
would facilitate the transport of newly formed proteins into
the spine head and the solated actin network there could
facilitate incorporation of these proteins into the plasma
and synaptic membranes. Such types of events could account
for the observed morphometric changes in spines (Fifkova and
Van Harreveld, 1977; Fifkova et al., 1983; Fifkova, 1985a).

Different actin-associated proteins and proteins
controlling the levels of free cytosolic Ca^{2+} are not
homogeneously distributed across the neuronal compartments
and across individual brain regions (Caceres et al., 1984;
Cumming and Burgoyne, 1983). Given the control that these

proteins have over the actin networks, such a differential
distribution may determine the kind of role that actin may
play in individual parts of the neuron and in individual
regions of the brain. Actin may serve as a matrix whose
capacity to generate plastic reactions may be determined by
the type of regulatory proteins.

Plasticity in dendritic spines may also involve other
than volumetric changes. Dendritic spines were found to be
very sensitive to variations in the normal sensory input and
to other interventions. Variations in the spine density
were observed in different brain regions after a variety of
interventions like visual deprivation (Boyce and Fifkova,
1980; Fifkova, 1974; 1979; 1980; Valverde, 1967), hibernation
(Boycott, 1982), chronic ethanol consumption (Tavares et al.,
1983), lesions (Cotman and Nadler, 1978), and the like. In
none of these experiments was the reduced number of spines
accompanied by spine degeneration. This could also be
attributed to the actin network of the spine. A modified
input to the spine may affect the physicochemical properties
of its cytoplasm inducing disengagement of the axospinous
synapse with a consequent retraction of the spines. The
importance of spines and their proper geometry for normal
cognitive functions was also demonstrated in mental
retardation of the Down's type (Marin-Padilla, 1972, 1976;
Purpura, 1974; Suetsugu and Mehraien, 1980), in the cerebral
cortex and hippocampus. An extensive spine loss was observed
together with the presence of spines with abnormally long
and thin stalks. Since the abnormal spines were contacted
by normal axon terminals, it can be surmised that the main
failure of normal synaptic transmission resides in dendritic
spines. The severity of these changes was proportional to
the severity of the syndrome. Pathological changes observed
in dendritic spines resemble those of animal experiments and
may share a common mechanism involving actin networks.

ACKNOWLEDGMENTS

The part of the research reviewed here that was carried
out in Dr. Fifkova's laboratory was supported in part by
Grants MH 27240-10 (from NIMH), AA 06196-03 (from ADAMHA),
AG 04804-02 (from NIA).

REFERENCES

Adelstein RS (1982). Calmodulin and the regulation of the
  actin-myosin interaction in smooth muscle and nonmuscle
  cells. Cell 30:349-350.
Aunis D, Perrin D (1984). Chromaffin granule membrane-F-
  actin interactions and spectrin-like protein of subcellular
  organelles: A possible relationship. J Neurochem 42:
  1558-1569.
Barnes CA (1979). Memory deficits associated with
  senescence: A neurophysiological and behavioral study in
  the rat. J Comp Physiol Psych 93:74-104.
Barylko B, Sobieszek A (1983). Phosphorylation and actin
  activation of brain myosin. EMBO J 2:369-374.
Berger TW, Alger B, Thompson RF (1976). Neuronal substrate
  of classical conditioning in the hippocampus. Science
  192:483-485.
Berger TW, Thompson RF (1978). Neuronal plasticity in the
  limbic system during classical conditioning of the rabbit
  nictitating membrane response. I. The hippocampus.
  Brain Res 145:323-346.
Berl S, Puszkin S, Nicklas WJ (1973). Actomyosin-like
  protein in brain. Science 179:441-446.
Berlin RD, Oliver JM, Walter RJ (1978). Surface functions
  during mitosis. Cell 15:327-341.
Blitz AL, Fine RE (1974). Muscle-like contractile proteins
  and tubulin in synaptosomes. Proc Natl Acad Sci USA 71:
  4472-4476.
Bourguignon LYW, Nagpal M, Balazovick K, Guerriero V,
  Means AR (1982). Association of myosin light chain kinase
  with lymphocyte membrane-cytoskeleton complex. J Cell
  Biol 95:793-797.
Boyce S, Fifkova E (1980). Synaptic changes in the visual
  cortex of monocularly deprived hooded rats. Soc Neurosci
  Abstr 6:492.
Boycott BB (1982). Some further comment concerning dendritic
  spines. Trends Neurosci 5:328-329.
Bradley P, Horn G (1979). Neuronal plasticity in the chick
  brain: Morphological effects of visual experience on
  neurons in hyperstriatum accessorium. Brain Res 162:148-
  153.
Brandon JG, Coss RG (1982). Rapid dendritic spine stem
  shortening during one-trial learning: The honeybee's first
  orientation flight. Brain Res 252:51-61.
Brochat KO, Stidwill RP, Burgess DR (1985). Phosphorylation
  controls brush border motility by regulating myosin

structure and association with the cytoskeleton. Cell 35: 561-571.

Brown MW, Horn G (1979). Neuronal plasticity in the chick brain: Electrophysiological effects of visual experience on hyperstriatal neurons. Brain Res 162:142-147.

Burgess JW, Coss RG (1982). Effects of chronic crowding stress on midbrain development: Changes in dendritic spine density and morphology. Dev Psychobiol 15:461-470.

Burgess JW, Coss RG (1983). Rapid effect of biologically relevant stimulation on tectal neurons: Changes in dendritic spine morphology after nine minutes are retained for twenty-four hours. Brain Res 266:217-233.

Burridge K (1976). Multiple forms of nonmuscle myosin. In Goldman R, Pollard TD, Rosenbaum J (eds), "Cell Motility, Book B," pp 739-747.

Burridge K, Bray D (1975). Purification and structural analysis of myosins from the brain and other nonmuscle tissues. J Mol Biol 99:1-24.

Caceres A, Bender P, Snavely L, Rebhun LI, Steward O (1983). Distribution and subcellular localization of calmodulin in adult and developing brain tissue. Brain Res 10:449-461.

Caceres A, Binder LI, Payne MR, Bender P, Rebhun L, Steward O (1984). Differential subcellular localization of tubulin and microtubule-associated protein MAP2 in brain tissue as revealed by immunocytochemistry with monoclonal hybridoma antibodies. J Neurosci 4:394-410.

Carlin RK, Grab DJ, Cohen RS, Siekevitz P (1980). Isolation and characterization of postsynaptic densities from various brain regions: enrichment of different types of postsynaptic densities. J Cell Biol 86:831-843.

Coleman TR, Mooseker MS (1985). Effects of actin filament cross-linking and filament length on actin-myosin interaction. J Cell Biol 101:1850-1857.

Condeelis J (1983). Rheological properties of cytoplasm: Significance for the organization of spatial information and movement. In McIntosh JR (ed), Spatial organization of eukaryotic cells, "Modern Cell Biology," Vol. 2, Alan R Liss: New York, pp 225-240.

Connolly JA (1984). Role of the cytoskeleton in the formation, stabilization, and removal of acetylcholine receptor clusters in cultured muscle cells. J Cell Biol 99:148-154.

Connolly JA, Graham AJ (1985). Actin filaments and acetylcholine receptor clusters in embryonic chick myotubes. Europ J Cell Biol 37:191-195.

Coss RG, Globus A (1978). Spine stems on tectal interneurons in jewel fish are shortened by social stimulation. Science 200:787-790.

Coss RG, Brandon JG, Globus A (1980). Changes in morphology of dendritic spines on honeybee calycal interneurons associated with cumulative nursing and foraging experiences. Brain Res 192:49-59.

Cotman CW, Kelly PT (1980). Macromolecular architecture of CNS synapses. In Cotman CW, Poste G, Nicholson GL (eds), "The Cell Surface and Neuronal Function," Elsevier-North Holland Publishing Co: Amsterdam, pp 505-533.

Cotman CW, Nadler JV (1978). Reactive synaptogenesis in the hippocampus. In Cotman CW (ed.), "Neuronal Plasticity," Raven Press: New York, pp 270-271.

Crick F (1982). Do dendritic spines twitch? Trends Neurosci 5:44-46.

Cumming R, Burgoyne R (1983). Compartmentalization of neuronal cytoskeletal proteins. Biosci Rep 3:997-1006.

Desmond NL, Levy WB (1983). Synaptic correlates of associative potentiation/depression: An ultrastructural study in the hippocampus. Brain Res 265:21-30.

Drenckhahn D, Kaiser HW (1983). Evidence for the concentration of F-actin and myosin in synapses and in the plasmalemmal zone of axons. Eur J Cell Biol 31:235-240.

Drenckhahn D, Frotcher M, Kaiser HW (1984). Concentration of F-actin in synaptic formations of the hippocampus as visualized by staining with fluorescent phalloidin. Brain Res 300:381-384.

Drenckhahn D, Kellner J, Mannherz HG, Groschel-Stewart U, Kendrick-Jones J, Scholley JM (1982). Absence of myosin-like immunoactivity in stereocilia of cochlear hair cells. Nature (London) 300:330-332.

Fifkova E (1974). Plastic and degenerative changes in visual centers. In Newton G, Riesen AH (eds), "Advances in Psychobiology," Wiley and Sons: New York, pp 59-131.

Fifkova E (1975). Two types of terminal degeneration in the molecular layer of the dentate fascia following lesions of the entorhinal cortex. Brain Res 85:169-175.

Fifkova E (1979). Effect of monocular deprivation on synaptic density of the visual cortex in hooded rats. Anat Rec 193:537.

Fifkova E (1980). Development of postdeprivation changes in the visual cortex of hooded rats. Anat Rec 196:56A.

Fifkova E (1985a). Actin in the nervous system. Brain Res Rev 9:187-215.

Fifkova E (1985b). A possible mechanism of morphometric changes in dendritic spines induced by stimulation. Cell Molec Neurobiol 5:47-63.

Fifkova E (1985c). Synaptic hypertrophy in the dentate fascia of the hippocampus. In Dimitrijevic M, Eccles JC (eds.), "Recent Achievements in Restorative Neurology," M Karger: Basel, pp 263-271.

Fifkova E, Anderson CL (1981). Stimulation-induced changes in dimensions of stalks of dendritic spines in the dentate molecular layer. Exp Neurol 74:621-627.

Fifkova E, Delay RJ (1982). Cytoplasmic actin in neuronal processes as a possible mediator of synaptic plasticity. J Cell Biol 95:345-350.

Fifkova E, Van Harreveld A (1977). Long-lasting morphological changes in dendritic spines of dentate granular cells following stimulation of the entorhinal area. J Neurocytol 6:211-230.

Fifkova E, Markham JA, Cullen-Dockstader K (1984). Association of the actin lattice with cytoplasmic organelles and the plasma membrane in dendrites and dendritic spines. Soc Neurosci Abstr 10:425.

Fifkova E, Markham JA, Delay RJ (1983). Calcium in the spine apparatus of dendritic spines in the dentate molecular layer. Brain Res 266:163-168.

Fifkova E, Anderson CL, Young SJ, Van Harreveld A (1982). Effect of anisomycin on stimulation-induced changes in dendritic spines of the dentate granule cells. J. Neurocytol 11:183-210

Fine RE, Blitz AL (1976). Chemical and functional studies of tropomyosin and troponin C from brain and other tissues. In Goldman R, Pollard TD, Rosenbaum J (eds), "Cell Motility, Book B," pp 785-795.

Flock A, Cheung HC, Flock B, Utter G (1981). Three sets of actin filaments in sensory cells of the inner ear. J Neurocytol 10:133-147.

Fujiwara K, Pollard TD (1976). Fluorescent antibody localization of myosin in the cytoplasm, cleavage furrow, and mitotic spindle of human cells. J Cell Biol 71:848-875.

Geinisman Y, Bondareff W, Dodge JT (1977). Age-related loss of dendritic branches and spines in the molecular layer of the rat dentate gyrus. Anat Rec 187:586.

Geinisman Y, Bondareff W, Dodge JT (1978). Dendritic atrophy in the dentate gyrus of the senescent rat. Amer J Anat 152:321-330.

Goodman SR, Zagon IS (1984). Brain spectrin: A review.

Brain Res Bull 13:813-832.

Grab DJ, Berzins K, Cohen RS, Siekevitz P (1979). Presence of calmodulin in postsynaptic densities isolated from canine cerebral cortex. J Biol Chem 254:8690-8696.

Griffith LM, Pollard TD (1982). The interaction of actin filaments with microtubules and microtubule associated proteins. J Biol Chem 257:9143-9151.

Hathaway DR, Adelstein RS, Klee CB (1981). Interaction of calmodulin with myosin light chain kinase and cAMP-dependent protein kinase in bovine brain. J Biol Chem 256:8183-8189.

Hathaway DR, Konicki MV, Coolican SA (1985). Phosphorylation of myosin light chain kinase from vascular smooth muscle by cAMP- and cGMP-dependent protein kinases. J Mol Cell Cardiol 17:841-850, 1985.

Hirokawa N, Tilney LG, Fujiwara K, Heuser JE (1982). Organization of actin, myosin, and intermediate filaments in the brush border of intestinal epithelial cells. J Cell Biol 94:425-443.

Isenberg G, Jockusch BM (1982). Capping, bundling, cross-linking: Three properties of actin binding proteins. In Sakai H, Mohri H, Borisy G (eds), "Biological Functions of Microtubules and Related Structures," Academic Press: New York.

Jones EG, Powell TPS (1970). An anatomical study of converging sensory pathways within the cerebral cortex of the monkey. Brain 93:793-820.

Karp G (1984). "Cell Biology," McGraw-Hill: New York pp 641-661.

Keller TCS, Mooseker MS (1982). CA^{++}-calmodulin-dependent phosphorylation of myosin and its role in brush border contraction in vitro. J Cell Biol 95:943-959.

Kerrick GL, Bourguignon LYW (1984). Regulation of receptor capping in mouse lymphoma T cells by Ca^{2+}-activated myosin light chain kinase. Proc Natl Acad Sci USA 81:165-169.

Kuczmarski ER, Rosenbaum JL (1979a). Chick brain actin and myosin. J Cell Biol 80:341-355.

Kuczmarski ER, Rosenbaum JL (1979b). Studies on the organization and localization of actin and myosin in neurons. J Cell Biol 80:356-371.

Kuznicki J, Cote GP, Bowers B, Korn ED (1985). Filament formation and actin-activated ATPase activity are abolished by proteolytic removal of a small peptide from the tip of the tail of the heavy chain of Acanthamoeba myosin II. J Biol Chem 260:1967-1973.

Lasek RJ, Hoffman PN (1976). The axonal transport of

cytoskeletal proteins. In Goldman R, Pollard R, Rosenbaum J (eds), "Cell Motility," Cold Spring Harbor Laboratory, Cold Spring Harbor: New York, pp 1021-1049.

Lazarides E, Nelson WJ (1983a). Erythrocyte and brain forms of spectrin in cerebellum: Distinct membrane-cytoskeletal domains in neurons. Science 220:1295-1296.

Lazarides E, Nelson WJ (1983b). Erythrocyte form of spectrin in cerebellum: Appearance at a specific stage in the terminal differentiation of neurons. Science 222: 931-933.

Letourneau PC (1981). Immunocytochemical evidence for colocalization in neurite growth cones of actin and myosin and their relationship to cell substratum adhesions. Dev Biol 85:113-122.

Levine J, Willard M (1981). Fodrin: Axonally transported polypeptides associated with the internal periphery of many cells. J Cell Biol 90:631-643.

Mangeat PH, Burridge K (1984). Immunoprecipitation of nonerythrocyte spectrin within live cells following micro-injection of specific antibodies: relation to cytoskeletal structures. J Cell Biol 98:1363-1377.

Marin-Padilla M (1972). Structural abnormalities of the cerebral cortex in human chromosomal aberrations. A Golgi study. Brain Res 44:625-629.

Marin-Padilla M (1976). Pyramidal cell abnormalities in the motor cortex of a child with Down's syndrome: A Golgi study. J Comp Neurol 167:63-82.

Markham JA, Fifkova E (1986). Actin filament within dendrites and dendritic spines during development. Brain Res 27:263-269.

Matthews DA, Cotman CW, Lynch G (1976). An electron microscopic study of lesion-induced synaptogenesis in the dentate gyrus of the adult rat. Brain Res 115:1-21.

McNaughton BL (1983). Activity dependent modulation of hippocampal synaptic efficacy: Some implications for memory processes. In Seifert W (ed), "Neurobiology of the Hippocampus," Academic Press: New York, pp 233-252.

Mooseker MS, Bonder EM, Conzelman KA, Fishkind DJ, Howe CL, Keller, III, TCS (1984). Brush border cytoskeleton and integration of cellular functions. J Cell Biol 99: 104s-112s.

Nafstadt PMJ (1967). An electron microscope study on the termination of the perforant path fibers in the hippocampus and fascia dentata. Zeitschrift fur Zellforschung und Mikroskopische Anatomie 76:532-542.

Painter RG, Ginsberg MH (1984). Centripetal myosin

redistribution in thrombin-stimulated platelets. Exp Cell Res 155:198-212.

Painter RG, Gaarde W, Ginsberg MH (1985a). Direct evidence for the interaction of platelet surface membrane proteins GPIIb and III with cytoskeletal components: Protein cross-linking studies. J Cell Biochem 27:277-290.

Painter RG, Prodouz KN, Gaarde W (1985b). Isolation of a subpopulation of glycoprotein IIb-III from platelet membranes that is bound to membrane actin. J Cell Biol 100:652-657.

Patterson MM, Berger TW, Thompson RF (1979). Neuronal plasticity recorded from cat hippocampus during classical conditioning. Brain Res 163:339-343.

Peng HB, Phelan KA (1984). Early cytoplasmic specialization at the presumptive acetylcholine receptor cluster: A meshwork of thin filaments. J Cell Biol 99:344-349.

Perrin D, Aunis D (1985). Reorganization of α-fodrin induced by stimulation in secretory cells. Nature 315: 589-591.

Pollard TD (1981). Cytoplasmic contractile proteins. J Cell Biol 91:156s-165s.

Pollard TD (1982). Structure and polymerization of Acanthanolba myosin II filaments. J Cell Biol 95:816-825.

Pollard TD (1986). Assembly and dynamics of the actin filament system. J Cell Biochem 31:87-95.

Pollard TD, Craig SW (1982). Mechanism of actin polymerization. Trends Biochem Sci 8:55-58.

Pollard TD, Maupin P (1982). Electron microscopy of actin and myosin. In Griffith ZG (ed), "Electron Microscopy in Biology," Vol 2, pp 2-28.

Pollard TD, Aebi U, Cooper JA, Fowler WE, Tseng P (1982). Actin structure, polymerization, and gelation. Cold Spring Harb Symp Quant Biol 46:513-524.

Pollard TD, Fujiwara K, Niederman R, Maupin-Szamier P (1976). Evidence for the role of cytoplasmic actin and myosin in cellular structure and motility. In Goldman R, Pollard TD, Rosenbaum J (eds), "Cell Motility, Book B," Cold Spring Harbor Laboratory, pp 689-724.

Purpura DP (1974). Dendritic spine "dysgenesis" and mental retardation. Science 186:1126-1128.

Puzskin S, Nicklas WJ, Berl S (1972). Actomyosin-like protein in the brain: Subcellular distribution. J Neurochem 19:1319-1333.

Rall W (1974). Dendritic spines, synaptic potency and neuronal plasticity. In Woody CD, Brown KD, Crow TJ, Knispel JD (eds), "Cellular Mechanism Subserving Changes in Neuronal Activity," University of Calfornia, Brain Research Institute.

Rall W (1978). Dendritic spines and synaptic potency. In Porter R (ed), "Studies in Neurophysiology," Cambridge University Press, pp 203-209.

Schliwa M (1981). Proteins associated with cytoplasmic actin. Cell 25:587-590.

Schliwa M, Pryzwansky KB, van Blerkom J (1982a). Implications of cytoskeletal interactions for cellular architecture and behavior. Phil Trans Roy Soc B 299: 199-205.

Schliwa M, van Blerkom J, Pryzwansky KB (1982b). Structural organization of the cytoplasm. Cold Spring Harb Symp Quant Biol 46:51-67.

Spudich JA, Pardee JD, Simpson PA, Yamamoto ER, Kuczmarski ER, Stryer L (1982). Actin and myosin: Control of filament assembly. Phil Trans Roy Soc B 299:247-261.

Steward O, Levy WB (1982). Preferential localization of polyribosomes under the base of dendritic spines in granule cells of the dentate gyrus. J Neurosci 2:284-291.

Stossel TP (1982). The structure of the cortical cytoplasm. Phil Trans Roy Soc B 299:275-289.

Stossel TP (1983). The spatial organization of cortical cytoplasm in macrophages. In McIntosh JR (ed), "Spatial organization of eukaryotic cells, Modern Cell Biology," Vol 2, Alan R Liss: New York, pp 203-223.

Suetsugu M, Mehraien P (1980). Spine distribution along the apical dendrites of the pyramidal neurons in Down's syndrome. Acta Neuropat 50:207-210.

Tavarco MA, Paula-Barbosa MM, Gray EG (1983). Dendritic spine plasticity and chronic alcoholism in rats. Neurosci Lett 42:235-238.

Taylor D, Condeelis J (1985). Cytoplasmic structure and contractility in amoeboid cells. Int Rev Cytol 56:57-144.

Trybus KM, Lowey S (1984). Conformational states of smooth muscle myosin: Effects of light chain phosphorylation and ionic strength. J Biol Chem 259:8564-8571.

Valverde F (1967). Apical dendritic spines of the visual cortex and light deprivation in the mouse. Exp Brain Res 3:337-352.

Van Harreveld A, Fifkova E (1975). Swelling of dendritic spines in the fascia dentata after stimulation of the perforant path. Exp Neurol 49:736-750.

Weeds A (1982). Actin-binding proteins-regulators of cell architecture and motility. Nature (Lond.) 296:811-816.

Winson J (1980). Raphe influences on neuronal transmission

from the perforant pathway through dentate gyrus. J
Neurophysiol 44:937-950.
Zagon IS, McLaughlin PJ, Goodman SR (1984). Localization
of spectrin in mammalian brain. J Neurosci 4:3089-3100.

Neuroplasticity, Learning, and Memory, pages 87–124
© 1987 Alan R. Liss, Inc.

THE CELLULAR BASIS OF LEARNING AND MEMORY: THE ANATOMICAL
SEQUEL TO NEURONAL USE

Ted L. Petit and Etan J. Markus

Division of Life Sciences, University of
Toronto, Scarborough Campus, Scarborough,
Ontario M1C 1A4, Canada

In 1949, Donald O. Hebb postulated one of the major
tenets on the neurobiology of ·learning and memory formation:
"repeated stimulation of specific receptors will lead slowly
to the formation of an 'assembly' of association-area cells
which can act briefly as a closed system after stimulation
has ceased; this prolongs the time during which the
structural changes of learning occur. The structural
changes that make lasting memory possible...[are]...that a
growth process accompanying synaptic activity makes the
synapse more readily traversed" (Hebb, 1949, p. 60 and 486).
This hypothesis has inspired considerable research aimed at
determining whether Hebb was correct, i.e., does neuronal
activation cause alterations in synaptic or neuronal
structure, and if so, what are the alterations and how do
they occur. This chapter will address this question by
examining the types of changes that occur in the cell
following neuronal activation (both "normal" activation
that occurs over time, and experimentally induced
activation), in an attempt to determine whether such
activation induces structural changes that would likely
increase the power of transmission across the synapse. We
will also discuss data that suggests that these activation
induced structural changes may be diminished in conditions
where learning and memory capacities are reduced. Finally,
we will briefly overview the mechanism by which synaptic
activation leads to neuronal structural changes.

CELLULAR PLASTICITY: THE DEVELOPMENTAL APPROACH

Cellular models of learning and memory, such as that proposed by Hebb, assume that some element of the neuron must be altered for the storage of new information. This process or ability of the neuron to change in response to events is referred to as neural plasticity. Nowhere is the process of neural plasticity more evident than in the developing animal. Not only are the reactive properties of the cell more robust, i.e., cells early in development show their greatest response to environmental stimulation, lesion induced synaptogenesis, etc., but also the growth of the cell is a "naturally occurring" plastic process. As a consequence, many researchers now consider normal development, and plasticity during the developmental period, a critical key in determining the events underlying information storage (e.g. Schmidt, 1985).

Thus, there are three major factors which make examining developmental events critical in our quest to understand the neuroanatomical basis of learning and memory. First, development is probably the most intensive period of natural learning for animals, during which time they are storing memories about their new world, and there is a concomitant increase in cognitive capacities; if learning and memory formation cause alterations in cellular anatomy, these alterations should be readily seen by examining animals at different developmental ages. Second, many of the cellular events seen in adult models of neuroanatomical plasticity, such as synaptogenesis and increases in dendritic structure, occur as a natural sequence and at a rapid rate during development. In a system where plastic processes are occurring with such frequency, their properties, mechanisms, etc., can be easily studied. Finally, it is important to examine the changes that occur in the cell during this period of normal neuronal use, or activation, in order to compare them to the changes seen in adult brains with the various experimentally induced models of learning. For example, certain neuroanatomical changes have been observed following long-term potentiation; if similar alterations are seen over time during development, then they likely represent the normal physiological response of the cell to activation. Conversely, with the massive amount of learning that occurs during development, if the neuroanatomical changes proposed to underlie memory formation are not seen during this period, it seems unlikely that they could underlie information storage.

The Behavioral Perspective

To determine the neural mechanisms underlying behavioral change, neural alterations must be studied in the context of learning. As would be expected based on the extensive research on the increasing cognitive capacities, knowledge, and memory formation in developing humans, the rat similarly undergoes marked changes in its behavioral repertoire as it develops. To study this in greater detail and to allow a correlation with later anatomical analyses of the motor-sensory neocortex, rats were examined on a battery of motor-sensory behavioral tests over their development (Markus and Petit, 1986). Male rats were tested on postnatal days 1 (P1), 3, 5, 7, 10, 15, 20, 30, 60, and 90. The behavioral battery, ranging from simple reflexive tests to tests of complex locomotor capacities, consisted of tactile induced (paw-touch) forelimb placing, chin-touch induced forelimb placing, body righting after being placed on their back, climbing an inclined plane, traversing narrow beams of different widths and textures, and keeping up with a revolving wheel.

Large variations were seen in the mastery of the different tasks. Reflex motor behaviors such as tactile induced placing and body righting reached a mature level at P7 - 10. Performance of more complex motor behaviors, such as climbing an inclined plane and different types of locomotion (traversing a narrow beam and keeping up with a revolving wheel) reached a mature level by the third postnatal week (see Fig. 1). Chin induced placing is intermediate, with a mature reaction appearing by approximately P15. These results are consistent with and extend previous reports (Altman and Sudarshan, 1975; Hicks and D'Amato, 1975; Donatelle, 1977; Bell and Lundenberg, 1985; Rabe et al., 1985). The observed differences in the development of various motor skills are not unexpected since they require different neural structures, levels of integration and degrees of prior experience.

Thus, during the period examined, there are clear changes in the behavioral capacities of the animal. Some behaviors mature around P7 - 10 and appear to reflect the maturation of lower centers and the reflexes that they

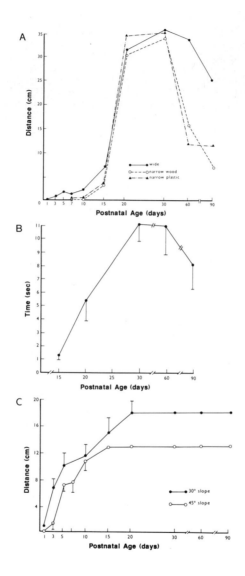

Figure 1. (A). The distance traversed by rats of different postnatal ages on paths of different widths and surface textures. (B). The amount of time animals of different postnatal ages were able to keep up with a turning wheel. (C). The distance traversed by animals of different postnatal ages in climbing inclined slopes.

mediate. Other motor-sensory behaviors, however, which animals master by P20 - 30, require the motor-sensory neocortex for their mediation, and involve prior experience and the formation of memories concerning motor-sensory skills (Hicks and D'Amato, 1975). To determine what cellular changes could underlie this increase in the behavioral capabilities of the animal, we conducted a series of studies examining the anatomical changes that occur in neurons of the motor-sensory cortex over the period of behavioral change.

Synaptogenesis and Synaptic Plasticity

The synapse is the point of contact where information is transferred between two neurons in most vertebrate systems. It seems likely, therefore, that if the passage of information from one cell to another, i.e., activation of the synapse, is to cause an alteration in the structure of the cell, such anatomical alterations are most likely to start or initially be most evident at the synapse, probably by altering the morphology of the synapse or inducing the formation of new synapses. One of the major events of early development is a marked increase in the number of (new) synapses. Studies on developing animals, therefore, allow an examination of the speed, mechanism, and process of synaptogenesis, the changes in the structure of new synapses over time (with usage), and the association between synaptogenesis and the increasing cognitive capacities of the animal.

We have recently completed an in-depth analysis of synapse formation and the way synaptic morphology changes over time during development in both the human (Petit et al., 1984) and rat (Markus and Petit, 1986; Markus, Petit and LeBoutillier, 1986). Although the data gathered from the human is important, the data from the rat is more complete (reflecting the greater access to tissue at specific developmental stages) and the tissue is better preserved since there is no delay between death and fixation. Therefore, the data from the rat will be discussed in detail, with reference made to the human where appropriate (the interested reader is referred to our paper on human tissue for more information [Petit et al., 1984]).

The rats discussed above were sacrificed (on P1, 3, 5, 7, 10, 15, 20, 30, 60 or 90). Additional rats were sacrificed at 28-29 months of age; rats at this age are considered "old" since the 50% survival rate of this strain of rats is 27 months (Janicke et al., 1985). Following fixation, tissue samples were taken from the dorsal motor-sensory neocortex and prepared for electron microscopy. One half of the tissue was stained with the routine osmium-lead citrate - uranyl acetate (osmium) method, while the other half was stained with the ethanol phosphotungstic acid (EPTA) technique. Synaptic density in the molecular layer was determined and the data corrected for section thickness and synaptic size. To determine if synapse size is altered over development, synapses were also systematically photographed and a series of measurements were taken of the synapses, including the presynaptic element length, area, and maximal dense projection height, the number and size of synaptic vesicles adjacent to the presynaptic element, synaptic cleft width, and the postsynaptic element length and area (see Fig. 2).

Synaptogenesis. Our data indicate a large increase in synaptic density (the number of synapses per unit area), commencing at approximately P10, peaking at P30 (see Fig. 3). Even a superficial examination of Fig. 3, with the realization of the extremely small area sampled per micrograph (a 3600 by 5680 nm area), indicates that massive numbers of new synapses are being formed each day. The peak in synaptic density at P30 is initially followed by a sharp decline, and then by a gradual decline or plateau into adulthood. These data are in agreement with most other synaptic density reports in the rat neocortex (Aghajanian and Bloom, 1967; Armstrong-James and Johnson, 1970; Woodward et al., 1971; Dyson and Jones, 1980; Stewart and Falk, 1985). The initial sharp decline in synaptic density following the peak at P30 supports the selective stabilization model (Changeux and Danchin, 1976) which suggests that during development many extra synapses are initially formed, some of which are later eliminated according to their use. Thus the above data, as well as research by others (e.g. LeVay, Wiesel and Hubel, 1980; Adams and Jones, 1982; Burry et al., 1984; Greenough, 1985; Thompson, 1985) indicates that synapses which are not used or do not make functional contacts will not be retained.

Synaptic Structural Plasticity. The formation of an

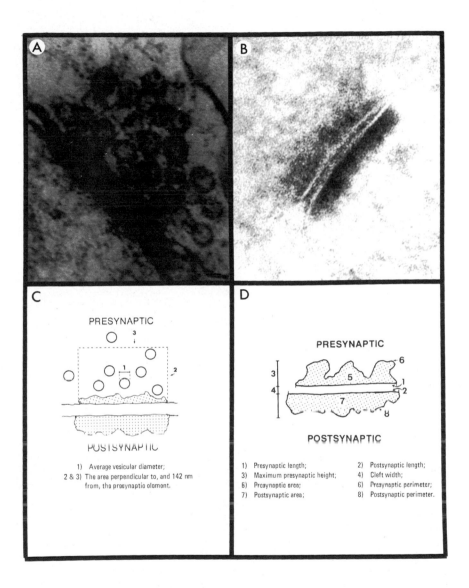

Figure 2. (A). An osmium stained synapse (28,000 X).
(B). An EPTA stained synapse (28,000 X). (C). Schematic
of an osmium stained synapse and the parameters measured.
(D). Schematic of an EPTA stained synapse and the
parameters measured.

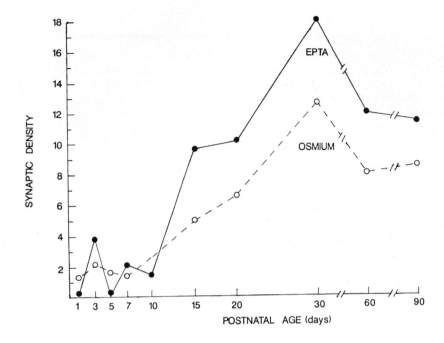

Figure 3. The density of synapses in the molecular layer of the motor-sensory neocortex of the rat over postnatal development.

identifiable synapse is only the beginning of a series of plastic changes in the structure of the synapse. Since non-functional or unused synapses disappear, the changes that occur in the structure of retained synapses are likely to be a result of either maturation or usage. If such changes are seen only during development, they may only reflect maturational processes. However, if similar but more marked changes are seen following developmental stimulation, or similar changes are seen with synaptic activation in adulthood (as will be discussed below), then these developmental changes are likely the result of neuronal activation, and may reflect the plastic process underlying information storage. This is particularly true if such changes would be expected to increase the efficacy of synaptic transmission at that synapse.

Our data indicate a number of changes in the structure of the synapse during development. There is a steady increase in the area of the presynaptic element with development. This increase is seen initially as an increase in length (to approximately P15), which is followed by an increase in the thickness of the presynaptic element. The presynaptic dense projections increase in both width and maximal height, beginning around P15. The postsynaptic element also shows a slight increase in length early in development, followed by an increase in element width thereafter. The observation that, other than showing a slight increase early in development, the length of the synaptic contact is relatively stable, is consistent with previous observations (Jones et al., 1974; Jones and Dyson, 1976; Hinds and Hinds, 1976; DeGroot and Vrensen, 1978; Dyson and Jones, 1980; Devon and Jones, 1981; Petit et al., 1984). Our findings of a developmental increase in the height of the presynaptic projections and thickness of the postsynaptic element are also in agreement with and extend earlier reports (Adinolfi, 1972; Jones and Dyson, 1976; DeGroot and Vrensen, 1978), as well as our observations in the developing human (Petit et al., 1984). Over the lifespan of the rat, we observed that synaptic vesicles decrease in size, but they also increase in number proportionately. In agreement with most other studies (Johnson and Armstrong, 1970; Hays and Roberts, 1973; DeGroot and Vrensen, 1978), we observed no effect of age on cleft width.

Although, as discussed above, there is a sharp increase in the number of synapses, there is no reduction in any measurement of synaptic size during this same period as would be expected if these numerous newly generated synapses were as small as new synapses formed early in development. These results suggest that a newly formed synapse rapidly develops to the structural level of surrounding synapses. The possibility that existing synapses grow in an exaggerated manner, thus statistically compensating for the small new synapses, is ruled out because there is no rise in the statistical variance. Thus, it would appear that new synapses are either formed at the structural size of surrounding synapses or are extremely plastic and grow to that size very rapidly.

In summary, data from the developing animal suggests that synapses can be labile structures. New synapses can

be formed in large numbers relatively quickly, and non-
functional synapses can be eliminated. Also certain
structural components of the synapse can be and are altered,
such that the thickness (and to a lesser extent the length),
of the pre- and postsynaptic elements, as well as the size
and number of synaptic vesicles, are plastic parameters of
the synaptic contact, whereas the width of the synaptic
cleft is not. Other researchers have reported a
developmental increase in the number of synapses with
perforations (small holes in their center, making the
synapses resemble donuts; Greenough et al., 1978; Muller
et al., 1981; Dyson and Jones, 1984). These perforations
may represent the first step in the splitting, or doubling,
of synapses. Finally, changes in the curvature of synapses
have been observed over development (Dyson and Jones, 1980;
Markus and Petit, in preparation). Thus, several aspects
of the synapse are known to undergo change during
development, and as such, most likely represent the plastic
components of the synapse.

Further support for this suggestion comes from
experiments which employ altered levels of environmental
stimulation during development. For example, the
environmental enrichment paradigm employs the placement of
weanling rats in large interconnected cages filled with
toys and other objects, which along with other features of
their environment are changed periodically (Bennett et al.,
1964). This paradigm, used in our laboratory as well as
others, results primarily in increased weight and size of
the cerebral cortex, particularly the occipital area, and
increased behavioral capabilities of the animals, such as
maze solving (e.g. Bennett et al., 1964; Rosenzweig et al.,
1972; Greenough, 1976; Petit and Alfano, 1979). Synaptic
analyses indicate that this experience results in an
increase of approximately 20% in the number of visual cortex
synapses in enriched rats (Turner and Greenough, 1984).
More detailed analyses have revealed that the length of
neocortical synapses are 14 to 52% greater in the enriched
rats, and that there are more perforated synapses
(Mollgaard et al., 1971; West and Greenough, 1972; Greenough
et al., 1978). Enlargement of the synapse has also been
observed in the visual system following the animals' first
exposure to light (Cragg, 1967). Imprinting, a form of
early learning, is also associated with an increase in the
length of the synapse as measured by the postsynaptic
density (Horn, 1985). Conversely, depriving the developing

brain of normal environmental stimulation results in fewer synapses, reduction in the size of synapses, alterations in the curvature of synapses, and reductions in the percent of perforated synapses (see Tieman, 1985). It would appear, therefore, that those aspects of the synapse that undergo change during normal development are also those components that are altered by differing levels of stimulation, learning, or neural activation during the developmental period.

Dendritic Plasticity

Since dendrites are the postsynaptic component of most synaptic contacts in neocortical cells, with the massive increase in synaptic number during development, it is important to determine what changes occur in dendrites during this developmental period. To examine how dendrites are altered during periods of behavioral change, we have recently completed an examination of the pattern of dendritic growth of layer V pyramidal cells in the litter-mates of the animals used for behavioral and synaptic analysis outlined above (Petit, LeBoutillier, Gregorio and Libstug, 1986).

The brains were processed with the rapid Golgi stain and cells from the motor-sensory cortex examined for maximal apical and basilar dendritic field, number of dendritic branches at 20 μm intervals from the cell body, number of apical and basilar branch types (branch order), length of dendritic branch segments, and dendritic spine density (see Fig. 4).

The dendritic structure of these neocortical cells undergoes major growth during this developmental period (see Fig. 5). Dendritic spine density increases markedly during early development, and there is also a large increase in the maximal dendritic field, number of dendritic branches, and length of dendritic branch segments during this period.

Dendrites leaving the cell body are produced until the end of the first week, at which time branching close to the cell body also ends. These data as well as others, suggests that once dendrites are formed, their branching takes place at the growing tip rather than through the proliferation of new branches along their trunks close to the cell body, i.e., new branches do not sprout from the trunk of a dendrite

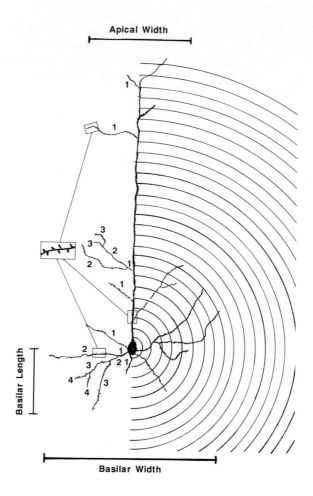

Figure 4.   Schematic drawing of a pyramidal cell showing
the measures taken of dendritic structure.

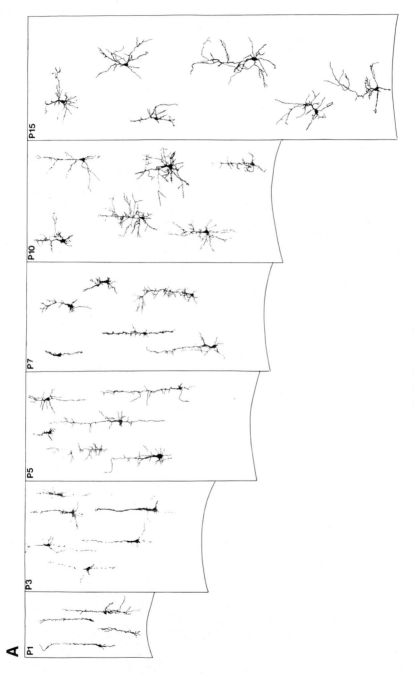

Fig. 5. (*Continued on next page*)

B

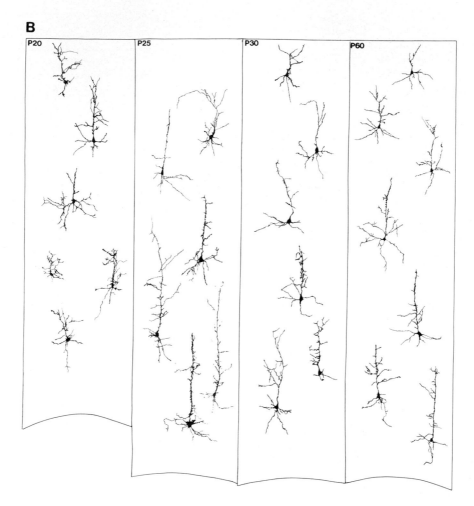

Fig. 5. (*Continued*)

Figure 5. Camera lucida drawings of neurons from the dorsal motor-sensory neocortex of the rat from each age examined, illustrating qualitatively the dendritic growth occurring during this period (A: from P1 to P15; B: from P20 to P60). 200 X.

which has branched at its tip. There is also little change
in the length of dendritic trunks with age, indicating that
once a dendrite has divided at its tip, the trunk does not
continue to increase in length. Any new dendritic material
potentially involved in information storage, therefore, is
likely added at the tip of the dendrite rather than to the
trunk or through the sprouting of new branches from the
trunk.

Spine density peaks around P25 - 30 on the proximal
portion of dendrites, followed by a decline, although no
significant decline was found in dendritic arborization in
the same cells. These results are consistent with Juraska
(1982), although a peak/decline has been observed in some
brain areas (Parnavelas and Uylings, 1980; Duffy and Rakic,
1983; Murphy and Magness, 1984; Lueba and Garey, 1984).
This decline in the number of spines per unit length of
dendrite coincides with the decline in synapses discussed
above, while the absence of a significant decline in
dendritic length or branching in the same cells suggests
that synapses and spines may be more labile, and can change
with little or no change in dendritic length.

In adulthood, measures of the distal portions of the
dendrite indicate an increase in the maximal dendritic
field, the number of distal concentric circle intersections,
the total dendritic length of the cell and the length of
terminal branches. Dendrites, therefore, clearly are
capable of growing into adulthood. Further, unlike during
earlier development when dendrites branch at 20 - 30 µm,
terminal branches grow to lengths of 40 - 50 µm and there
is no increase in the number of higher order dendritic
branches; this indicates that growth during adulthood is
comprised principally of adding length to existing terminal
branches. Our data are consistent with and extends that
reported by others (Parnavelas and Uylings, 1980; Uylings
and Parnavelas, 1981). Similarly, while there is a plateau
or decline in the density of dendritic spines on proximal
dendrites in adulthood, there is an increase in spine density
on the terminal portions of the dendrite. The increased
spine density and dendritic length of the distal portions of
the dendritic field point to the plastic properties of this
portion of the dendrite into adulthood, and are consistent
with findings in other brain regions (Lueba and Garey, 1984;
Dardenness et al., 1984).

   In summary, there are several components of dendritic structure which show plastic properties and morphological changes during development (i.e., there are increases in the number of dendritic spines and in the length and branching of dendrites).

   As with synapses, further support for the assumption that the features discussed above are the plastic components of the dendrite comes from research altering the environmental stimulation received by the animal. It now appears well established that environmental stimulation or enrichment in young animals leads to increases in the number of dendritic spines and the amount of dendritic arborization, while the converse occurs in animals deprived of stimulation (see Greenough, 1975; 1976; 1984; 1985 for reviews). Ultrastructural examinations of dendritic spines indicate that stimulation can cause alterations in the size and shape of the spine head and neck (Freire, 1978; Bradley and Horn, 1979; Brandon and Coss, 1982).

   In the adult, our results suggest that any new dendritic structure associated with the formation of new memories is most likely to occur at the tips of dendrites. Also, dendritic spines can be, and are, produced in adulthood and it is evident that spines (which are no longer functional?) can also be eliminated, as synapses are. Finally, dendritic spines appear to be more labile than dendritic branches and, as such, may represent either the first part of the dendrite to change, or the most easily changed part.

Behavioral - Anatomical Integration

   When attempting to determine what cellular anatomical alterations may form the basis for the changes in the behavioral repertoire, it is important to note that the development of complex motor behaviors (which require both prior experience and memory formation as well as use of the motor-sensory cortex) is closely associated with the anatomical changes discussed above in that structure. For example, a peak in the animal's behavioral capabilities is reached at P20 - 30, which closely coincides with the peak in synaptic density at P30. The period from birth to P30 is also a period of marked increases in the size of synapses as well as the number of dendritic spines and length and branching of dendritic segments. It is possible that any one, or all, of these cellular changes could underlie the observed behavioral changes. It is not possible to make a finer distinction from the developmental paradigm, and, further, it must be realized that these systems are not independent. Since dendrites (particularly dendritic spines) are the most common postsynaptic element, any change in synaptic number would probably be reflected in changes in dendritic properties. As mentioned above, however, certain cellular properties (such as synapses and dendritic spines) appear to be more labile than others (such as dendritic length and branching). Possibly synapses may appear to be more labile not only because they are the actual contact point where information is transferred between cells, but also because they are examined at a much higher magnification such that even small structural changes would be evident. Therefore, it seems most likely that synaptic activation induced by learning causes changes initially in the most microscopic, immediate or labile components of the cell, such as synapses, and only after a period of time do these changes become evident in the more grossly observable dendritic structure.

Caution must be used, however, in making direct connections between behavioral and cellular events. For example, not all of the behaviors examined are mediated by the motor-sensory cortex. Reflex behaviors, which are mediated by lower centers, developed well before the observed changes in cellular anatomy in the neocortex. Also, synaptic density and some motor behaviors show a decline after P30; the rates of the decline are not similar, however, which suggests that the behavioral decline is not a result of synaptic loss.

CELLULAR PLASTICITY IN THE ADULT FOLLOWING NEURONAL ACTIVATION

The morphological alterations discussed above occur in the developing animal concomitant with increasing behavioral capacities which depended in part on the previous formation of memories. If similar morphological changes occur in adult cells following neuronal use, it would seem reasonable to conclude that these aspects of the cell comprise the plastic components of the neuron.

Several studies have suggested that the adult synapse may be modifiable, and consequently may play a key role in learning and memory processes. The types of changes that occur in synapses following repetitive use, and the time course of these changes, are not fully characterized, however (e.g. Bailey and Chen, 1983; Desmond and Levy, 1983; Chang and Greenough, 1984; Horn et al., 1985). The rat hippocampus is an ideal structure for examining these effects since its synaptic connections are well known. For example, the axons of CA3 pyramidal cells make synaptic contact with the proximal portion of the apical dendritic field of CA1 pyramids via the Schaffer collaterals. Further, kainic acid is known to induce high rates of repetitive activation of CA3 pyramids, which in turn drive CA1 cells through their Schaffer collateral synaptic contacts (after a prolonged period this repetitive activation can become cytotoxic, presumably by exceeding the calcium buffering power of the cell; therefore our use of this paradigm was limited to brief periods of time [Olney et al., 1979; Griffiths et al., 1983; Sloviter and Damiano, 1981; Ben-Ari et al., 1979]).

To examine the morphological effects of repetitive activation in the adult and compare them to the plastic changes seen during development, we employed systemic administration of kainic acid as a neurochemical tool to drive CA3 to CA1 synapses for varying periods of time, and the anatomical consequences of this synaptic use subsequently were studied in detail. The advantage of using this protocol is that neurochemical stimulation avoids artifact due to damage (or damage related neuronal firing) from electrodes or in vitro manipulation.

Adult male Wistar rats were injected intraperitoneally with kainic acid and sacrificed 30 min, 1, 2, or 4 hr post-injection. Additional animals not used for anatomical analysis, were monitored electrophysiologically through bipolar wire electrodes previously implanted in the CA1 and CA3 regions of the hippocampus. For anatomical analysis, Golgi stained CA1 pyramidal cells and synapses in the terminal field of the Schaffer collaterals (the zone of activated synapses) were analyzed as described above, with the additional categorization of synapses as concave, straight, or convex relative to the presynaptic terminal (see Fig. 6).

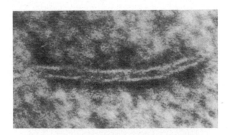

CONCAVE SYNAPSE

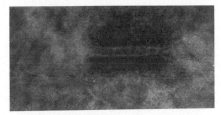

STRAIGHT SYNAPSE

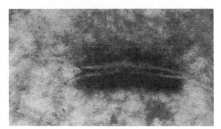

CONVEX SYNAPSE

Figure 6. Electron micrographs of EPTA stained synapses showing the morphological characterization of concave, straight, and convex synapses.

Electrophysiological recordings confirmed that kainic acid causes repetitive activation of CA3 neurons within approximately 15 min of injection, with a concomitant activation of CA1 pyramids. Cellular activity is initially within bursts separated by periods of normal activity. By approximately 30 min following injection, continuous repetitive activation is recorded from both CA3 and CA1 electrodes, and continues throughout the 4 hr period examined.

An examination of the number of synapses of each shape following different periods of stimulation indicated that straight synapses undergo a transient increase at 2 hr followed by a decline to control levels, while concave synapses showed an increase at 2 and 4 hr (see Fig. 7). These data are consistent with previous suggestions of a conversion of synapses from a convex, through straight, to a concave shape with repetitive activation (Desmond and Levy, 1983). However, it is important to note that there is also an increase in the total number of synapses associated with repetitive activation, which reaches significance at 2 hr (see Fig. 7). Thus the results indicate that the repetitive firing of neurons induces both the formation of new synapses, and a change in the number and relative proportions of synaptic shape subtypes that is consistent with a conversion in synaptic shape.

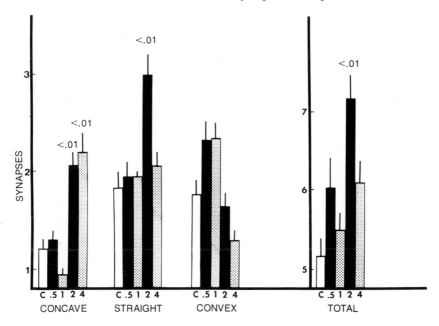

Figure 7. The number of concave, straight, and convex synapses, and total synapses per 15,000 X field in control (C) animals, and those injected with kainic acid 30 min (.5), 1, 2, or 4 hr prior to sacrifice.

The measures of synaptic size indicated a consistent, but non-significant reduction of every synaptic parameter in convex synapses in every group. Concave synapses, however, showed consistent increases in their size following repetitive activation. Increases were observed in maximal height, area, and perimeter of the presynaptic element of concave synapses at 2 hr (see Fig. 8). In contrast to the alterations in the size of the presynaptic element, there were no significant or consistent changes in the dimensions of the postsynaptic element. These results indicate that repetitive synaptic use in this brain area induces increases in the number and presynaptic size of concave synapses.

The finding in our study of significant increases in the size of the presynaptic element suggests that this may be a critical site for plastic changes in synaptic morphology following the present protocol. Other studies have noted increases in the length of the synapse or post-synaptic element as well as the thickness of the post-synaptic density following neuronal use such as stimulation or training (Vrensen and Nunes Cardozo, 1981; Desmond and Levy, 1983; Bailey and Chen, 1983; Horn et al., 1985). Further, Bailey and Chen (1983) found that synapses increase in size in Aplysia which have been sensitized, but decrease in size in those animals that have been habituated. Thus, while different studies have examined different aspects of synaptic structure, the data appear to be consistent with those from young animals which indicated that both the pre- and postsynaptic elements can be labile components of the synapse. The component of the synapse which is most likely to show a morphological change may vary depending on the brain area, species, and experience. Also, similar to data gathered from the developing brain, an increase in perforated synapses has also been reported following visual training in adult rabbits (Vrensen and Nunes Cardozo, 1981).

Alterations in the shape of synapses following stimulation have been reported previously, although the shape change varies in different brain regions and species (Pysh and Wiley, 1972; Desmond and Levy, 1983). Given Bailey and Chen's (1983) data on differential size changes following habituation vs. sensitization, and the differential size change in our concave vs. convex synapses, it remains a possibility that concave and convex synapses may represent two different functional types of synapses (e.g. excitatory and inhibitory) which are altered in

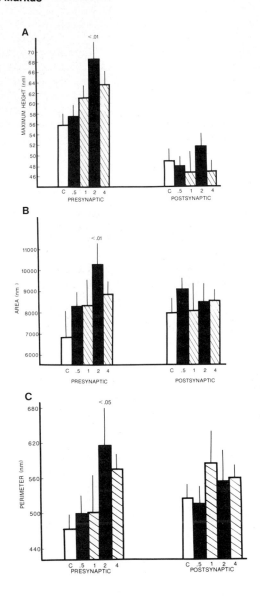

Figure 8. (A). The maximum height; (B). area; and (C). perimeter, of the presynaptic and postsynaptic element in concave synapses in control [C] animals, and those injected with kainic acid and sacrificed 30 min (.5), 1, 2, and 4 hr later.

different directions by the stimulus paradigm employed.
Thus, the data presently suggests that synapses can either
increase or decrease in size following relevant stimuli,
depending on the type of stimulation, or perhaps the
synapse's functional role.

The overall effect of the stimulation was to produce
an increase in the total number of synapses. This is
consistent with other findings using a variety of
stimulation paradigms, including behavioral manipulations
(Lee et al., 1980; Vrensen and Nunes Cardozo, 1981; Chang
and Greenough, 1984; Tweedle and Hatton, 1984). Although
the earliest significant increase in synaptic size or number
occurred at 2 hr, an examination of total synapses in Fig.
7, and structural changes in Fig. 8 suggests that these
changes begin within 30 min of injection. Since kainic acid
induced activity does not begin until approximately 15 min
after injection, and is sporadic until approximately 30 min,
it seems clear that activation can very rapidly induce
changes in synaptic morphology. Other researchers have
found increased numbers of synapses following electrical
stimulation leading to long-term potentiation within 10 – 15
min (Lee et al., 1980; Chang and Greenough. 1984).

In contrast to the alterations seen at the electron
microscopic level in synapses, relatively smaller alterations
were seen in measures taken on the Golgi stained cells.
There were no significant changes in the number of dendritic
spines per micron, although some increases were seen in
dendritic length at 2 hr. An increase in synaptic number
without a concomitant increase in dendritic spine density
suggests that synaptic activation may initially induce
increases in the number of synapses per spine.

The morphological changes observed at the electron
microscopic level, therefore, appear to be either less
obvious or extensive at the light microscopic level, or may
precede large light microscopically observable alterations
in the dendritic structure of the cell within this brief
period. Other researchers conducting examinations of
dendritic spine morphology in adult animals at the electron
microscopic level have noted alterations in the size and
shape of the dendritic spine head and neck following
stimulation paradigms such as long-term potentiation (see
Fifkova, 1985; and the chapter in this book for reviews).
Also, data gathered from environmental enrichment in adult

animals indicates that the dendritic structure of the cell
can be increased following stimulation (Green et al., 1983).
Thus, the shape of the dendritic spine appears to be rapidly
altered, although changes in the number of spines and length
of dendritic segments may be more delayed in their response
to stimulation.

In summary, these findings indicate that both synaptic
size and number are very quickly altered with neuronal use.
The number of synapses rapidly increases, and there may be
changes in the shape and proportion of different types of
synapses. The morphology of the synapse and dendritic spine
also changes, with large increases in the size of the pre-
or postsynaptic terminal in certain synaptic types,
depending on the protocol, species and brain area examined.
Changes in the number of dendritic spines and dendritic
length appear to occur over a longer period of time.

NEURONAL STRUCTURAL CHANGES: WHAT DO THEY MEAN?

In both developing and adult animals, therefore, the
same components of the cell are changed by activation:
synaptic number, size, shape, and possibly perforations;
dendritic spine number and spine head and neck shape; and
dendritic branch length. These alterations have been
observed in different species and brain areas, and following
the use of different protocols such as normal development,
neural stimulation in the adult, behavioral training, long-
term potentiation, imprinting, environmental enrichment,
different states of hydration, epileptic discharges, etc.
This consistency in neuronal response suggests that these
aspects of cellular plasticity are not simply the result
of maturation during development or some aberrant response
to our (or other researchers') protocols. Rather, the
universal nature of these findings suggests that these
cellular components are plastic during adulthood and are
capable of responding to external events with an alteration
in their structure. Further, and most important, the
observed changes in neuronal anatomy form a series of events.
This series of events appears to begin with changes in the
shape of the synapse and increases in the size of the pre-
or postsynaptic thickenings, as well as increases in the
size of the spine head and changes in the shape of the
spine neck. This appears to be followed by the formation of
new synapses, perhaps by a division (initially seen as

synaptic perforations?) of existing synapses. Finally, new
dendritic spines and new dendritic branch length are added
to the cell. Given the universal agreement of the data
collected in this area, it would seem reasonable to conclude
that this series of events constitutes the neuron's
structural response to repetitive activation above routine
levels, and that such a series of events likely forms the
cellular basis of learning and memory processes.

The question remains as to what these structural
changes would mean to neuronal functioning. Would they,
as Hebb suggested, increase the power of synaptic
transmission from the pre- to the postsynaptic neuron? It
seems reasonable to conclude that increases in the number
of synapses would increase the efficacy and power of
transmission between interconnected neurons and, as such,
could form a basis for learning and memory. Also, an
increase in the size of the synapse, particularly the
presynaptic terminal, would lead to an increase in the
number of front-line synaptic vesicles available for
release. It would also increase the number of available
calcium channels, which would in turn increase the magnitude
of the vesicular release. These structural changes in the
synapse, along with the increased number of synapses, would
result in an increase in the total number of synaptic quanta
available for release per impulse in affected neurons. The
alteration in the curvature of the synapse may allow new
areas of the membrane, and their associated transmitter
receptors, previously hidden within the membrane to now
become exposed; such an increase has been observed in
glutamate receptors following long-term potentiation (Baudry
et al., 1980). Finally, alterations in the shape of
dendritic spines and spine necks would alter their cable
properties and increase the power of synapses located on
them (see Fifkova, 1985).

LESSONS FROM NEURONS THAT DO NOT LEARN

Neurons do not always develop or function normally,
and sometimes their aberrations result in learning and
memory impairments in individuals. Our research on the
cellular changes that normally accompany increasing
cognitive capacities over development and neuronal
activation in adulthood suggest that alterations in the
morphology of synapses and dendrites may allow a rapid

mechanism for the storage of engrams. If such changes do
form the basis for learning and memory, they should be
disrupted or altered in conditions which are associated
with learning and memory deficiencies.

To examine this possibility in detail, we conducted,
in collaboration with our colleagues Drs. Brian Scott and
Larry Becker, a series of studies examining the neurobiology
of Down's syndrome (Petit et al., 1984; Scott et al., 1982,
1983). Down's syndrome is characterized biologically by the
presence of an extra chromosome 21, and behaviorally by
moderate to severe mental retardation. Despite the research
on Down's syndrome, there is little understanding of how the
extra chromosome 21 produces the mental retardation.
Further, Down's syndrome is an interesting form of mental
retardation for researchers interested in the neurobiology
of learning and memory since the intellectual deficiency
does not result from trauma, anoxia, vascular disorders, or
other problems which would easily explain the learning
deficits.

We made quantitative determinations of synaptic density
and synaptic structure in normal human sensorimotor
neocortex at a number of early developmental ages, along
with a comparative evaluation of synaptic development in
Down's syndrome nervous tissue. Tissue preparation and
quantitative analyses were carried out as described earlier.
In addition, synaptic contacts were divided into three
categories: primitive contacts which resembled desmosomes,
gap junctions, or perhaps very immature synapses; and two
types of mature synapses based on whether synaptic vesicles
were present or had undergone postmortem degeneration.

The results indicated that the number of synapses
increased in normals and Down's syndrome fetuses at
approximately the same rate, with some divergence by birth,
yielding slightly fewer synapses in Down's tissue by that
time. The most prominent differences, however, were in
synaptic structure. At the later stages of gestation there
was a higher percentage of primitive and a lower percentage
of mature synaptic contacts in Down's tissue. Further,
quantitative measures of the synapses indicated that during
the later stages of gestation the length and thickness of
both the pre- and postsynaptic elements were reduced in
Down's syndrome. Dr. Becker's group examined the dendritic
properties of these neurons (Takashima et al., 1981; Scott

et al., 1983). They found no detectable differences in the number of dendritic spines between normals and Down's neurons preterm, but a slight reduction in the number of spines became apparent around birth and this increased to marked reductions in spine density by four months postnatal. The diverging curves recording spine density, beginning around birth, are consistent with our findings on synaptic density. Reductions in the development of dendrites or dendritic spines have also been reported in other forms of mental retardation (e.g. Marin-Padilla, 1972; Huttenlocher, 1974; Purpura, 1974).

A reduced density of synapses and dendritic spines together with smaller, more immature synaptic contacts would suggest reduced integrative capacities and less efficacy in synaptic transmission in Down's syndrome neurons. Further, and perhaps more important, our detailed analyses of synaptic development and plasticity discussed above indicate that synaptic size and number, as well as dendritic spine number, are plastic properties of the cell, and that this plasticity is an integral process allowing neurons to alter their anatomy with use during development and adulthood. The results from the Down's syndrome tissue suggest that there is some deficit in the normal plastic properties of those synapses, resulting in a reduced growth of synapses over the developmental period. While these reductions in synaptic plasticity were observed during development, definitive conclusions must await studies of stimulation-induced synaptic plasticity in Down's neurons. However, the finding that neurons from mentally retarded individuals do not show the same degree of plasticity in these cell structures over development adds further credence to the suggestion that this plasticity is integral to learning and memory processes. A reduction in their plastic properties would yield neurons with deficient capacities to respond to events by altering their structure, and would conceivably contribute to the learning and memory deficits seen in Down's syndrome.

THE PROCESS OF ENGRAM FORMATION

As discussed above, we and others have shown that activation of a synapse between two neurons induces morphological changes in those two neurons which would make future transmission across that synapse or between those

cells more effective. The question remains as to how these
morphological changes come about, i.e., what is the
mechanism by which electrophysiological events trigger
anatomical changes.

When examining the numerous events that occur during
synaptic activation in search of some process that could
trigger morphological changes, the primary factor appears
to be the entry of calcium into the cell. In resting cells,
the concentration of intracellular calcium is maintained at
extremely low levels. However, during stimulation, voltage
dependent calcium channels open and calcium enters the pre-
and postsynaptic cell, resulting in increased levels of
intracellular calcium (e.g., Hagiwara, 1981). Meanwhile,
inside the neuron there is an internal cytoskeleton made up
of contractile proteins which govern neuronal shape, the
primary ones being tubulin (neurotubules), and actin myosin
(neurofilaments). These intraneuronal structures resemble
those in other body cells, such as muscle cells, which
allow a rapid change in cellular shape and size when
activated. These cytoskeletal elements are responsible for
the growth and expansion of neural processes during
development.

In a series of experiments, we have shown that a
disruption of this cytoskeleton results in a disruption of
the cell's normal ability to grow new dendritic structure
during development, or induces a contraction of dendritic
processes in adulthood (Petit and Isaacson, 1977; Petit and
Moore, 1979; Petit et al., 1980; 1985). From this and
similar research on neurofilaments, it seems clear that
these cytoskeletal structures control cellular shape and
allow neuronal processes to alter their shape. These
contractile structures have been intensively studied in the
dendritic spine by Fifkova, who observed a very dense
network of actin and myosin in the spine head and a
longitudinal organization within the spine stalk (Fifkova
and Delay, 1982; Fifkova, 1985). Further, these networks
are known to be activated by increased levels of free
cytoplasmic calcium (Condeelis, 1983; Stossel, 1983).
Therefore, the large influx of calcium which accompanies
synaptic activation is capable of activating intracellular
contractile proteins responsible for alterations in cell
shape. Calcium may also activate the proteinase calpain,
which would in turn disrupt fodrin. Fodrin normally links
the cytoskeleton to the cell membrane, such that a calcium

activated disruption of fodrin would free the neuronal
membrane from the filaments, allowing a reorganization of
neuronal structure (Siman et al., 1984). It seems,
therefore, that the neuronal activation induced influx of
calcium may be the major trigger for changes in the shape
of synapses and dendritic spines (Fifkova and VanHarreveld,
1977; Fifkova and Anderson, 1981; Fifkova et al., 1983;
Fifkova, 1985).

We know, however, that the repetitive use of synapses
produces not only a change in neuronal shape, but increases
in several aspects of the structure of those cells as well.
Any increase in the synaptic or dendritic structure of the
cell would require the production of additional proteins
found in these structures. It now appears that the influx
of calcium which accompanies neural activation is also the
major trigger for increasing neural structure. The influx
of calcium ions interacts with ATP and cyclic AMP causing a
cascading series of events which lead to the production of
new proteins and possibly the phosphorylation of existing
proteins. Thus, synaptic activation induced increases in
intracellular calcium may not only cause changes in the
shape of synapses, but may also trigger the formation of
new proteins which underlie structural increases of neural
components.

Support for the role of calcium in learning and memory
comes from several sources (e.g. Klein and Kandel, 1978;
1980; Lynch, 1985; Alkon, 1985). Our laboratory has
employed lead, a potent calcium blocker, in examinations of
neural and behavioral development and plasticity. As would
be expected from a disruption of calcium's functions, lead
disrupts the normal development of synapses and dendrites
and is associated with a diminution of learning and memory
capacities (see Petit and Alfano, 1983; Petit et al., 1983
for reviews). Lead also disrupts normal neural plastic
processes in the adult; for example it has been shown to
reduce lesion induced synaptogenesis in the hippocampus
(Alfano et al., 1983). Thus, research from both the
examination of the normal role of calcium as well as from
the use of calcium blockers support the suggestion of its
pivotal role in the cellular processes underlying learning
and memory.

CONCLUSIONS

All of the above research points to a mechanism by which the repetitive use of neurons can cause alterations in their shape (see Fig. 9). These alterations can be rapid and underlie not only the electrophysiological consequences of repetitive activation such as long-term potentiation, but would also be a reasonable substrate for the formation of memories. This model depends on repeated activation of neurons above routine levels, and allows the neuron a mechanism for turning transient signals into relatively long-term changes in structure. These morphological alterations, in turn, could potentially increase the protein network available for transmitter release, the number of transmitter receptors, the shape and cable properties of the dendritic spine, and ultimately the total number of synapses, spines, and dendritic surface of the neuron. More contact points allows more complex networks and greater integration and storage of information.

In viewing all of this data on anatomical changes in the context of their role in learning and memory storage, it is important to keep in mind the importance of forgetting. Just as the formation of, or increases in, neural structures are crucial in learning, it seems likely that a decrease in the size, or the observed elimination of structures such as synapses and dendritic spines would be a reasonable substrate for forgetting. Such reductions in synapses and dendritic structure following previous increases have been observed in several preparations (Bennett et al., 1974; Katz and Davies, 1984; Tweedle and Hatton, 1984).

It seems likely, therefore, that the process outlined in this chapter, involving the continual addition and elimination (turnover) of synapses forms the basis of learning and forgetting over the lifetime of an individual. It would also appear reasonable to conclude that this process or sequence of events may form the cellular substrate of learning and memory.

ACKNOWLEDGMENTS

This research was supported by grants from the Natural Sciences and Engineering Research Council of Canada, and the Ontario Mental Health Foundation to T.L.P.

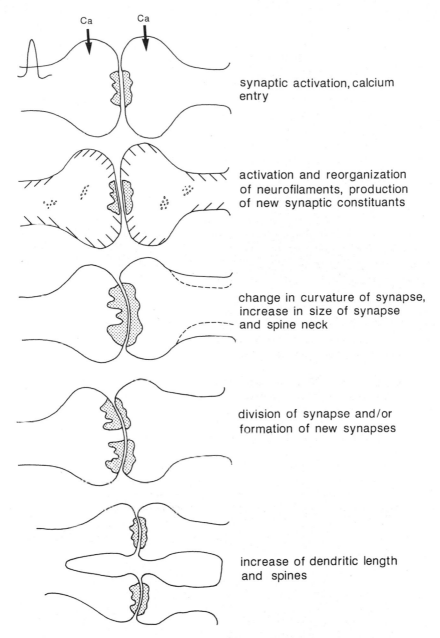

Figure 9. The proposed sequence underlying the cellular anatomical basis of learning and memory.

REFERENCES

Adinolfi AM (1972). Morphogenesis of synaptic junctions in layers I and II of the somatic sensory cortex. Exp Neurol 34:372-383.
Aghajanian GK, Bloom FE (1967). The formation of synaptic junctions in the developing rat brain: A quantitative electron microscopic study. Brain Res 6: 716-727.
Alfano DP, Petit TL, LeBoutillier JC (1983). Development and plasticity of the hippocampal cholinergic system in normal and early lead exposed rats. Dev Brain Res 10: 117-124.
Altman J, Sudarshan K (1975). Postnatal development of locomotion in the laboratory rat. Anim Behav 23:896-920.
Armstrong-James M, Johnson R (1970). Quantitative studies of postnatal changes in rat superficial motor cortex. An electron microscopical study. Z Zellforsch 110:559-568.
Bailey CH, Chen M (1983). Morphological basis of long-term habituation and sensitization in Aplysia. Science 220: 91-93.
Baudry M, Oliver M, Creager R, Wieraszko A, Lynch G (1980). Increase in glutamate receptors following repetitive electrical stimulation in hippocampal slices. Life Sci 27:325-330.
Bell FJ, Ludenberg PK (1985). Effects of commercial soy lecithin preparation on development of sensorimotor behavior and brain biochemistry in the rat. Dev Psychobiol 18:59-66.
Bennett EL, Diamond MC, Krech D, Rosenzweig MR (1964). Chemical and anatomical plasticity of brain. Science 146: 610-619.
Bennett EL, Rosenzweig MR, Diamond MC, Morimoto H, Herbert M (1974). Effects of successive environments on brain measures. Physiol Behav 12:621-631.
Bradley P, Horn G (1979). Neuronal plasticity in the chick brain: morphological effects of visual experience on neurons in hyperstriatum accessorium. Brain Res 162:148-153.
Brandon JG, Coss RG (1982). Rapid dendritic spine stem shortening during one-trial learning: The honeybee's first orientation flight. Brain Res 252:51-61
Burry RW, Kniss DA, Scribner LR (1984). Mechanisms of synapse formation and maturation. In Jones DG (ed): "Current Topics in Research on Synapses, Vol 1," New York: Alan R. Liss, pp 1-52.
Chang FL, Greenough WT (1984). Transient and enduring

morphological correlates of synaptic activity and efficacy change in the rat hippocampal slice. Brain Res 309:35-46.

Changeux JP, Danchin A (1976). Selective stabilization of developing synapses as a mechanism for the specificity of neuronal networks. Nature 264:705-712.

Condeelis J (1983). Rheological properties of cytoplasm: Significance for the organization of spatial information and movement. In McIntosh JR (ed): "Spatial Organization of Eukaryotic Cells, Modern Cell Biology, Vol 2," New York: Alan R. Liss, pp 225-240.

Cragg BG (1967). Changes in visual cortex on first exposure of rats to light. Nature 215:251-253.

Dardenness R, Jarreau PH, Meininger V (1984). A quantitative golgi analysis of the postnatal maturation of dendrites in the central nucleus of the inferior colliculus of the rat. Dev Brain Res 16:159-169.

DeGroot D, Vrensen G (1978). Postnatal development of synaptic contact zones in the visual cortex of rabbits. Brain Res 147:362-369.

Desmond NL, Levy WB (1983). Synaptic correlates of associative potentiation/depression: An ultrastructural study in the hippocampus. Brain Res 265:21-30.

Devon RM, Jones DG (1981). Synaptic parameters in the developing rat cerebral cortex: A comparison of anaesthetized and unanaesthetized states. Dev Neurosci 4:351-362.

Donatelle JM (1977). Growth of the corticospinal tract and the development of placing reaction in the postnatal rat. J Comp Neur 175:207-232.

Duffy CJ, Rakic P (1983). Differentiation of granule cell dendrites in the dentate gyrus of the rhesus monkey: A quantitative Golgi study. J Comp Neurol 214:224-237.

Dyson SE, Jones DG (1980). Quantitation of terminal parameters and their inter-relationships in maturing central synapses: A perspective for experimental studies. Brain Res 183:43-59.

Dyson SE, Jones DG (1984). Synaptic remodelling during development and maturation: Junctional differentiation and splitting as a mechanism for modifying connectivity. Dev Brain Res 13:125-137.

Fifkova E (1985). A possible mechanism of morphometric changes in dendritic spines induced by stimulation. Cell Molec Neurobiol 5:47-63.

Fifkova E, Anderson CL (1981). Stimulation induced changes in dimensions of stalks of dendritic spines in the dentate molecular layer. Exp Neurol 74:621-627.

Fifkova E, Delay RJ (1982). Cytoplasmic actin in neuronal processes as a possible mediator of synaptic plasticity. J Cell Biol 95:345-350.

Fifkova E, Van Harreveld A (1977). Long-lasting morphological changes in dendritic spines of dentate granular cells following stimulation of the entorhinal area. J Neurocytol 6:211-230.

Fifkova E, Markham JA, Delay RJ (1983). Calcium in the spine apparatus of dendritic spines in the dentate molecular layer. Brain Res 266:163-168.

Freire M (1978). Effects of dark rearing on dendritic spines in layer IV of the mouse visual cortex. A quantitative electron microscopical study. J Anat 126: 193-201.

Green EJ, Greenough WT, Schlumpf BE (1983). Effects of complex or isolated environments on cortical dendrites of middle-aged rats. Brain Res 264:233-240.

Greenough WT (1975). Experiential modification of the developing brain. Amer Scientist 63:37-46.

Greenough WT (1976). Enduring brain effects of differential experience and training. In Rosenzweig MR, Bennett EL (eds): "Neural Mechanisms of Learning and Memory," Cambridge, Mass.: M.I.T. Press, pp 225-278.

Greenough WT (1984). Structural correlates of information storage in the mammalian brain: a review and hypothesis. Trends in Neurosci 7:229-233.

Greenough WT (1985). The possible role of experience-dependent synaptogenesis, or synapses on demand, in the memory process. In Weinberger NM, McGaugh JL, Lynch G (eds): "Memory Systems of the Brain," New York: Guilford Press, pp 177-206.

Greenough WT, West RW, DeVoogd TJ (1978). Subsynaptic plate perforations: Changes with age and experience in the rat. Science 202:1096-1098.

Hagiwara S (1981). Calcium channels. Ann Rev Neurosci 4: 69-125.

Hays BP, Roberts A (1973). Synaptic junction development in the spinal cord of an amphibian embryo: An electron microscope study. Z Zellforsch 137:251-269.

Hicks SP, D'Amato CJ (1975). Motor-sensory cortex cortico-spinal system and developing locomotion and placing in rats. Am J Anat 143:1-42.

Hinds JW, Hinds PL (1976). Synapse formation in the mouse olfactory bulb, 2. Morphogenesis. J Comp Neur 169:41-62.

Horn G, Bradley P, McCabe BJ (1985). Changes in the structure of synapses associated with learning. J

Neurosci 5:3161-3168.
Huttenlocher PR (1974). Dendritic development in neocortex of children with mental defect and infantile spasms. Neurol 24:203-210.
Janicke B, Wrobel D, Schulze G (1985). The effects of various drugs on performance capacity of old rats. Pharmacopsychiat 18:136-137.
Johnson R, Armstrong M (1970). Morphology of supraficial postnatal cerebral cortex with special reference to synapses. Z Zellforsch 110:540-558.
Jones DG, Dittmer MM, Reading LC (1974). Synaptogenesis in guinea pig cerebral cortex: A glutaraldehyde - epta study. Brain Res 70:245-259.
Jones DG, Dyson SE (1976). Synaptic junctions in under- nourished rat brain - an ultrastructural investigation. Exp Neurol 51:529-535.
Juraska JM (1982). The development of pyramidal neurons after eye opening in the visual cortex of hooded rats: A quantitative study. J Comp Neurol 212:208-213.
Katz HB, Davies CA (1984). Effects of differential environments on the cerebral anatomy of rats as a function of previous and subsequent housing conditions. Exper Neurol 83:274-287.
Klein M, Kandel ER (1978). Presynaptic modulation of voltage dependent Ca current: Mechanisms for behavioral sensitization in Aplysia californicia. Proc Natl Acad Sci 75:3512-3516.
Klein M, Kandel ER (1980). Mechanism of calcium current modulation underlying presynaptic facilitation and behavioral sensitization in Aplysia. Proc Natl Acad Sci 77:6912-6916.
Leuba G, Garey J (1984). Development of dendritic patterns in the lateral geniculate nucleus of monkey: a quantitative golgi study. Dev Brain Res 16:285-299.
Lee KS, Schottler F, Oliver M, Lynch C (1980). Brief bursts of high frequency stimulation produce two types of structural change in rat hippocampus. J Neurophysiol 44:247-258.
LeVay S, Wiesel TN, Hubel DH (1980). The development of ocular dominance columns in normal and visually deprived monkeys. J Comp Neurol 205:1-51.
Lynch G (1985). What memories are made of. The Sciences 25:38-43.
Marin-Padilla M (1972). Structural abnormalities of the cerebral cortex in human chromosomal aberrations: A Golgi study. Brain Res 44:625-629.

Markus EJ, Petit TL, LeBoutillier JC (1986). Changes in synaptic morphology during development and aging. Submitted.

Markus EJ, Petit TL (1986). Neocortical synaptogenesis and behavior: Development and aging of the motor-sensory system in the rat. Submitted.

Mollgaard K, Diamond MC, Bennett EL, Rosenzweig MR, Linder B (1971). Qualitative synaptic changes with differential experience in rat brain. Internat J Neurosci 2:113-128.

Muller L, Pattiselanno A, Vrensen G (1981). The postnatal development of the presynaptic grid in the visual cortex of rabbits and the effect of dark rearing. Brain Res 205:39-48.

Murphy EH, Magness R (1984). Development of the rabbit visual cortex: A quantitative golgi analysis. Exp Brain Res 53:304-314.

Parnavelas JG, Uylings HBM (1980). The growth of non-pyramidal neurons in the visual cortex of the rat: A morphometric study. Brain Res 193:337-382.

Petit TL, Alfano DP (1979). Differential experience following developmental lead exposure: Effects on brain and behavior. Pharmacol Biochem Behav 11:165-171.

Petit TL, Alfano DP (1983). The neurobiological and behavioral effects of lead. In Dreosti IE, Smith RM (eds): "Neurobiology of the Trace Elements," Clifton, N.J.: Humana Press, pp 50-74.

Petit TL, Alfano DP, LeBoutillier JC (1983). Early lead exposure and the hippocampus. Neurotoxicol 4:79-94.

Petit TL, Biederman GB, McMullen PA (1980). Neurofibrillary degeneration, dendritic dying back and learning-memory deficits following aluminum administration: Implications for brain aging. Exp Neurol 67:152-162.

Petit TL, Isaacson RL (1977). Deficient brain development following colcemid treatment in postnatal rats. Brain Res 132:380-385.

Petit TL, LeBoutillier JC (1984). Synaptic development in the human fetus: A morphometric analysis of normal and Down's syndrome neocortex. Exper Neurol 83:13-23.

Petit TL, LeBoutillier JC, Gregorio A, Libstug H (1986). The pattern of dendritic development in the cerebral cortex of the rat. Submitted.

Petit TL, Moore WL (1979). Behavioral effects of Colcemid-induced deficient brain development in rats. Physiol Psychol 7:139-142.

Purpura DP (1974). Dendritic spine "dysgenesis" and mental retardation. Science 186:1126-1128.

Pysh JJ, Wiley RG (1972). Morphologic alterations of synapses in electrically stimulated superior cervical ganglia of the cat. Science 176:191-193.

Rabe A, French JH, Sinha B, Fersko R (1985). Functional consequences of prenatal exposure to lead in immature rats. Neurotoxicol 6:43-54.

Rosenzweig MR, Bennett EL, Diamond MC (1972). Chemical and anatomical plasticity of brain: Replications and extensions. In Gaito J (ed), "Macromolecules and Behavior, 2nd ed.," New York: Appleton-Century-Crofts, 1972.

Schmidt JT (1985). Activity-dependent synaptic stabilization in development and learning: How similar the mechanisms? Cell Molec Neurobiol 5:1-3.

Scott BS, Becker LE, Petit TL (1983). Neurobiology of Down's syndrome. Prog Neurobiol 21:199-237.

Scott BS, Petit TL, Becker LE, Edwards BA (1982). Abnormal electric membrane properties of Down's syndrome DRG neurons in cell culture. Dev Brain Res 2:257-270.

Siman R, Baudry M, Lynch G (1984). Brain fodrin: Substrate for calpain I, an endogenous calcium activated protease. Proc Natl Acad Sci 81:3572-3576.

Steward O, Falk PM (1985). Polyribosomes under developing spine synapses: Growth specializations of dendrites at sites of synaptogenesis. J Neurosci Res 13:75-88.

Stossel TP (1983). The spatial organization of cortical cytoplasm in macrophages. In McIntosh JR (ed): Spatial Organization of Eukaryotic Cells, Modern Cell Biology, Vol 2," New York: Alan R. Liss, pp 203-223.

Takashima S, Becker LE, Armstrong DL, Chan F (1981). Abnormal neuronal development in the visual cortex of the human fetus and infant with Down's syndrome. A quantitative and qualitative Golgi study. Brain Res 225: 1-21.

Thompson WJ (1985). Activity and synapse elimination at the neuromuscular junction. Cell Molec Neurobiol 5:167-182.

Tieman SB (1985). The anatomy of geniculocortical connections in monocularly deprived cats. Cell Molec Neurobiol 5:35-45.

Turner AM, Greenough WT (1985). Differential rearing effects on rat visual cortex synapses. I. Synaptic and neuronal density and synapses per neuron. Brain Res 329: 195-203.

Tweedle CD, Hatton GI (1984). Synapse formation and disappearance in adult rat supraoptic nucleus during different hydration states. Brain Res 309:373-376.

Uylings HBM, Parnavelas JG (1981). Growth and plasticity
   of cortical dendrites. In Feher D, Joo F (eds):
   "Advances in Physiological Sciences, Vol. 36. Cellular
   Analogues of Conditioning and Neural Plasticity",
   Budapest: Pergamon Press, pp 57-64.
Vrensen G, Nunes Cardozo J (1981). Changes in size and
   shape of synaptic connections after visual training: An
   ultrastructural approach of synaptic plasticity. Brain
   Res 218:79-97.
West RW, Greenough WT (1972). Effect of environmental
   complexity on cortical synapses of rats: Preliminary
   results. Behav Biol 7:279-284.
Woodward DJ, Hoffer BJ, Siggins GR, Bloom FE (1971). The
   ontogenetic development of synaptic junctions: Synaptic
   activation and responsiveness to neurotransmitter
   substance in the rat cerebellar Purkinje cells. Brain
   Res 34:73-97.

Neuroplasticity, Learning, and Memory, pages 125–150
© 1987 Alan R. Liss, Inc.

A PROTEINASE INHIBITOR MODEL OF AGING:
IMPLICATIONS FOR DECREASED NEURONAL PLASTICITY

Gwen O. Ivy

Division of Life Sciences
University of Toronto, Scarborough Campus
Scarborough, Ontario, M1C 1A4

The process of aging leads gradually to numerous
morphological, biochemical and physiological alterations in
living cells. In higher organisms, such physical changes in
the nervous system often are correlated with behavioral
abnormalities and with various neurological deficits. The
search for mechanisms underlying the physical and behavioral
changes with age has gained momentum in recent years, both
because of the rapidly growing proportion of aged
individuals in the world and because of the advent of
technologies which allow us to probe the intricacies of
cellular machinery in ways never before possible.
    The search has been continuously hampered, however, by
the difficulties of studying the cellular mechanisms of
aging in old animals. By the time an animal has accumulated
various manifestations of aging, it is virtually impossible
to determine if the anomalies all arose from a single event
or if certain anomalies themselves caused the evolution of
others. The primary cause of aging is thus likely to remain
obscure until a reasonable model is developed in which the
different manifestations of aging are induced in healthy
young animals, therefore allowing determination of their
relationship to each other over time.

REQUIREMENTS OF A MODEL

    Any model of aging must reproduce its prominent
hallmarks, of which there are several. In the nervous
system the most dramatic is an increase in lipofuscin, or
age pigment, in the perikarya of selective cell populations

including the large and medium sized pyramidal cells of
cerebral cortex, pyramidal and granule cells of hippocampus,
Purkinje cells of cerebellum and scattered larger neurons of
other brain regions (reviewed in Brizzee & Ordy, 1981, and
Kemper, 1984). Additional hallmarks of aging which the
model should be able to create are amyloid and neurofilament
accumulation in cerebral and hippocampal cortex, cell death
in cerebellum and hippocampus (reviewed in Kemper, 1984),
dendritic atrophy and loss of synapses in neocortex and
hippocampus (Feldman, 1977; McWilliams & Lynch, 1983;
Scheibel & Scheibel, 1975, 1977), changes in various enzyme
and neurotransmitter levels (reviewed in Selkoe & Kosik,
1984), and dolichol accumulation across various brain
regions (reviewed in Wolfe et al, 1986). In addition to
producing morphological and biochemical changes, the model
should also produce a modification in the physiological
properties of neural tissue. Aged brains are less
responsive to various stimuli than are young brains. This
decreased neural plasticity with age has been measured in
several ways, four of which are discussed below.

One of the most demonstrable forms of neural plasticity
relates to the effect of experience on dendritic field
expanse. Neurons of the visual cortex of adult rats which
were raised from birth in complex environments have more
extensive dendritic fields than do those of rats raised in
environments containing fewer sensory stimuli (Greenough &
Volkmar, 1983). The effect of an enriched environment on
dendritic field expanse appears to be greater in young
compared to middle-aged rats (Juraska et al, 1980; Uylings
et al, 1978). This phenomenon may relate to regressive
changes such as the generalized dendritic atrophy found in
neocortex and hippocampus of aged animals.

Another age-related indication of anatomical plasticity
is the capacity to develop new dendritic spines. In young
adults, electrical stimulation that induces long term
potentiation (LTP) causes an increase in dendritic spines
(Lee et al, 1980, 1981). The new spines develop within 10
to 15 minutes after stimulation of a hippocampal slice in
vitro (Chang & Greenough, 1984). Similar increases in spine
number have been described in the visual cortex of rats
raised in complex compared to simple environments (Turner &
Greenough, 1985). Further, there is strong evidence that
new spine formation is involved in the learning or memory of
specific behaviors that utilize the modified neurons. For
example, rats can learn to reach into a chamber for bits of
sweetened food and, when doing so, will display a preference

for the use of one forepaw (Peterson, 1934). Individual rats can then be trained to alter their preferred forepaw and the ensuing shift in forepaw preference has been shown to last for several months (Peterson, 1951). Larsen and Greenough (1981) examined neurons in layer V of the area of sensory-motor cortex associated with the forepaw in both hemispheres of rats trained with either their original preferred forepaw, or reversal trained. In both groups, the oblique branches of the apical dendrites of neurons of sensorimotor cortex in the hemisphere opposite the current preferred forepaw (i.e., the cortical area involved in the reaching) were more profuse. That this area is directly involved in the performance of the learned task is indicated by the fact that specific lesions of the area contralateral to the preferred paw cause a preference shift to the other paw (Peterson and Devine, 1963).

While definitive work with aged rats remains to be done, several lines of evidence indicate that there is a lower probability that new spines will be produced by electrical or environmental stimulation in' old 'than in young animals. First, increases in numbers of spines are known to correlate with dendritic field extent (Turner & Greenough, 1985), and the dendritic field has been shown to be less modifiable in older animals. Second, increases in numbers of spines accompany both induction of LTP in hippocampus and deafferentation-induced reinnervation (described below), and both of these phenomena are less robust in older animals. Third, overall decreases in numbers of spines have been extensively documented in hippocampus and in cerebral cortex of aged brains (Bondareff, 1979; Feldman & Dowd, 1974; 1975; Geinisman & Bondareff, 1976; McWilliams & Lynch, 1983) and this is correlated with a pronounced dendritic atrophy in these regions.

A third example of decreased plasticity with age is a restriction in axonal sprouting. After a large lesion of the entorhinal cortex in rats, the distal portion of the dendritic trees of granule cells of the dentate gyrus is almost completely deafferented. Entorhinal axons cannot, of course, regenerate, but intact axons from the contralateral hippocampus that normally terminate on the proximal dendrites of the granule cells can "sprout" axon collaterals which grow up and innervate the recently vacated outer dendrites (reviewed in Gall et al, 1986). In a neonatal rat, the new innervation is complete over the whole extent of the dendritic tree. Sometime after the fifteenth postnatal day of life, however, the sprouting axons no longer can reach the most distal portions of the dendrites (Gall and Lynch, 1981).

In related studies of hippocampal sprouting, McWilliams and Lynch (1983; 1984) have shown that the extent of sprouting of associational inputs to the dentate gyrus following commissurotomy is severely reduced during aging. If the commissural input to the dentate gyrus is removed in a young adult rat, the associational axons grow to reinnervate the deafferented zone. A measure used to indicate such sprouting is the density of synapses in the denervated region, and this shows a marked age-related variation. In 35–day old (young adult) rats, only 8 days are required before synaptic bouton densities are replaced to approximately pre-lesion levels. This same replacement takes a week longer in 60–day old (adult) rats. On the other hand, in 3 to 12 month old (adult) rats there is negligible synaptic replacement by 8 days post-lesion, and less than 50% recovery of lost synapses by post-lesion day 15. Finally, in 18 to 24 month old (old to aged) rats, there is virtually no synaptic replacement 15 days after commissurotomy

These results indicate that the ability to form new synapses declines sharply with age. Such a decrease in postsynaptic plasticity may not be due to the decreased ability of dendrites to form new synapses; rather, it may result from a failure of new axonal growth to reach the deafferented dendrites in the first place. These alternatives cannot be separated at present, but the faulty mechanisms underlying decreased pre- or postsynaptic plasticity may be similar, as described below.

A fourth form of neuronal plasticity which demonstrates decremental changes with age is long term synaptic potentiation. The amplitude of the LTP has been shown to be correlated with the speed of maze learning in rats (Barnes, 1979), thus indicating that this physiological form of neural plasticity is related to learning. Moreover, after high-frequency stimulation of hippocampal afferent fibers in rats, responses at hippocampal synapses are enhanced more slowly and undergo a faster rate of decay in old animals. Such synaptic changes have been shown to be related to rates of acquisition and forgetting of spatial information in rats (reviewed in Barnes & McNaughton, 1985) and may thus underlie at least some of the behavioral deficits found in aged humans and animals.

POSSIBLE COMMON MECHANISMS UNDERLYING THE
MANIFESTATIONS OF AGING AND DECREASED NEURAL PLASTICITY

Despite considerable interest in the mechanisms
underlying different forms of neural plasticity, little is
known about why plasticity decreases with age. An
intriguing possibility is suggested by my work: changes in
specific aspects of cellular metabolism underlie several of
the morphological and biochemical manifestations of aging
(Ivy et al, 1984, 1985, 1986a,b; Wolfe et al, 1986) and also
may cause decreased neural plasticity with age.
    The first three examples of neural plasticity discussed
in the previous section, morphological alterations in
dendrites and spines following environmental or electrical
stimulation or deafferentation, are very likely to involve
changes in the membrane and cytoskeletal elements that
comprise these structures. There is substantial evidence
(see Lynch & Baudry, 1984) that cytoplasmic calcium-
activated thiol proteinases of the family called "calpain"
(Murachi et al, 1981) are involved. Calpain is known to
break down the integral membrane protein brain spectrin, as
well as tubulin, microtubule associated proteins and
neurofilament proteins (Klein et al, 1981; Schlaepfer &
Zimmerman, 1981; Siman et al, 1984), which could easily
account for the degradation of spines, since these proteins
are major building blocks of these structures. In addition,
at least some of these proteins may be degraded further by
lysosomal enzymes prior to recycling of the building blocks,
and there is evidence that calpain is required for the
fusion of lysosomes with vessicles containing membrane-
derived elements (Libby et al, 1980). Thus, both cytoplasmic
and lysosomal proteinases are likely to be involved in the
molecular remodeling of the postsynaptic region. It is also
likely that protein synthesis is involved in the formation
of new spines during (at least) development (Hwang &
Greenough, 1984) and deafferentation-induced reinnervation
(Steward, 1983), and thus that anabolic as well as catabolic
mechanisms underlie the observed plastic changes in spines.
However, general perturbations in protein synthesis are not
likely to account for the specific decreases in neural
plasticity during aging, as will be discussed below.
    With regard to the decreased synapse replacement
following deafferentation in old rats, it should be noted
that before the formation of dendritic spines or
postsynaptic specializations, the axons must grow and
contact the vacant dendrites. The observed decrease in

lesion-induced synaptic replacement with age may thus not be due to dendritic failure but may be an inherent property of axons, or of their environment, which is actively reflected in the morphology of the dendrites. Axonal growth is, indeed, restricted in older animals, although the factors responsible for this decreased plasticity are not understood. It is possible, for example, that astrocytes (which are not prominent during the unrestricted neonatal period of axonal growth) form a physical or chemical barrier to growth at later ages. In aged brains, astrocytes have been shown to be greatly hypertrophied (Landfield, 1977), as they are after a lesion, thus possibly providing a bad environment for axonal growth in aged animals.

Alternatively, axons may acquire an intrinsic restriction of growth during the aging process. In this regard, a decline in axonal transport is known to accompany aging (reviewed in McMartin, 1983), and such a decline would likely indicate a decreased ability to repair and replace axonal neurofilaments, microtubules and cell membranes. The aged axon might thus have a decreased ability to grow following deafferentation. Interestingly, both slow and fast anterograde as well as retrograde transport appears to be mediated by neurofilaments and microtubules (reviewed in McMartin, 1983). Since calpain is likely to be involved in the metabolic turnover of both of these cytoskeletal elements (Schlaepfer & Zimmerman, 1981), calpain may be responsible for this form of decreased neuronal plasticity with age, as well.

Finally, with regard to the fourth form of neural plasticity, there is evidence that induction of LTP is accompanied by a postsynaptic increase in calpain activity caused by calcium influx (Lynch et al, 1982; reviewed in Lynch & Baudry, 1984). As cited above, both LTP and learning are perturbed in aged animals, but concomitant changes in calpain activity have not yet been described.

A MODEL OF AGING

Several forms of neural plasticity that are known to decrease with age involve changes in membrane and cytoskeletal proteins and these changes may be mediated by proteolytic enzymes or by the protein synthetic machinery. A reasonable approach to developing a model for aging might thus involve inhibitors of calpain or of other enzymes related to the catabolism of these proteins, or,

alternatively, inhibitors of protein synthesis. The value
of such a model would be indicated by its ability to
reproduce both the morphological and biochemical
manifestations of aging, and the several forms of decreased
neural plasticity mentioned above.

For several years, my research has been directed toward
developing a model of aging using inhibitors of protein
catabolism. The inhibitors initially were selected because
of the likelihood that they would effect changes in neural
plasticity. Thus far, I have been able to show that
inhibition of calpain or of lysosomal thiol proteinases
produces several morphological and biochemical
manifestations of aging.

The experiments were carried out on Sprague-Dawley rats
(40-60 days of age). The rats were implanted with Alzet
osmotic mini-pumps attached to a cannula which led into the
lateral ventricle. The pumps administered leupeptin (8, 20,
40 or 60 mg/ml), chloroquine (40 mg/ml), aprotinin (40
mg/ml), sodium chloride (9mg/ml) or artificial CSF at a
steady rate of $0.5\mu l$ per hour for two weeks, at which time
most animals were sacrificed. Some rats implanted with
leupeptin-filled pumps (40mg/ml) were allowed to survive for
1 to 10 weeks after the pumps were exhausted, while other
rats had their pumps replaced regularly at two week
intervals. Yet other rats received daily intraventricular
injections of leupeptin ($0.5mg/5\mu l$), chloroquine ($0.5mg/5\mu l$)
or sodium chloride ($0.045 mg/5\mu l$) for three consecutive
days, and two rats received single intraventricular
injections of leupeptin ($0.5 mg/5\mu l$) and were sacrificed 8
hours later.

These inhibitors were chosen for the following reasons.
Leupeptin is a small peptide that reversibly binds to thiol
proteinases and thereby inhibits their activity; calpain is
a calcium activated cytoplasmic thiol proteinase that is
inhibited by leupeptin (Toyo-oka et al, 1978) and cathepsins
B, H and L are lysosomal thiol proteinases that leupeptin
inhibits (Barrett, 1980). Chloroquine causes a pronounced
elevation of intralysosomal pH and thus indirectly blocks
all of the acidic proteinases (Bhattacharyya et al, 1983;
Wibo & Poole, 1974). This drug was used to determine whether
certain effects of leupeptin were caused by its inhibition
of the lysosomal or of the cytoplasmic thiol proteinases. To
determine whether inhibition of still other, non-lysosomal
families of proteinases could cause manifestations of aging,
the serine proteinase inhibitor, aprotinin, was
administered. Aprotinin inhibits proteinases which function

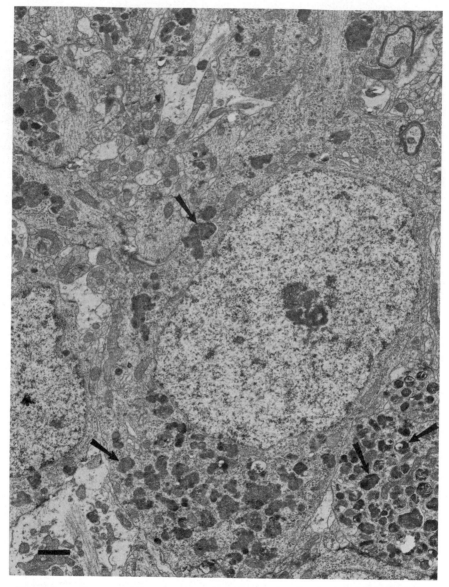

Fig. 1. Low-power electron micrograph of cells in dentate gyrus of hippocampus of a rat treated with intraventricular infusion of leupeptin for 2 weeks. Note the numerous electron-dense residual bodies, or "ceroid", which fill the cytoplasm of these cells (arrows). Scale bar equals 1 micron.

optimally at a pH range of 7–9 and such enzymes are not thought to exist in lysosomes (Barrett, 1980).

Thus, several different inhibitors of protein catabolism, with different modes of action, were utilized in an attempt to determine if any or all of them might cause changes in the brains of young rats that resembled the effects of aging.

Induction of Lipofuscin–like Ceroid

The first evidence that administration of proteinase inhibitors caused manifestations of aging in young rat brain came from electron microscopic examination of dentate gyrus granule cells in leupeptin–treated animals. Figure 1 is an electron micrograph which shows a dense accumulation of substances resembling lipofuscin, or age pigment, in the cytoplasm of these cells. The majority of the induced substance is of a rough or fine granular nature, often associated with intact or disrupted lysosomes, vacuoles and membranous inclusions. Fingerprint profiles are also quite common (Figure 2). These characteristics encompass the various morphological categories of lipofuscin from aged animals as defined by Miyagishi et al (1967).

A wide variety of lysosomally associated substances, termed "ceroids", accumulate in different lysosomal storage disorders as the result of a genetically defective lysosomal enzyme (Hers & Van Hoof, 1973). Ceroids can also be induced to accumulate experimentally by administration of various drugs and toxic substances (reviewed in Oliver, 1981). In most instances, however, the fine morphology of the genetically or experimentally induced ceroids is substantially different from that of the lipofuscin which accumulates during normal aging. To determine if the accumulation of lipofuscin–like ceroid (CL) following leupeptin administration was due to inhibition of lysosomal or of cytoplasmic proteinases, the general lysosomal enzyme inhibitor chloroquine was administered. Chloroquine caused a buildup of intracellular ceroids which resembled those of several different lysosomal storage disorders. The most prominent ceroid morphology was membranous whorls, like those found in Tay Sachs disease but, importantly, lipofuscin–like ceroid was also induced. On the other hand, treatment with the serine proteinase inhibitor, aprotinin, did not produce an intracellular buildup of ceroid; this drug does not act on lysosomal enzymes. Thus, it is likely

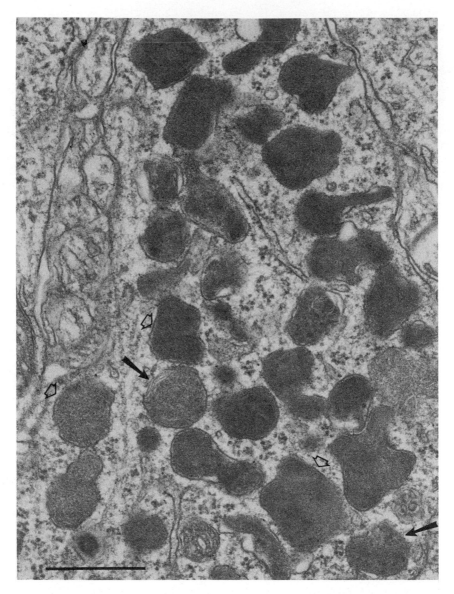

Fig. 2. Electron micrograph showing the fine morphology of the residual bodies induced by leupeptin. The induced ceroid is commonly of a granular nature (open arrows) and often contains fingerprint profiles (solid arrows), as is the case with lipofuscin that accumulates during normal aging. Scale bar equals 1 micron.

that the accumulation of lipofuscin-like ceroid in
leupeptin-treated brains is due to inhibition of lysosomal
thiol proteinases.

Interestingly, the leupeptin-induced CL found in the
present experiments also has a strong morphological
similarity to the substance which accumulates in the brains
of patients with the infantile form of Neuronal Ceroid
Lipofuscinosis (NCL) disease (Zeman, 1976; Ikeda & Goebel,
1979; Goebel & Armstrong, personal communication). The
precise genetic lesion in NCL diseases is not known;
however, on the basis of results with leupeptin, Ivy et al
(1984) have proposed that the defect may lie in the
lysosomal proteinases. Support for this hypothesis comes
from studies showing that the biochemical composition of
ceroids which accumulate in a sheep model of NCL disease is
largely proteinaceous (Palmer et al, 1986).

The induction of CL by leupeptin is clearly dose and
time dependent. For example, CL is absent or barely
detectable in animals treated with 8 mg/ml leupeptin for two
weeks, but is prominent after 20mg/ml and is massive at
higher doses of the drug. Further, the leupeptin-induced
accumulation of CL has a rapid onset. In a series of
animals sacrificed at various times after intraventricular
injection of leupeptin, there was an increase in CL by 8
hours and a substantial accumulation by 72 hours. The
effect of leupeptin is at least partly reversible, since
animals allowed to survive for 8-10 weeks after exhaustion
of the pumps had appreciably less CL than did rats examined
at 10-14 days post implantation or at one week after
cessation of infusion.

In several of the rats which received an infusion of
leupeptin (40mg/ml) over two weeks, the CL in the granule
cells of the dorsal leaf of hippocampal dentate gyrus was
quantified by taking measurements from electron micrographs.
The CL content per granule cell in three of the leupeptin
treated rats ranged from 21-31% of the cytoplasm.
Preliminarily, the CL content was 16-24% and 7-15% of the
cytoplasm of these cells in rats which survived for 3 weeks
or 10 weeks, respectively, after exhaustion of a leupeptin
filled pump. This compared to a range of 3-8% of the
cytoplasm of granule cells in saline treated rats.
Interestingly, cells aging in tissue culture have been shown
to die after about 30% of their cytoplasm is occupied by
lipofuscin (Collins & Brunk, 1978). It is not known if the
death is a direct result of lipofuscin accumulation, or is
indirect, perhaps resulting from the general clogging up of

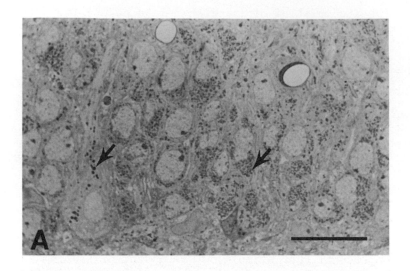

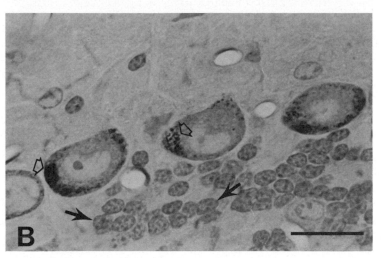

Fig. 3. A. One micron thick plastic section of cells in the
dentate gyrus of a leupeptin-treated rat. Ceroid-lipofuscin
bodies (arrows) are densely stained by toluidine blue.
B. One micron thick plastic section from the cerebellum of
a leupeptin treated rat stained with the PAS method and
hematoxylin. Ceroid-lipofuscin is intensely stained by PAS
in Purkinje perikarya (open arrows). Granule cells, in
contrast (solid arrows), are not obviously affected by
leupeptin treatment. Scale bars equal 25 microns.

cellular machinery by the large mass of the residues.

The leupeptin-induced CL has a number of histochemical properties in common with those of the lipofuscin pigment which accumulates during normal aging. It is stained by toluidine blue (Figure 3A), the PAS technique (Fig. 3B), Nile blue sulfate, oil red O, Sudan black B and Schmorl's method. Together they indicate that, like lipofuscin, leupeptin-induced CL contains high concentrations of glycoproteins and lipids. These results were found, in light microscopic preparations, at all levels of the neuroaxis of leupeptin-treated rats. Further, regional variations in the density of the induced substance were apparent. For example, cerebellar Purkinje cells and neocortical pyramidal cells were heavily affected, as were dentate gyrus granule cells and pyramidal cells of the CA3 region of hippocampus. These same cell populations are also heavily affected by lipofuscin accumulation during normal aging (reviewed in Brizzee & Ordy, 1981).

In sum, the leupeptin-induced ceroid-lipofuscin is similar to the lipofuscin which accumulated in cells during normal aging with regard to fine morphology, histochemical properties and brain distribution. Further, as one might expect from administration of an enzyme inhibitor, the ceroid-lipofuscin accumulation is larger with higher doses of leupeptin and with longer times of administration and it also disappears gradually when the inhibitor is removed. Leupeptin probably causes the buildup of ceroid-lipofuscin by inhibiting lysosomal enzymes.

Neurofilament Accumulation

Another morphological feature that can be found in aged brains is that of neurofibrillary tangles. These are accumulations of neurofilaments which, in humans, have a characteristic paired helical filament organization. Neurofibrillary tangles are known to exhibit a marked birefringence in polarized light after Congo red staining (Wisniewski & Terry, 1973) and to stain particularly well with Thioflavin S (Terry, 1985). Preliminary evidence with Congo red and Thioflavin S stains on leupeptin-treated rat brains indicates abnormal birefringent properties in several brainstem and basal forebrain areas, as well as fluorescent particles within large pyramidal cells of frontal cortex. At present, it is difficult to interpret these findings.

More recent experiments using antibodies to

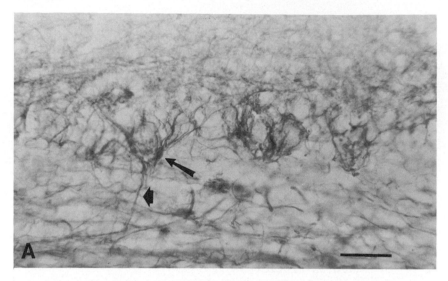

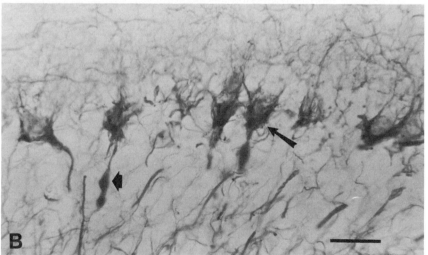

Fig. 4. Immunocytochemical staining of cerebellum with antibodies to neurofilament subunit 68 kd in a CSF-treated rat (A) and a leupeptin-treated rat (B). Note the increased staining intensity of basket cell terminals (long arrows) and the bulbous anti-neurofilament positive protrusions in the proximal axons of Purkinje cells (short arrows) in the leupeptin-treated rat. Scale bars equal 50 microns.

neurofilament subunits have shown that leupeptin induces an abnormal accumulation of neurofilaments which is particularly notable in the cerebellum (Ivy et al, 1986a,b). The Purkinje cells display large protrusions in their proximal axons which react positively with antibodies to both neurofilament subunit 68 and 200 kd (Fig. 4a). The axons of basket interneurons, which occupy the internal portion of the molecular layer are generally increased in thickness, as revealed by immunocytochemistry with anti-neurofilament proteins. After prolonged treatment with leupeptin, additional cytoskeletal abberations appear. After 12 to 16 weeks, accumulations of neurofilaments appear in Purkinje cell dendrites and, in some regions of cerebellum, there is a dramatic loss of Purkinje cells which is marked by the remnants of dense basket cell terminals surrounding Purkinje perikaryal ghosts. Similar changes in the distribution of neurofilaments are seen during normal aging of the cerebellum in humans and rodents. Roots (1983) has reported neurofilament accumulation in synaptic terminals of goldfish brainstem after leupeptin administration. This effect of leupeptin is probably due to its inhibition of calpain rather than of lysosomal enzymes, since calpain is potent in degrading neurofilaments (Schlaepfer & Zimmerman, 1981). However, the effects of chloroquine remain to be tested, thus determining the likelihood that inhibition of lysosomal proteinases are responsible for the effects of leupeptin.

Cell Death

        Neuronal loss with age is well documented in several parts of the nervous system and in numerous species (see Brizzee & Ordy, 1978, for review). For example, an age-related decrease in the number of Purkinje cells with age has been reported in human (Ellis, 1920; Corsellis, 1976) and rat (Inukai, 1928; Rogers et al, 1984), and a similar decrease with age has been reported among rat hippocampal pyramidal cells (Landfield et al, 1977; Brizzee & Ordy, 1978). Leupeptin can also induce the death of cerebellar Purkinje cells (Ivy et al, 1984, 1986b) and, possibly, of hippocampal pyramidal and granule cells (unpublished results). As both of these populations of neurons accumulate large amounts of lipofuscin before death and as the Purkinje cells also evidence neurofibrillary pathology, it is impossible to determine the direct cause of death. However, it is significant that the population of cells affected by inhibitors of thiol proteinases are the same as those affected in normal aging. This may indicate that the biochemical mechanisms underlying aging include or cause perturbed protein turnover and, since certain cell types are particularly susceptible to such perturbations, they thus may be employed as models for studying the time course of the effects.

Dolichol Accumulation

Dolichols are long-chain alcohols of the polyisoprenol group which have been shown by Leonard Wolfe and his collaborators to increase in a linear manner in both rodents and humans. Thus, they provide a major biochemical correlate of aging. Moreover, they are present in abnormally high concentrations in the brains of patients with NCL disease or with Alzheimer's disease (Ng Ying Kin et al, 1983; reviewed in Wolfe et al, 1986).

The brains of rats which had been treated for two weeks with leupeptin, chloroquine, aprotinin or saline were processed for dolichol accumulation. In most brain regions, leupeptin and chloroquine, but not aprotinin or saline, caused significant accumulation of dolichols (Ivy et al, 1984a,b; 1986b; Wolfe et al, 1986). In summary, these biochemical results mimic the morphological findings: inhibition of thiol proteinases leads to the accumulation of CL, neurofilaments and dolichols, and to selective cell death in the CNS. It remains to be determined if treatment with leupeptin can lead to other manifestations of aging and to decreased neural plasticity as well.

A CRITICAL EVALUATION OF THE MODEL AND
DIRECTIONS FOR FUTURE RESEARCH

The search for clues to the aging process has involved numerous comparisons of enzyme properties in young and old animals. A large proportion of the early work on enzyme properties was directed toward proving or disproving Orgel's Error Catastrophy hypothesis (1963, 1970). According to this theory, errors in the protein synthetic machinery result in defective proteins which, in turn, become part of the protein synthetic machinery and cause an accumulation of more errors. The cascade of errors eventually leads to

cellular catastrophe. This hypothesis is supported by a
number of studies showing that enzymes from old animals
often have a lower specific activity and a different UV
spectrum and heat sensitivity than enzymes of younger
animals. Further, old enzymes display a different
immunologic response to antisera produced to the
corresponding young enzyme (reviewed in Rothstein, 1985). No
less numerous, however, are studies in which various enzymes
were found to be unaltered in aged animals. These results
are inconsistent with the Error Catastrophe hypothesis,
since errors in basic protein synthetic processes such as
transcription or translation would be expected to create
errors in all proteins (reviewed in Rothstein, 1985). Thus,
enzyme modifications during aging must take place
post-translationally in some proteins but not others.

There has been considerable interest in the nature of
the changes in enzymes which occur during aging. It has
been possible to rule out an addition or deletion of amide,
ester, phosphate, sulfate or methyl groups by studies
utilizing isoelectric focusing techniques to detect changes
in the electric charges of several enzymes (Rothstein,
1985). As an alternative, Reiss and Rothstein (1974) and
Rothstein (1975) have proposed that differences in old
enzymes result from conformational changes taking place in
the molecule. According to their theory, the "dwell time"
of enzymes in an old cell is longer, due to a decrease in
protein degradation. The increased dwell time causes some
enzymes to become subtly denatured, just as they would if
left at room temperature in a test tube overnight. Since
some enzymes are inherently more stable than others,
different classes of enzymes would lose more or less of
their activity by the following day, and enzymes that are
inherently very stable would be unaltered.

Available evidence supports the idea that an increasing
proportion of certain enzymes exist in varying states of
denaturation in old animals (reviewed in Resnick, et al,
1985; and Rothstein, 1985). There is also support for the
hypothesis on which this premise was based; protein turnover
has been shown to become slower with age in a variety of
species (Lavie et al, 1981; Prasanna & Lane, 1979; Resnick
et al, 1981; Resnick & Gershon, 1979; Sharma et al, 1979).
It is not known, however, what causes the increased dwell
time within the cell which in turn leads to structural
changes in the more "fragile" enzymes.

Altered, inactive enzyme molecules that accumulate in
cells with age have been shown to be normal intermediates of

protein degradation (Resnick et al, 1981), as though the
catabolic process were interfered with at some point before
completion. Resnick and colleagues (1981) have proposed that
the defective enzymes have undergone oxidative damage to
thiol (sulfhydryl) groups and thus are indigestible by the
proteolytic disposal system. According to the hypothesis,
such defective, indigestible enzyme molecules would
accumulate in cells, gradually losing activity over time and
decreasing the proportion of active enzymes in aged cells.

My results suggest an alternative explanation, namely
that the change which occurs during aging is in enzyme
molecules within the proteolytic pathway, rather than their
substrates (as proposed by Resnick et al, (1981). Oxidative
damage to protein and lipid moities is thought to be caused
by free radicals that are generated during the normal
metabolic processes of living cells, and is a main tenet of
the Free Radical hypothesis of aging (reviewed in Halliwell,
1981). Since thiol groups are among the first to be damaged
by free radicals, the present results are consistent with
the hypothesis that oxidative damage to thiol proteinases
occurs progressively during aging, and that this damage has
the most drastic consequences for cellular homeostasis.
Damage to thiol groups in various proteins which are not
part of the proteolytic pathway may be of relatively little
consequence to the functioning of the cell in terms of its
lifespan. On the other hand, the effects of damage to thiol
proteinases become manifest as the hallmarks of aging.

In summary, according to the theory of aging proposed
here, defects in thiol proteinase molecules, possibly caused
by free radical damage, gradually accumulate in cells with
age. Specific enzymes which may be affected are the calcium
activated cytoplasmic proteinase, calpain, and the lysosomal
thiol proteinases, which include cathepsins B, H and L.
Decreases in the efficacy of these enzymes with age lead to
the accumulation of lipofuscin and dolichols,
neurofibrillary pathology and selective cell death.
Decreased neural plasticity may be a secondary phenomenon,
resulting from the anatomical and biochemical changes in
neurons, or may be a direct result of decreased proteinase
activity.

A related but opposing theory of aging has been proposed
by some of my colleagues, on the basis of extensive studies
of calpain activity across species and in different regions
of mammalian brain. Lynch, Larsen and Baudry (1986), focus
on the extensive atrophy and degeneration which occurs
during brain aging and point out that 1) those species with

higher brain concentrations of calpain live shorter lives and 2) specific neuronal populations that have higher relative concentrations of calpain within a mammalian brain may be at greater risk for damage to their cytoskeletal proteins if "mistakes" in calcium regulation occur during aging. There is evidence that alterations in calcium buffering capacity do occur over the course of normal aging (reviewed in Khachaturian, 1984). Thus, the authors suggest that since higher calpain concentrations are correlated with shorter lifespans among species and since neurons with high calpain levels appear to exhibit a greater proportion of age related pathologies, transient increases in calcium concentration that occur during aging affect these species and neurons more than others. Increased calcium does this by causing increased calpain activity which, in turn, leads to selective neuronal atrophy and degeneration.

It is difficult to reconcile their hypothesis with my data, which indicate that several manifestations of aging can be produced by <u>inhibition</u> of calpain. On the other hand, how can my data be reconciled with evidence that species and cell types showing high calpain levels have shorter lives? In fact, these data are neither surprising nor inconsistent with my hypothesis. The normal metabolic requirements of a cell and, by extrapolation, an organism, are reflected in its biochemical makeup. If certain neurons contain greater concentrations of calpain, it is because they normally use this amount of the enzyme for maintaining homeostasis. Any decrease of enzyme activity by overall decreases in turnover time or damage to thiol groups would result in greater catastrophe to cells which normally use more of the enzyme to maintain themselves.

I thus suggest here, that decreased, rather than increased, calpain activity is responsible for at least some of the manifestations of aging, and that calpain disturbance is a subset of the larger malfunction of cellular thiol proteinases. Consistent with this hypothesis is the recent finding that in senescent humans and in individuals with the premature aging conditions, Werner's Syndrome and Progeria, levels of the lysosomal thiol proteinase cathepsin B are severely decreased (Gracy et al, 1985). Further, Peterson and colleagues (1986) have recently shown that cytosolic free calcium levels are significantly decreased in cells from aged humans and from patients with Alzheimer's disease. This decreased cytoplasmic calcium level could cause a decrease in calpain activity. If calpain is necessary for the fusion of lysosomes with the substances they should

degrade (Libby et al, 1980), then decreased calpain activity
could, in turn, lead to decreased lysosomal enzyme function.
However, since aging does not appear to be a condition
analogous to chloroquine administration (i.e., total
inhibition of all classes of lysosomal enzymes), then either
calpain facilitates only the fusion of lysosomes with
vessicles containing proteins, or the decreased calpain
activity affects primarily cytoplasmic degradation. At
present, the effect of decreased calcium concentration on
aged cells is not clear. The best way to account for damage
to thiol proteinases in general appears to be the free
radical theory.

To conclude, in this chapter I have attempted to
develop an animal model of aging based on inhibition of the
activity of thiol proteinases. The model was originally
suggested by evidence that administration of leupeptin to
young rats produces several of the morphological and
biochemical markers of aging. The model is consistent with
evidence that decreased protein turnover during aging leads
to a buildup of defective enzymes and that aged cells
contain decreased calcium levels. The future utility of the
model depends on its ability to create additional
manifestations of aging. In particular, I have argued that
treatment with leupeptin should also result in decreased
neural plasticity. The effect should be manifest
anatomically, in decreased dendritic branching and spine
plasticity following experience or electrical stimulation,
and in decreased axonal sprouting and spine formation
following lesions. The treatment should also cause
decreased physiological ability to develop LTP and to learn,
and should produce a number of the behavioral signs of
aging. It is possible that the anatomical and biochemical
manifestations of aging or of leupeptin treatment would
contribute to decreased plasticity, since if neurons are
loaded with age pigment or have neurofibrillary pathology,
they cannot be expected to function normally. Suffice it to
say for now that one cannot easily dismiss the findings that
leupeptin administration to young rats produces several of
the morphological and biochemical markers of aging. It
remains to be determined if leupeptin can cause a decrease
in neuroplastic phenomena as well.

REFERENCES

Barrett AJ (1980). The many forms and functions of cellular

proteinases. Fed Proc 39:9-14.

Barnes CA (1979). Memory deficits associated with senescence: A neurophysiological and behavioral study in the rat. J Comp Physiol Psyc 93:74-104.

Barnes CA, McNaughton BL (9185). An age comparison of the rates of acquisition and forgetting of spatial information in relation to long-term enhancement of hippocampal synapses. Behav Neurosci 99:1040-1048.

Bhachatarrya TK, Chatterjee TK, Ghosh JJ (1983). Effects of chloroquine on lysosomal enzymes, NADPH-induced lipid peroxidation, and antioxidant enzymes of rat retina. Biochem Pharmachol 32:2965-2968.

Bondareff W (1979) Synaptic atrophy in the scenescent hippocampus. Mech Age Develop 9:163-171.

Brizzee KR, Ordy JM (1981). Cellular features, regional accumulation, and prospects of modification of age pigments in mammals. In Sohal RS (ed): "Age Pigments", New York: Elsevier, pp 102-155.

Brunk UT, Collins VP (1981). Lysosomes and age pigments in cultured cells. In Sohal RS (ed): "Age Pigments", New York: Elsevier, pp 243-264.

Chang F-L F, Greenough WT (1984). Transient and enduring morphological correlates of synaptic activity and efficacy change in the rat hippocampal slice. Brain Res 309:35-46.

Collins VP, Brunk U (1978). Quantitation of residual bodies in cultured glial cells during stationary and logarithmic growth phases. Mech Age Develop 8:139-152.

Corsellis JAN (1976). Some observations on the Purkinje cell population and on brain aging in the human population. In "Neurobiology of aging, Aging Vol 3." Terry RD, Gershon S (eds), New York: Raven Press, pp 205-209.

Ellis RS (1920). Norms for some structural changes in the cerebellum from birth to old age. J Comp Neurol 32: 1-35.

Feldman ML, Dowd C (1974). Aging in rat visual cortex: light microscopic observations in layer V pyramidal apical dendrites. Anat Rec 178:355.

Feldman ML, Dowd C (1975). Loss of dendritic spines in aging cerebral cortex. Anat Embryol 148:279-301.

Gall C, Ivy G, Lynch G (1986). Neuroanatomical plasticity: its role in the organization and reorganization of the nervous system. In Tanner JM, Faulkner F (eds): "Human growth: A comprehensive treatise" 2nd Edition, New York: Plenum Press, pp 411-436.

Gall CM, Lynch G (1981). Fiber architecture of the dentate gyrus following removal of the entorhinal cortex in rats of different ages: Evidence that two forms of axonal sprouting occur after lesions in the immature rat. Neuroscience 6:903-910.

Geinisman Y, Bondareff W (1976). Decrease in the number of synapses in the senescent brain: A quantitative electron microscopic analysis of the dentate gyrus molecular layer in the rat. Mech Ageing Develop 5:11-23.

Gracy RW, Yuksel KU, Chapman ML, Cini JK, Jahani M, Lu hs, Oray B, Talent JM (1985). Impaired protein degradation may account for the accumulation of "abnormal" proteins in aged cells. In "Modification of proteins during aging", New York: Alan R. Liss, pp 1-18.

Greenough WT, Volkmar FR (1983). Pattern of dendritic branching in occipital cortex of rats reared in complex environments. Exp Neurol 40:491-504.

Halliwell B (1981). Free radicals, oxygen toxicity and aging. In Sohal RS (ed): "Age Pigments", New York: Elsevier, pp 2-62.

Hers HG, Van Hoof F (1973). "Lysosomes and storage diseases". New York: Academic Press.

Hwang H-M, Greenough WT (1984). Spine formation and synaptogenesis in rat visual cortex: a serial section developmental study. Soc Neurosci Abs 10:579.

Ikeda K, Goebel HH (1979). Ultrastructural pathology of lymphocytes in neuronal ceroid lipofuscinosis. Brain and Develop 1:285-292.

Inukai T (1928). On the loss of Purkinje cells with advancing age, from cerebellar cortex of the albino rat. J Comp Neurol 45:1-31.

Ivy GO, Schottler F, Baudry M, Lynch G (1984a). Inhibitors of Lysosomal Enzymes: Accumulation of lipofuscin-like dense bodies in the brain. Science 226:985-987.

Ivy GO, Wolfe LS, Houston K, Baudry M, Lynch G (1984b). Lysosomal enzyme inhibitors cause the accumulatiion of ceroid lipofuscin and dolichols in rat brain. Soc Neurosci Abs 10:885.

Ivy GO, Do JT, Baudry M, Lynch G (1986a). Neurofilamentous swellings in proximal axons of Purkinje cells induced by a thiol proteinase inhibitor. Soc Neurosci Abs 12:1507.

Ivy GO, Schottler F, Baudry M, Lynch G (1986b). Leupeptin causes several manifestations of aging in brain and liver of young rats. In "Third Tokyo symposium: liver and aging, liver and brain". New York: Elsevier, in press.

Juraska JM, Greenough WT, Elliot C, Mack K, Berkowitz R (1980). Plasticity in adult rat visual cortex: an examination of several cell populations after differential rearing. Behav Neural Biol 29:157–167.

Kemper T (1984). Neuroanatomical and neuropathological changes in normal aging and in dementia. In Albert ML (ed). "Clinical neurology of aging". London: Oxford, pp 9–52.

Klein I, Lehotay D, Godek M (1981). Characterization of a calcium activated protease that hydrolyses a microtubule-associated protein. Arch Biochem Biophys 208:520–527.

Khachaturian ZS (1984). Towards theories of brain ageing. In Kay, Burrows (eds): "Handbook of studies on psychiatry and old age", New York, Elsevier, pp7–30.

Landfield PW, Rose G, Sandles L, Wohlstadter TC, Lynch G (1977). Patterns of astroglial hypertrophy and neuronal degeneration in the hippocampus of aged, memory-deficient rats. J Gerontol 1:3–12.

Larson JR, Greenough WT (1981). Effects of handedness training on dendritic branching of neurons in forelimb area of rat motor cortex. Soc Neurosci Abs 7:65.

Lavie L, Reznick AZ, Gershon D (1981). Decreased protein and puromycinylpeptide degradation in livers of senescent mice. Biochem J 202:47–63.

Lee KS, Oliver M, Schottler F, Lynch G (1981). Electron microscopic studies of brain slices: The effects of high frequency stimulatioon on dendritic ultrastructure. In Kerkut GA, Wheal HV (eds) "Electrophysiology of isolated mammalian CNS preparations". New York: Academic Press.

Lee KS, Schottler F, Oliver M, Lynch G (1980). Brief bursts of high frequency stimulaton produce two types of structural change in rat hippocampus. J Neurophys 44:247–258.

Libby P, Bursztajn S, Goldberg AL (1980). Degradation of the acetylcholine receptor in cultured muscle cells: selective inhibition and the fate of undegraded receptors. Cell 19:481–491.

Lynch G, Baudry, M (1984). The biochemistry of memory: A new and specific hypothesis. Science 224:1057–1063.

Lynch G, Halpain S, Baudry M (1982). Effects of high-frequency stimulation on glutamate receptor binding studied with an in vitro slice preparation. Brain Res 115:23–41.

Lynch GS, Larson J, Baudry M (1986). Proteases, neuronal stability and brain aging: An hypothesis. In Crook T, Bartus R, Ferris S, Gershon, S (eds): "Treatment development strategies for Alzheimers disease", Madison, Wisconsin: Mark Powley Associates.

McMartin D (1983). Effects of age on axoplasmic transport

in peripheral nerves. In Cervos-Navarro J, Sarkander H -I (eds): "Brain Aging: Neuropathology and Neuropharmacology", New York: Raven Press, pp 351-362.

McWilliams JR, Lynch G (1983). Rate of synaptic replacement in denervated rat hippocampus declines precipitously in the juvenile period to adulthood, Science 221:572-574.

McWilliams JR, Lynch G (9184). Synaptic density and axonal sprouting in rat hippocampus: Stability in adulthood and decline in late adulthood. Brain Res. 294:152-156.

Miyagishi T, Takahata N, Iizuka R (1967). Electron microscopic studies on the lipopigments in the cerebral cortex of nerve cells of senile and vitamin E-deficient rats. Acta Neuropathol 9:7-17.

Murachi T, Tanaka K, Hatanaka M (1981). Intracellular calcium dependent protease (calpain) and its high molecular weight endogenous inhibitor (calpastatin). Biochem Internat 2:651-656.

Ng Ying Kin NMK, Palo J, Haltia M, Wolfe L (1983). High levels of brain dolichols in neuronal ceroid-lipofuscinosis and senescence. J Neurochem 40:1463-1473.

Oliver C (1981). Lipofuscin and ceroid accumulation in experimental animals. In Sohal RS (ed): "Age Pigments", New York: Elsevier, pp 335-354.

Orgel LE (1963). The maintenance of the accuracy of protein synthesis and its relevance to ageing. Proc Natl Acad Sci USA 49:517-519.

Orgel LE (1970). The maintenance and accuracy of protein synthesis and its relevance to ageing: a correction. Proc Natl Acad Sci USA 67:1476-77.

Palmer DN, Barns G, Husbands DR, Jolly RD (1986). Ceroid-lipofuscinosis in sheep (II). The major component of the lipopigment in liver, kidney, pancreas and brain is low molecular weight protein. J Biol Chem, in press.

Peterson C, Ratan RR, Shelanski ML, Goldman JE (1986). Cytosolic free calcium and cell spreading decrease in fibroblasts from aged and Alzheimer donors. Proc Natl Acad Sci USA 83: 7999-8001.

Peterson GM (1934). Mechanisms of handedness in the rat. Comp Psyc Monographs 9:1-67.

Peterson GM, Devine JV (1963). Transfer of handedness in the rat resulting from small cortical lesions after limited forced practice. J Comp Physiol Psyc 56:752-756.

Prasanna HR, Lane RS (1979). Protein degradation in aged nematodes (Turbatrix aceti). Biochem Biophys Res Commun 86:552-554.

Reiss U, Rothstein M (1974). Heat-labile isozymes of

isocitrate lyase from aging Turbatrix aceti. Biochem
Biophys Res Commun 61:1012-1015.

Reznick AZ, Dovrat A, Rosenfelder L, Shpund S, Gershon D
(1985). Defective enzyme molecules in cells of aging
animals are partially denatured, totally inactive, normal
degradation intermediates. In "Modification of proteins
during aging", New York: Alan R. Liss, pp 69-81.

Reznick AZ, Gershon D (1979). The effect of age on the
protein degradation system in the nematode, Turbatrix
aceti. Mech Ageing Develop 11:403-412.

Reznick AZ, Lavie L, Gershon HE, Gershon D (1981).
Age-associated accumulation of altered FDP aldolase B in
mice. FEBS Lett 128:221-225.

Rogers J, Zornetzer SF, Bloom, FE, Mervis RE (1984).
Scenescent microstructural changes in rat cerebellum.
Brain Res 292: 23-32.

Roots B (1983). Neurofilamant accumulation induced in
synapses by leupeptin. Science 221:971-972.

Rothstein M (1975). Aging and the alteration of enzymes: a
review. Mech Ageing Develop 4:325-337.

Rothstein M (1985). The alteration of enzymes in aging. In
"Modification of proteins during aging", New York: Alan R
Liss, pp 53-67.

Scheibel ME, Scheibel AB (1975). Structural changes in the
aging brain. In Brody H, Harman D, Ordy JM (eds):
"Aging", New York: Raven Press.

Scheibel ME, Scheibel AB (1977). "Differential changes
with aging in old and new cortices. In Nandy K, Sherwin I
(eds): "The aging brain and senile dementia". New York:
Plenum Press. pp 39-58.

Schlaepfer WW, Zimmerman U-JP (1981). Calcium mediated
breakdown of glial filaments and neurofilaments in rat
optic nerve and spinal cord. Neurochem Res 6.243 255.

Selkoe D, Kosik K (1984). Neurochemical changes with aging.
In Albert ML (ed); "Clinical Neurology of Aging", New
York: Oxford University Press, pp 53-75.

Siman R, Baudry M, Lynch G (1984). Brain fodrin: substrate
for the endogenous calcium activated protease calpain I.
Proc Natl Acad Sci USA 81: 3276-3280.

Sharma HK, Prasanna HR, Lane RS, Rothstein M (1979). The
effect of age on enolase turnover in the free-living
nematode, Turbatrix aceti. Arch Biochem Biophys
194:275-283.

Steward O (1983). Polyribosomes at the base of dendritic
spines of CNS neurons: Their possible role in synapse
construction and modification. Cold Spring Harbor

Symposia on Quantitatitive Biology, 48:745–759.

Terry R (1985) Symposium on Alzheimer's dementia. FASEB meeting, Anaheim, Calif.

Toyo-oka T, Shimizu T, Masaki T (1978) Inhibition of proteolytic activity of calcium activated neutral protease by leupeptin and antipain. Biochem Biophys Res Commun 82: 484–491.

Turner AM, Greenough WT (1985). Differential rearing effects on rat visual cortex synapses. I. Synaptic and neuronal density and synapses per neuron. Brain Res 329:195–203.

Uylings HBM, Kuypers K, Veltman WAM (1978). Environmental influences on neocortex in later life. Prog Brain Res 48:261–274.

Wibo M, Poole B (1974) Protein degradation in cultured cells. II The uptake of chloroquine by rat fibroblasts and the inhibition of cellular protein degradation by cathepsin B1. J Cell Biol 63:430–440.

Wisniewski HKM, Terry RD (1973). Morphology of the aging brain, human and animal. In Forel DH (ed) "Progress in Brian Research", Amsterdam: Elsevier, 40:167–187.

Wolfe LS, Ivy GO, Witkop CJ (1986). Dolichols, lysosomal membrane turnover and relationships to the turnover of ceroid and lipofuscin in inherited diseases, Alzheimer's and aging. In: Twelfth Nobel Conference: Structure, biosynthesis and function of isoprenoid compounds in eucaryotic cells. Sodergarn, Sweden: Chimica Scripta, in press.

Zeman W (1976) The neuronal ceroid-lipofuscinoses. In Zimmerman HM (ed) "Progress in neuropathology III". New York: Grune and Straton, pp203–223.

Zimmerman U-J P, Schlaepfer WW (1984) Calcium-activated neutral protease (CANP) in brain and other tissues. Prog Neurobiol 23:63–78.

Neuroplasticity, Learning, and Memory, pages 151–172
© 1987 Alan R. Liss, Inc.

IDENTIFICATION OF AN ESSENTIAL MEMORY TRACE CIRCUIT IN THE
MAMMALIAN BRAIN

Richard F. Thompson

Department of Psychology
Stanford University
Stanford, California 94305

Some years ago we selected classical conditioning of
the eyelid closure response as a model system in which to
analyze the neuronal substrates of basic associative
learning and memory. We adopted this paradigm, and the
rabbit as the experimental animal of choice, for two key
reasons: (1) There is an extensive literature on the
properties and parameters of this basic form of associative
learning in both humans and animals (particularly the
rabbit) (Black and Prokasy, 1972; Gormezano, 1972), (2) It
obeys the basic "laws" and exhibits the basic phenomena of
associative learning in a similar manner in humans and in
other mammals.

When we began this work about sixteen years ago, we
had no idea that we would be led to the cerebellum as the
key structure that appears to store the essential memory
trace. With the advantage of hindsight, it is perhaps
not so surprising. The conditioned eyelid closure response
is a very precisely timed movement -- over the entire
effective CS-US onset interval where learning occurs, from
about 100 msec to over a sec., the learned response develops
such that the eyelid closure is maximal at the time of onset
of the US. In this sense it is a maximally adaptive
response. It is also a very precisely timed "skilled"
movement, perhaps the most elementary form of learned
skilled movement.

LEARNED SKILLED MOVEMENTS

There is an extensive theoretical literature concerning
the possibility that the "memory traces" for learned,
skilled movements are stored in the cerebellum: "We can
say that normally our most complex muscle movements are
carried out subconsciously and with consummate skill.....
It is my thesis that the cerebellum is concerned in this
enormously complex organization and control of movement,
and that throughout life, particularly in the earliest
years, we are engaged in an incessant teaching program for
the cerebellum. As a consequence, it can carry out all
these remarkable tasks that we set it to do in the whole
repertoire of our skilled movements in games, in techniques,
in musical performances, in speech, dance, song and so on."
(Eccles, 1977, p. 328).

There is general agreement that the cerebellum is
involved in the production and control of movements,
including skilled, learned movements, but less agreement
regarding possible loci of memory storage for learned
movements. On one side are the now-classic theories of
how the cerebellar cortex might serve as the site for
storage of memory traces that code learned movements or
motor programs (Albus, 1971; Eccles, 1977; Ito, 1972; Marr,
1969). The opposing view holds that the cerebellum is a
computational network involved in the control and regulation
of movement, including skilled movements, but that the
memory traces are not stored there.

Evidence for the involvement of the cerebellum in
skilled movements is incontravertable. Particularly
impressive are studies using primates trained to make
highly skilled, precise movements. This literature has
been reviewed in depth (Brooks and Thach, 1981; Ito, 1984).
In general, when a monkey performs an "intentional" skilled
movement, as in moving a lever rapidly in a particular
manner following a visual or auditory stimulus, one of the
earliest signs of neuronal activity is in the dentate
nucleus; lateral Purkinje cells show alterations at about
this time or a bit later (Thach, 1978). Next are neural
changes in interpositus and in motor cortex (Thach, 1970).
These statements are of course based on means of samples
with considerable overlaps. The majority of dentate neurons
fire in relation to the stimulus onset and a smaller
proportion fire in relation to the onset of movement,

whereas interpositus neurons, while often preceding the movement in terms of onset latencies, tend to fire more in relation to the movement itself. Interestingly, the "stimulus evoked" dentate response occurs in the trained animal and disappears if the learned behavior is extinguished (Chapman et al., 1982). Cooling of the dentate nucleus in monkeys trained to perform a prompt arm-wrist flexion task causes the execution of the task to be delayed by 90 to 250 msec (Brooks et al., 1973; Brooks, 1979; Meyer-Lohmann et al., 1977). Furthermore, cooling of the dentate in a monkey that has just learned a new variation of an arm-wrist task reverts the animal's arm movements back to prelearning levels of performance (Horvath et al., 1968).

A common hypothetical functional description would have the "intention" to move possibly originate in association areas of the cerebral cortex, which activate neurons in the pontine nuclei, projecting to the cerebellum as mossy fibers, and also activate basal ganglia. A next event is activation of dentate neurons by mossy fibers, and also activation of Purkinje neurons, which act in turn to modulate dentate neurons. The dentate neurons then activate motor cortex via the thalamus, which in turn activates descending pathways to motor neurons and also pontine mossy fibers to cerebellum. Interpositus neurons are also activated by mossy fibers, and influenced by Purkinje cells although it is not clear at exactly what points in the above sequence. Once behavioral movement begins, feedback from the periphery is of course provided to these central systems. The climbing fiber system is not thought to play a direct role in movement initiation or control because of the very slow discharge frequency of inferior olivary neurons (1-2/sec). Instead, it may play some role as a "corrective" signal when errors occur or provide some other kind of information. The motor cortex and the interpositus provide two descending motor systems, the interpositus by way of the magnocellular red nucleus and rubral pathways. This schema is of course greatly oversimplified; most regions that connect have reciprocal connections, e.g., the nucleocortical fibers in the cerebellum (Chan-Palay, 1977), and other neuronal systems are also involved (see Brooks and Thach, 1981, for detailed discussion). Where the motor program memory traces for such skilled movements are located in these networks is not yet known, but the possibility they are stored in cerebellar cortex seems a reasonable working hypothesis and is not contradicted in any strong manner by current evidence.

Lisberger (1982) stressed the point that if a given structure is the locus of learned motor program storage neurons there, particularly principal cells, must show patterns of activity that correlate in some consistent manner with behavioral performance. Correlated neuronal activity is thus necessary, but of course not sufficient to establish the locus of storage. This requirement is certainly met in the literature noted above for signaled skilled movements.

The issue of what constitutes evidence necessary and sufficient to establish conclusively the locus of storage of an essential memory trace is complex and not completely known since to date no memory traces have been so localized in the mammalian brain. However, we feel our evidence for eyelid conditioning now provides a strong case for localization of the essential memory trace at least to a structure, the cerebellum (see below). Indeed, we feel our evidence is the most convincing yet developed for localization of an associative memory trace in the mammalian brain.

ADAPTATION OF THE VESTIBULO-OCULAR REFLEX (VOR)

A similar case can be made for another kind of behavioral plasticity, namely adaptation of the vestibulo-ocular reflex (VOR) to altered visual input (Ito, 1984, 1985; Miles and Lisberger, 1981). In brief, gain control can be altered by using lenses or by moving the visual field and the head. The VOR shows a persisting (hours to days) adaptation to the changed gain. It appears to differ fundamentally from associative learning and memory in at least one important way: There is no sign of long-term retention, i.e., there is no savings with repeated training sessions; neither the rate of adaptation nor the rate of recovery increases with repeated exposures (Ito, 1984; Miles, and Lisberger, 1981; Watanabe, 1985). Such savings with repeated training sessions is universally characteristic of associative learning and even of nonassociative learning processes like habituation.

There is currently a vigorous debate regarding the locus of essential neuronal plasticity that codes adaptation of the VOR. Ablation of the cerebellar flocculus abolishes adaptation of the VOR in all mammalian species tested. The issue is thus not whether the cerebellum is essential but rather whether the plasticity is established in the cerebellum or in brain-stem structures that either must project through the cerebellum (i.e., afferent systems for which the cerebellum is a mandatory efferent) or for which the cerebellum plays a facilitatory role. We do not wish to venture into the details of this debate here, other than to observe that Ito's case for localization of the plasticity to the cerebellar flocculus in the rabbit seems very strong (Ito, 1984).

Recent evidence that bears on our own work strongly supports Ito's view that plasticity can in fact be established in the flocculus of the rabbit using an electrical stimulation analogue of VOR adaptation: Electrical stimulation of the vestibular nerve (activating mossy fibers to flocculus) and of the inferior olive (climbing fibers to flocculus) conjointly (many seconds at 1-4 Hz) in the high decerebrate rabbit (Ito, 1984). This produced both a brief (10 min.) and prolonged (1 h) depression in the floccular Purkinje cell response to vestibular nerve stimulation. The same result was obtained with direct stimulation of parallel fibers and climbing fibers and with conjoint application of glutamate and climbing fiber stimulation in decerebrate rabbit and with conjoint parallel fiber and white matter stimulation (Purkinje cell EPSPs) in guinea pig in vitro cerebellar slice (Ito, 1985; Sakurai, 1985). Ito has termed this phenomenon long-term depression (LTD).

Insofar as the putative mechanism of LTD is concerned, Ekerot and Kano (1985) suggested that the critical event is the climbing fiber-evoked depolarizing plateau-like potential which, in distal Purkinje cell dendrites, may have a duration of several hundred msec. It is presumed to represent influx of Ca^{++} ions into Purkinje cell dendrites (Llinas and Sugimori, 1980). If Purkinje cells are inhibited (stimulation of "off beam" parallel fibers inducing inhibition via stellate and basket cells) simultaneously with climbing fiber activation, the plateau-like potential does not develop, nor does LTD (Ekerot and Kano, 1985). This result implies that Ca^{++} influx may be necessary for LTD and argues against the possibility that an extracellular factor released by climbing fiber

terminals is critically involved. In terms of
neurotransmitter action, Ito presents evidence suggesting
that quisqualate-sensitive glutamate receptors may be
specifically involved in LTD (Ito, 1984).

ESSENTIAL CIRCUITRY FOR LEARNING OF DISCRETE, ADAPTIVE
BEHAVIORAL RESPONSES

   Recent evidence from our laboratory based primarily on
eyelid conditioning as a model system overwhelmingly favors
an essential role for the cerebellum in both learning and
memory of discrete, adaptive behavioral responses learned
to deal with aversive events, thus supporting the general
spirit of earlier theories of the role of the cerebellum
in motor learning (Albus, 1971; Eccles, 1977; Ito, 1972;
Marr, 1969) (see Figure 1).

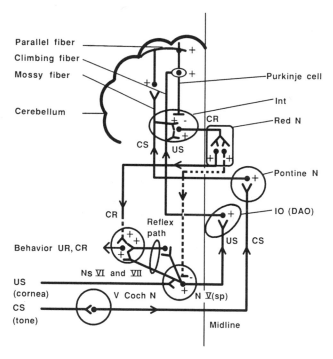

Fig. 1. (*Continued on next page*)

Figure 1. Simplified schematic of hypothetical memory trace circuit for discrete behavioral responses learned as adaptations to aversive events. The US (corneal airpuff) pathway seems to consist of somatosensory projections to the dorsal accessory portion of the inferior olive (DAO) and its climbing fiber projections to the cerebellum. The tone CS pathway seems to consist of auditory projections to pontine nuclei (Pontine N) and their mossy fiber projections to the cerebellum. The efferent (eyelid closure) CR pathway projects from the interpositus nucleus (Int) of the cerebellum to the red nucleus (Red N) and via the descending rubral pathway to act ultimately on motor neurons. The red nucleus may also exert inhibitory control over the transmission of somatic sensory information about the US to the inferior olive, so that when a CR occurs (eyelid closes), the red nucleus dampens US activation of climbing fibers. Evidence to date is most consistent with storage of the memory traces in localized regions of cerebellar cortex and possibly interpositus nucleus as well. Pluses indicate excitatory and minuses inhibitory synaptic action. Additional abbreviations: N V (sp), spinal fifth cranial nucleus; N VI, sixth cranial nucleus; N VII, seventh cranial nucleus; V Coch N, ventral cochlear nucleus. (Reprinted by permission of Science, 1986).

As noted below, this conclusion is not limited to eyelid conditioning in the rabbit but appears to hold for the learning of any discrete behavioral response learned to deal with an aversive event by mammals. It is thus a category of associative learning and might be described as "procedural" learning, i.e., learning how.

Some years ago we adopted the general strategy of recording neuronal unit activity in the trained animal (rabbit eyelid conditioning) as an initial survey and sampling method to identify putative sites of memory storage. As noted, a pattern of neuronal activity that correlates with the behavioral learned response (specifically one that precedes the behavioral response in time within trials), and that predicts the form of the learned response within trials and the development of learning over trials, is a necessary requirement for identification of a storage locus. We mapped a number of brain regions and systems thought to be involved in

learning and memory. Neuronal activity of pyramidal cells
in the hippocampus exhibited all the requirements described
above, but the hippocampus itself is not necessary for
learning and memory of such discrete behavioral responses
(Thompson et al., 1983). Recent evidence argues strongly
that long-lasting neuronal plasticity is established in the
hippocampus in these learning paradigms (Disterhoft et al.,
in press; Mamounas et al., 1984). Thus, "memory traces"
are formed in the hippocampus during learning but these
"higher order" traces are not necessary for learning of the
basic association between a neutral tone or light CS and
the precisely timed, adaptive behavioral response. However,
the hippocampus can become essential when appropriate task
demands are placed on the animal even in eyelid conditioning
(Thompson et al., 1983). Yet the hippocampus is not an
essential part of the memory trace circuit; that is, the
hippocampus is not necessary and sufficient for basic
associative learning and memory of discrete responses.
Indeed, decorticate and even decerebrate mammals can learn
the conditioned eyelid response (Norman et al., 1974;
Oakley and Russel, 1977) and animals that are first trained
and then acutely decerebrated retain the learned response
(Mauk and Thompson, in press). The essential memory trace
circuit is below the level of the thalamus.

In the course of mapping the brain stem and cerebellum
we discovered localized regions of cerebellar cortex and a
region in the lateral interpositus nucleus where neuronal
activity exhibited the requisite memory trace properties --
patterned changes in neuronal discharge frequency that
preceded the behavioral learned response by as much as 60
msec (minimum behavioral CR onset latency approx. 100 msec),
predicted the form of the learned behavioral response (but
not the reflex response) and grew over the course of
training, i.e., predicted the development of behavioral
learning (McCormick et al., 1981; McCormick, 1983; McCormick
and Thompson, 1984). We undertook a series of lesion
studies and found that large lesions of lateral cerebellar
cortex and nuclei, electrolytic lesions of the lateral
interpositus-medial dentate nuclear region and lesions of
the superior cerebellar peduncle ipsilateral to the learned
response all abolished the learned response completely and
permanently, but had no effect on the reflex UR and did
not prevent or impair learning on the contralateral side of
the body (McCormick et al., 1981, 1982; Lavond et al., 1981).
After our initial papers were published, Yeo, Glickstein

and associates replicated our basic lesion result for the interpositus nucleus, using light as well as tone CSs and a periorbital shock US (we had used corneal airpuff US), thus extending the generality of the result (Yeo et al., 1984).

Electrolytic or aspiration lesions of the cerebellum cause degeneration in the inferior olive; this lesion-abolition of the learned response could be due to olivary degeneration rather than cerebellar damage, per se. We made kainic acid lesions of the interpositus -and observed-a lesion as small as a cubic millimeter in the lateral anterior interpositus permanently and selectively abolished the learned response with no attendant degeneration in the inferior olive (Lavond et al., 1986). Additional work suggests that the lesion result holds across CS modalities, skeletal response systems, species, and perhaps with instrumental contingencies as well (Yeo et al., 1984; Donegan et al., 1983; Polenchar et al., 1985). Electrical microstimulation of the interpositus nucleus in untrained animals elicits behavioral responses by way of the superior cerebellar peduncle, e.g., eyeblink, leg-flexion, the nature of the response being determined by the locus of the electrode (McCormick and Thompson, 1984). Collectively, these data build a case that the memory traces are afferent to the efferent fibers of the superior cerebellar peduncle, i.e., in interpositus, cerebellar cortex or systems for which the cerebellum is a mandatory efferent.

The essential efferent CR pathway appears to consist of fibers exiting from the interpositus nucleus ipsilateral to the trained side of the body in the superior cerebellar peduncle, crossing to relay in the contralateral magnocellular division of the red nucleus and crossing back to descend in the rubral pathway to act ultimately on motor neurons (Lavond et al., 1981; McCormick et al., 1982; Haley et al., 1983; Madden et al., 1983; Chapman et al., 1985; Rosenfield et al., 1985) (see Figure 1). Possible involvement of other efferent systems in control of the CR has not yet been determined, but descending systems taking origin rostral to the midbrain are not necessary for learning or retention of the CR, as noted above.

Recent lesion and microstimulation evidence suggests that the essential US reinforcing pathway, the necessary and sufficient pathway conveying information about the US to the cerebellar memory trace circuit, is climbing fibers from the dorsal accessory olive (DAO) projecting via the inferior cerebellar peduncle (see Figure 1). Thus, lesions of the appropriate region of the DAO prevent acquisition and produce normal extinction of the behavioral CR with continued paired training in already trained animals (McCormick et al., 1985). Electrical microstimulation of this same region elicits behavioral responses and serves as an effective US for normal learning of behavioral CRs; the exact behavioral response elicited by DAO stimulation is learned as a normal CR to a CS (Mauk and Thompson, in press). The inferior olive-climbing fiber system also plays an important role in adaptation of the vestibulo-ocular reflex, as noted above, and in recovery from motor abnormalities issued by labyrinthine lesions (Llinas et al., 1975).

Lesion and microstimulation data suggest that the essential CS pathway includes mossy fiber projections to the cerebellum via the pontine nuclei (see Figure 1). Thus, sufficiently large lesions of the middle cerebellar peduncle prevent acquisition and immediately abolish retention of the eyelid CR to all modalities of CS (Solomon et al., 1986) whereas lesions in the pontine nuclear region can selectively abolish the eyelid CR to an acoustic CS (Steinmetz et al., 1986a,b). Consistent with this result is current anatomical evidence from our laboratory for a direct contralateral projection from the ventral cochlear nucleus to this same region of the pons (Thompson et al., 1986) and electrophysiological evidence of a "primary-like" auditory relay nucleus in this pontine region (Logan et al., 1986).

Electrical microstimulation of the mossy fiber system serves as a very effective CS, producing rapid learning, on average more rapid than with peripheral CSs, when paired with, e.g., a corneal airpuff US (Steinmetz et al., 1985a). If animals are trained with a left pontine nuclear stimulation CS and then tested for transfer to right pontine stimulation, transfer is immediate (i.e., 1 trial) if the two electrodes have similar locations in the two sides, suggesting that at least under these conditions the traces are not formed in the pontine nuclei but rather in the cerebellum, probably beyond the mossy fiber terminals (Steinmetz et al., in press). Finally, appropriate forward pairing of mossy fiber stimulation as a CS and climbing fiber stimulation as a US yields <u>normal behavioral learning</u> of the response elicited by climbing fiber stimulation

(Steinmetz et al., 1985b). Lesion of the interpositus abolishes both the CR and the UR in this paradigm. All of these results taken together would seem to build an increasingly strong case for localization of the essential memory traces to the cerebellum, particularly in the "reduced" preparation with stimulation of mossy fibers as the CS and climbing fibers as the US. In the normal animal trained with peripheral stimuli, the possibility of trace formation in brain stem structures has not yet been definitively ruled out.

We initially suggested that the memory traces might be formed in cerebellar cortex (McCormick et al., 1981); as Eccles and others have stressed, there is a vastly greater neuronal machinery there than in the interpositus nucleus. However, we have not yet found any cerebellar cortical lesion that permanently abolishes the CR. Yeo et al., (1985), using more complex stimulus and training conditions (that yield less robust learning), reported that complete removal of the cortex of Larsell's lobule H VI permanently abolished the eyelid CR. Complete removal of H VI did not abolish the CR in three separate studies in our laboratory (McCormick and Thompson, 1984; Woodruff-Pak et al., 1985a,b). Recently, we repeated exactly the stimulus and training conditions of Yeo et al. and found that complete removal of H VI causes only transient loss of the CR; all animals eventually relearned (Lavond et al., 1986). But these results do not rule out multiple parallel cortical sites (and interpositus as well?). Cortical lesions to date may not have removed all such sites; thus the flocculus has not been lesioned and it has recently been found that electrical microstimulation of the flocculus can elicit eyeblinks in the rabbit (Nago et al., 1984). In general, the larger the cerebellar cortical lesion the more pronounced and prolonged is the transient loss of the CR. Further, cerebellar cortical lesions prior to training can prevent learning in some animals (McCormick, 1983). The possibility of multiple cortical sites is consistent with the organization of somatosensory projections to cerebellum (Kassel et al., 1984; Shambes et al., 1978).

In current work we have compared electrical stimulation of the dorsolateral pontine nucleus (DLPN) and lateral reticular nucleus (LRN) as CSs. When paired with a peripheral US (corneal airpuff), both yield normal and rapid learning (Steinmetz et al., 1986a, in press;

Knowlton et al., 1986). The DLPN projects almost exclusively to an intermediate region of cerebellar cortex whereas the LRN projects in significant part to the interpositus nucleus (Bloedel and Courville, 1981; Brodal, 1975; Chan-Palay, 1977). Under these conditions, a lesion limited to the general region of cerebellar cortex receiving projections from the DLPN completely and permanently abolishes the CR to the DLPN stimulation CS but not to the LRN stimulation CS (Knowlton et al., 1986). We have thus created a situation where a relatively restricted region of cerebellar cortex is necessary for the CR, which will be most helpful for further analysis of mechanisms of memory trace formation. More generally, these results suggest that the particular region(s) of cerebellar cortex necessary for associative memory formation depend upon the patterns of mossy fiber projections to the cerebellum activated by the CS. We hypothesize that the memory traces are formed in regions of cerebellar cortex (and interpositus nucleus?) where CS-activated mossy fiber projections and US-activated climbing fiber projections converge.

Recordings from Purkinje cells in the eyelid conditioning paradigm are consistent with the formation of memory traces in cerebellar cortex. Prior to training, a tone CS causes a variable evoked increase in frequency of discharge of simple spikes in many Purkinje cells (Foy and Thompson, 1986; Donegan et al., 1985). Corneal airpuff onset commonly evokes complex climbing fiber spikes in activated Purkinje cells. Following training, the majority of Purkinje cells that develop a change in frequency of simple spike discharge that correlates with the behavioral response (as opposed to being stimulus evoked) show decreases in frequency of discharge of simple spikes that precede and "predict" the form of the behavioral learned response, although increases in "predictive" discharge frequency also occur fairly frequently. In a well-trained animal, the corneal airpuff US onset almost never evokes complex climbing fiber spikes. This last is reminiscent of a recent report that activation of red nucleus can depress somatosensory activation of the inferior olive (Weiss et al., 1985). In a trained animal (eyelid CR), there is a marked activation of interpositus neurons that is maximal at about the time of onset of the US, which would presumably so activate neurons in the red nucleus. Thus, climbing fiber activation of Purkinje cells could function as an "error signal," i.e., when the CR fails to occur, somewhat analogously to the role hypothesized by Ito for climbing fibers in VOR adaptation. Such a system could provide a mechanism to account for the behavioral learning phenomenon of blocking. (In blocking, training is first established to a CS_1; subsequent training trials with simultaneous CS_1 and CS_2, followed by US, yield much less learning to CS_2 than if no prior CS_1-US training were given).

Conjoint electrical stimulation of mossy fibers and climbing fibers can yield normal learning of behavioral responses, as noted above. The properties of these learned responses appear identical to those of the same conditioned responses learned with peripheral stimuli (e.g., eyelid closure, leg flexion). The temporal requirements for such conjoint stimulation that yields behavioral learning are essentially identical to those required with peripheral stimuli; there is no learning at all if CS onset does not precede US onset by more than 50 msec, best learning if CS precedes US by 200-400 msec, and progressively poorer learning with increasing CS precedence (Gormezano, 1972). Further, normal learning occurs if the mossy fiber CS consists of only 2 pulses, 5 msec apart, at the beginning of a 250 msec CS-US onset interval (Logan et al., 1985). These temporal requirements are very different than those reported for LTD induced by conjoint stimulation (see above). This may or may not imply a different mechanism than LTD, network properties may impose the timing requirements for behavioral learning.

OVERVIEW

Here we summarize the arguments for localization of the essential memory trace(s) for this category of basic associative learning to the cerebellum (see Figure 1).

Argument. The memory trace is afferent to the efferent fibers of the superior cerebellar peduncle exiting from the interpositus nucleus.

Evidence. Microstimulation of the interpositus nucleus evokes discrete, phasic behavioral responses, the nature of the response determined by electrode location. The region eliciting eyelid closure is the same region that, when lesioned, abolishes the eyelid CR and where neurons develop a "model" of the amplitude time course of the behavioral CR (see above). Further, such microstimulation of interpositus nucleus, presumably principal cells (i.e., cells of origin of superior cerebellar peduncle fibers), cannot be used as an effective US for learning nor can it serve to maintain a CR learned with a corneal airpuff US (Chapman et al., 1985). By the same token, stimulation of the appropriate region of the mangocellular division of the red nucleus elicits eyelid closure (the same region that when lesioned abolishes the CR) but such stimulation is completely ineffective as a US (Chapman and Thompson, 1986). These results stand in marked contrast to the fact that microstimulation of the appropriate region of the dorsal accessory olive serves as a very effective US for learning of the eyeblink response (see above).

Lesion of the efferent circuit at the interpositus nucleus, the existing fibers of the superior cerebellar peduncle, at the decussation of the peduncle, in the magnocellular red nucleus and in the descending rubral pathway abolishes the CR to all modalities of CS but does not abolish the UR (when corneal airpuff is used as the US). Finally, a neuronal "model" of the learned behavioral response develops in the interpositus nucleus -- a within-trial increase in neural activity that correlates closely with the amplitude time course of the behavioral CR (but not the UR) and precedes it substantially in time -- develops over training and predicts the learned response both within trials and over the trials of training (see above).

Collectively, this evidence builds a strong case that the memory trace is formed in the interpositus nucleus, the cerebellar cortex, or in systems afferent to the cerebellum for which the cerebellum is a mandatory efferent. The immediate afferents are two systems: climbing fibers coming exclusively from the inferior olive and mossy fibers coming largely from the pontine nuclei but from other sources as well.

Argument. The memory trace is not in the inferior olive.

Evidence. Lesions of most of the inferior olive have no effect on the CR. The only critical locus (for the eyeblink CR) is in the rostromedial portion of the dorsal accessory olive. A lesion here causes extinction of the CR with continued paired training (see above). Since the CR is present after the lesion, the essential memory trace cannot be here. Further, convergence of information from the CS and US must occur at the site(s) of trace formation. There does not appear to be any auditory input to this part of the inferior olive (Gellman et al., 1983).

<u>Argument</u>. The memory traces are formed in the cerebellum.

<u>Evidence</u>. Here, the evidence is somewhat more indirect but, we feel, relatively strong.

The most direct evidence would come from identification of the essential CS pathway to the cerebellum and demonstration that the principal cells at each nuclear relay do not show learning-related changes. We have just recently developed evidence that the auditory CS pathway involves primarily direct projections from the <u>ventral</u> cochlear nucleus to the contralateral ventral pontine nuclear region and from there to the cerebellum via mossy fibers in the middle cerebellar peduncle (see above). In earlier work using a signal detection paradigm in eyelid conditioning with an acoustic CS and unit recording, we developed very strong evidence that the memory trace is not formed in the ventral cochlear nucleus (Kettner and Thompson, 1985). In current preliminary single unit recording from the auditory pontine region, we see no signs of learning-related changes in unit responses to the auditory CS. Thus, in well-trained animals, the units respond with typical primary-like patterns (e.g., very short onset latency) that do not correlate at all with the learned behavioral response, in marked contrast to units in cerebellar cortex and interpositus.

The fact that normal behavioral conditioned responses can be established with electrical micro-stimulation of pontine nuclei/mossy fibers as a CS and dorsal accessory olive/climbing fibers as a US argues strongly for trace formation in the cerebellum. The two systems converge at but not before the cerebellum.

The transfer data provide another strong line of evidence: If an animal is trained with CS_1 in, e.g., the left pontine nuclei and then tested for transfer to a CS_2 on the right pontine nuclei, transfer is immediate (1 trial) if the electrodes are in the same locus on each side. In this paradigm, the corneal airpuff US is always delivered to the right eye, which activates the left inferior olive, which projects only to the right cerebellum. The only conceivable way that such immediate transfer can occur is if CS_1 and CS_2 activate a very large proportion of memory trace elements (neurons where the trace has developed) in common.

When learning develops to CS_1, the trace is either formed in the pontine nuclei at or near the site of stimulation, or elsewhere in the brain stem, or in the cerebellum. But wherever it is formed, lesion of the interpositus nucleus or of the middle cerebellar peduncle (mossy fibers) abolishes the CR. Hence the CR pathway must go to the cerebellum. Direct stimulation of the mossy fibers themselves in the middle cerebellar peduncle is also a very effective CS. Here there is no "fibers of passage problem" -- they are all one kind of fibers of passage, mossy fibers projecting to cerebellum. The stimulus also of course activates the cells of origin antidromically: This does not occur with peripheral CSs and is unphysiological. So with a CS_1 in the pontine nuclei, the mandatory CS pathway is via mossy fibers to the cerebellum.

When CS_2 is in the same locus in the pontine nuclei on the other side of the brain, the immediate transfer that occurs is very hard to explain if the trace for CS_1 were established in the pontine nuclei or elsewhere in the brain stem, since CS_2 does not activate these elements. But CS_1 and CS_2 activate many elements in common in the cerebellum, since a given region of pontine nuclei projects to the same regions of both left and right cerebellar hemispheres (more heavily contralateral). It is possible that CS_2 activates fibers of passage from the contralateral pontine nuclei activated as the CS pathway by CS_1. If so, then the common elements could be the mossy fiber terminals in the cerebellum. But the transfer is immediate and complete, which on a probabilistic basis argues against this possibility, which would thus localize the memory trace to cerebellar neurons beyond the mossy fiber terminals.

Finally, it is worth emphasizing that if in fact the memory traces are formed in the cerebellum and not in regions afferent to the cerebellum, as all our evidence argues, then our electrophysiological data showing learning-induced changes in Purkinje cell responses argues very strongly that neuronal plasticity does in fact develop in the cerebellar cortex.

ACKNOWLEDGEMENTS

Supported in part by National Science Foundation grant BNS 8117115, Office of Naval Research grant N00014-83-K-0238, the Sloan Foundation and the McKnight Foundation. I thank my many and valued collaborators on the work reported here (see references).

REFERENCES

Albus JS (1971). A theory of cerebellar funtion. Math Biosci 10:25-61.

Black AH, Prokasy WF (eds) (1972). "Classical Conditioning II: Current Research and Theory." New York: Appleton-Century-Crofts.

Bloedel JR, Courville J (1981). Cerebellar afferent systems. In Brookhart JM, Mountcastle VB, Brooks VB, Geiger SR (eds): "Handbook of Physiology," vol. 2. Baltimore: Am Physiol Soc, pp 735-829.

Brodal P (1975). Demonstration of a somatotopically organized projection onto the paramedian lobule and the anterior lobe from the lateral reticular nucleus: An experimental study with the horseradish peroxidase method. Brain Res 95:221-239.

Brooks VB (1979). Control of intended limb movements by the lateral and intermediate cerebellum. In Asanuma H, Wilson VJ (eds): "Integration in the Nervous System." Tokyo: Igaku Shoin, pp 321-357.

Brooks VB, Kozlovskaya IB, Atkin A, Horvath FE, Uno M (1973). Effects of cooling dentate nucleus on tracking-task performance in monkeys. J Neurophysiol 36:974-995.

Brooks VB, Thach WT (1981). Cerebellar control of posture and movement. In Brookhart JM, Mountcastle VB, Brooks VB, Geiger SR (eds): "Handbook of Physiology," vol 2. Bethesda, MD: Am Physiol Soc, pp 877-946.

Chan-Palay V (1977). "Cerebellar Dentate Nucleus." New York: Springer.

Chapman CE, Spidalieri G, Lamarre Y (1982). A study of sensorimotor properties of dentate neurons during conditioned arm movements in the monkey. Soc Neurosci

Abstr 8:830.

Chapman CE, Spidalieri G, Lamarre Y (1986). Activity of dentate neurons during arm movements triggered by visual, auditory, and somesthetic stimuli in the monkey. J Neurophysiol 55(2):203-226.

Chapman PF, Steinmetz JE, Thompson RF (1985). Classical conditioning of the rabbit eyeblink does not occur with stimulation of the cerebellar nuclei as the unconditioned stimulus. Soc Neurosci Abstr 11:835.

Chapman PF, Thompson RF (1986). Stimulation of red nucleus as unconditioned stimulus does not lead to classical conditioning of eyeblink response in rabbit. Soc Neurosci Abstr 12:753.

Disterhoft JF, Coulter DA, Alkon DL (in press). Conditioning-specific membrane changes of rabbit hippocampal neurons measured in vitro. Proc Natl Acad Sci.

Donegan NH, Foy MR, Thompson RF (1985). Neuronal responses of the rabbit cerebellar cortex during performance of the classically conditioned eyelid response. Soc Neurosci Abstr 11:835.

Donegan NH, Lowry RW, Thompson RF (1983). Effects of lesioning cerebellar nuclei on conditioned leg-flexion responses. Soc Neurosci Abstr 9:331.

Eccles JC (1977). An instruction-selection theory of learning in the cerebellar cortex. Brain Res 127:327-352.

Ekerot CF, Kano M (1985). Long-term depression of parallel fibre synapses following stimulation of climbing fibres. Brain Res 342:357-360.

Foy MR, Thompson RF (1986). Single unit analysis of Purkinje cell discharge in classically conditioned and untrained rabbits. Soc Neurosci Abstr 12:518.

Gellman R, Houk JC, Gibson AR (1983). Somatosensory properties of the inferior olive of the cat. J Comp Neurol 215:228-243.

Gormezano I (1972). Investigations of defense and reward conditioning in the rabbit. In Black AH, Prokasy WF (eds): "Classical Conditioning II: Current Research and Theory." New York: Appleton-Century-Crofts, pp 151-181.

Haley DA, Lavond DG, Thompson RF (1983). Effects of contralateral red nuclear lesions on retention of the classically conditioned nictitating membrane/eyelid response. Soc Neurosci Abstr 9:643.

Horvath F, Atkin EA, Kozlovskaya I, Fuller DRG, Brooks VB (1968). Effects of cooling the dentate nucleus on alternating bar-pressing performance in moneky. Int J Neurol 7:252-270.

Ito M (1972). Neural design of the cerebellar motor control system. Brain Res 40:81-84.

Ito M (1984). "The Cerebellum and Neural Control." New York: Raven.

Ito M (1985). Cerebellar plasticity as the basis for motor learning. In Eccles D (ed): "Recent Achievements in Restorative Neurology 1: Upper Motor Neuron Functions and Dysfunctions." Basel: Karger, pp 222-234.

Kassel J, Shambes GM, Welker W (1984). Fractured cutaneous projections to the granule cell layer of the posterior cerebellar hemisphere of the domestic cat. J Comp Neurol 225:458-468.

Kettner RE, Thompson RF (1985). Cochlear nucleus, inferior colliculus, and medial geniculate responses during the behavioral detection of threshold-level auditory stimuli in the rabbit. J Acoust Soc Am 77(6):2111-2127.

Knowlton B, Beekman G, Lavond DG, Steinmetz JE, Thompson RF (1986). Effects of aspiration of cerebellar cortex on retention of eyeblink conditioning using stimulation of different mossy fiber sources as conditioned stimuli. Soc Neurosci Abstr 12:754.

Lavond DG, McCormick DA, Clark GA, Holmes DT, Thompson RF (1981). Effects of ipsilateral rostral pontine reticular lesions on retention of classically conditioned nictitating membrane and eyelid response. Physiol Psychol 9(4):335-339.

Lavond DG, Steinmetz JE, Yokaitis MH, Lee J, Thompson RF (1986). Retention of classical conditioning after removal of cerebellar cortex. Soc Neurosci Abstr 12:753.

Lisberger SG (1982). Role of the cerebellum during motor learning in the vestibulo-ocular reflex: Different mechanisms in different species? Trends in Neurosci 5(12):437-441.

Llinas R, Walton K, Hillman DE (1975). Inferior olive: its role in motor learning. Science 190:1230-1231.

Llinas R, Sugimori M (1980). Electrophysiological properties of in vitro Purkinje cell dendrites in mammalian cerebellar slices. J Physiol 305:197-213.

Logan CG, Steinmetz JE, Woodruff-Pak DS, Thompson RF (1985). Short-duration mossy fiber stimulation is effective as a CS in eyelid classical conditioning. Soc Neurosci Abstr 11:835.

Logan CG, Steinmetz JE, Thompson RF (1986). Acoustic related responses recorded from the region of the pontine nuclei. Soc Neurosci Abstr 12:754.

Madden J IV, Haley DA, Barchas JD, Thompson RF (1983).
Microinfusion of picrotoxin into the caudal red nucleus
selectively abolishes the classically conditioned
nictitating membrane/eyelid response in the rabbit.
Neurosci Abstr 9:830.

Mamounas LA, Thompson RF, Lynch G, Baudry M (1984).
Classical conditioning of the rabbit eyelid response
increases glutamate receptor binding in hippocampal
synaptic membranes. Proc Nat Acad Sci USA 81(8):2548-
2552.

Marr D (1969). A theory of cerebellar cortex. J Physiol
202:437-470.

Mauk MD, Steinmetz JE, Thompson RF (1984). Classical
conditioning using stimulation of the inferior olive as
the unconditioned stimulus. Proc Nat Acad Sci USA 83:
5349-5353.

Mauk MD, Thompson RF (in press). Retention of classically
conditioned eyelid responses following acute decerebration.
Brain Res.

McCormick DA, Lavond DG, Clark GA, Kettner RE, Rising CE,
Thompson RF (1981). The engram found? Role of the
cerebellum in classical conditioning of nictitating
membrane and eyelid responses. B Psychon Soc 18(3):
103-105.

McCormick DA, Guyer PE, Thompson RF (1982). Superior
cerebellar peduncle lesions selectively abolish the
ipsilateral classically conditioned nictitating membrane/
eyelid response in the rabbit. Brain Res 244:347-350.

McCormick DA (1983). "Cerebellum: Essential Involvement
in a Simple Learned Response." Doctoral Dissertation,
Stanford University.

McCormick DA, Thompson RF (1984). Cerebellum: Essential
Involvement in the Classically Conditioned Eyelid
Response. Science 223:296-299.

McCormick DA, Steinmetz JE, Thompson RF (1985). Lesions of
the inferior olivary complex cause extinction of the
classically conditioned eyeblink response. Brain Res 359:
120-130.

Meyer-Lohmann J, Hore J, Brooks VB (1977). Cerebellar
participation in generation of prompt arm movements.
J Neurophysiol 40:1038-1050.

Miles FA, Lisberger SG (1981). Plasticity in the vestibulo-
ocular reflex: A new hypothesis. Ann Rev Neurosci 4:273-
299.

Nagao S, Ito M, Karachot L (1984). Sites in the rabbit

flocculus specifically related to eye blinking and neck muscle contraction. Neurosci Res 1:149-152.

Norman RJ, Villablanca JR, Brown KA, Schwafel JA, Buchwald JS (1974). Classical conditioning in the bilaterally hemispherectomized cat. Exp Neurol 44:363-380.

Oakley DA, Russel IS (1977). Subcortical storage of Pavlovian conditioning in the rabbit. Physiol Behav 18: 931-937.

Polenchar BE, Patterson MM, Lavond DG, Thompson RF (1985). Cerebellar lesions abolish an avoidance response in rabbit. Behav Neural Biol 44:221-227.

Rosenfield ME, Devydaitis A, Moore JW (1985). Brachium conjunctivum and rubrobulbar tract: Brainstem projections of red nucleus essential for the conditioned nictitating membrane response. Physiol Beh 34:751-759.

Sakurai M (1985). Long-term depression of parallel fiber-Purkinje cell synapses in vitro. Neurosci Lett Suppl 22:S26.

Shambes GM, Gibson JM, Welker W (1978). Fractured somatotopy in granule cell tactile areas of rat cerebellar hemispheres revealed by micromapping. Brain Behav Evol 15:94-140.

Solomon PR, Lewis JL, LoTurco JJ, Steinmetz JE, Thompson RF (1986). The role of the middle cerebellar peduncle in acquisition and retention of the rabbit's classically conditioned nictitating membrane response. B Psychon Soc 24(1):75-78.

Steinmetz JE, Lavond DG, Thompson RF (1985a). Classical conditioning of the rabbit eyelid response with mossy fiber stimulation as the conditioned stimulus. B Psychon Soc 23(3):245-248.

Steinmetz JE, Lavond DG, Thompson RF (1985b). Classical conditioning of skeletal muscle responses with mossy fiber stimulation CS and climbing fiber stimulation US. Soc Neurosci Abstr 11:982.

Steinmetz JE, Rosen DL, Chapman PF, Lavond DG, Thompson RF (1986a). Classical conditioning of the rabbit eyelid response with a mossy fiber stimulation CS. I. Pontine nuclei and middle cerebellar peduncle stimulation. Behav Neurosci 100:871-880.

Steinmetz JE, Logan CG, Rosen DJ, Lavond DG, Thompson RF (1986b). Lesions in the pontine nuclear region selectively abolish classically conditioned eyelid responses in rabbits. Soc Neuro Abstr 12:753.

Steinmetz JE, Rosen DJ, Woodruff-Pak DS, Lavond DG, Thompson RF (in press). Rapid transfer of training occurs when direct mossy fiber stimulation is used as a conditioned stimulus for classical eyelid conditioning. Neurosci Res.

Thach WT (1970). Discharge of cerebellar neurons related to two maintained postures and two prompt movements. I: Nuclear cell output. J Neurophysiol 33:527-536.

Thach WT (1978). Correlation of neural discharge with pattern and force of muscular activity, joint position, and direction of the intended movement in motor cortex and cerebellum. J Neurophysiol 41:654-676.

Thompson RF, Berger TW, Madden J IV (1983). Cellular processes of learning and memory in the mammalian CNS. Ann Rev Neurosci 6:447-491.

Thompson JK, Lavond DG, Thompson RF (1986). Preliminary evidence for a projection from the cochlear nucleus to the pontine nuclear region. Soc Neurosci Abstr 12:754.

Watanabe E (1985). Role of the primate flocculus in adaptation of the vestibulo-ocular reflex. Neurosci Res 3:20-38.

Weiss C, McCurdy ML, Houk JC, Gibson AR (1985). Anatomy and physiology of dorsal column afferents to forelimb dorsal accessory olive. Soc Neurosci Abstr 11:182.

Woodruff-Pak DS, Lavond DG, Thompson RF (1985a). Trace conditioning: Abolished by cerebellar nuclear lesions but not lateral cerebellar cortex aspiration. Brain Res 348: 249-260.

Woodruff-Pak DS, Lavond DG, Logan CG, Steinmetz JE, Thompson RF (1985b). The continuing search for a role of the cerebellar cortex in eyelid conditioning. Neurosci Abstr 11:333.

Yeo CH, Hardiman MJ, Glickstein M (1984). Discrete lesions of the cerebellar cortex abolish the classically conditioned nictitating membrane response of the rabbit. Beh Brain Res 13:261-266.

Yeo CH, Hardiman MJ, Glickstein M (1985). Classical conditioning of the nictitating membrane response of the rabbit: II: Lesions of the cerebellar cortex. Exp Brain Res 60:99-113.

Neuroplasticity, Learning, and Memory, pages 173–197

LONG-TERM POTENTIATION PHENOMENA: THE SEARCH FOR THE
MECHANISMS UNDERLYING MEMORY STORAGE PROCESSES

Ronald J. Racine and Edward W. Kairiss

Dept. of Psychology, McMaster University
Hamilton, Ontario, Canada and University
of Otago, P.O. Box 56, Dunedin, New Zealand

One of the most familiar uses of model phenomena in
the neurosciences is their application to the study of
memory mechanisms. Sechenov (1883) observed that
decapitated frogs would often show a sustained flexion of
the limbs in response to pinching the toes of the hindlimb.
This effect could last up to 30 minutes, and Sechenov
attributed it to a persisting trace in the spinal cord.
Romanes (1885), working with jellyfish, found that
repetitive stimulation of the umbrella could lead to
responses of increased amplitude. He spoke of a "memory"
for the event.

The need for model phenomena is clear. "Real" learning
involves complex and diffuse patterns of activation. It is
difficult to identify the cells that participate in the
construction of the memory trace, or engram. Certain model
phenomena simplify the plastic events to the extent that the
relevant cells, or even synapses, can be identified.

The most promising memory model to date is the so-called
long-term potentiation (LTP) phenomenon (or phenomena).
Potentiation refers to an increase in amplitude of the
responses evoked in a neural pathway following activation
of that pathway. The system is usually monosynaptic,
although potentiation effects have also been reported in
multisynaptic systems. Although there is no consensus as
to the temporal criteria these effects should satisfy in
order to call them "long-term", we do know that short-term
effects such as post-tetanic potentiation rarely last for
more than about 5 minutes (e.g., Magleby, 1973a,b; Magleby

and Zenzel, 1975a,b; 1976). Consequently, descriptions of LTP have included effects lasting anywhere from 10 minutes to several weeks. In this paper, we will consider a phenomenon as long-term if it lasts for 30 minuites or more.

Eccles and McIntyre (1951) provided the first description of a long-lasting potentiation effect. They found that activation of a disused (previously transected) spinal cord pathway could produce a potentiation that lasted for hours. In normal spinal cord, Beswick and Conroy (1965) found that prolonged stimulation could produce similarly long-lasting potentiation effects. These effects did not receive much attention, however, until they had been reported to occur in forebrain tissue. Also, the forebrain effects were found to persist for days or weeks rather than hours. The first report of LTP in the hippocampus appears to be in an abstract by Lomo in 1966. The most influential papers were those of Bliss and Lomo (1973) and Bliss and Gardner-Medwin (1973). These workers reported that repetitive stimulation of the perforant path could produce long-lasting increases in the amplitudes of responses evoked in the dentate gyrus. The increases were seen both in the population EPSPs, a field measure of the strength of synaptic drive, and in the population spike, a field measure of the number of cells generating action potentials (Lomo, 1971). The amplitudes remained increased for hours in acute preparations, and for days in chronic preparations.

The primary value of a model phenomenon is that it is amenable to experimental manipulation. It should facilitate the investigation into the underlying mechanisms, and into the "rules" that apply to the induction of the phenomenon. Also important are the attempts to validate the model, or to obtain some indication that the two phenomena, memory and the memory model, are based upon the same mechanisms. More of this type of evidence has been obtained for LTP than for any other memory model. We will first discuss some of this research and then proceed to a discussion of possible mechanisms.

THE LINKS WITH MEMORY

If LTP is based upon the same mechanisms as those involved in engram formation, then one could expect some

correlations between memory and LTP phenomena. Before
describing some of these, it should be pointed out that a
lack of correlation would not disprove the validity of the
model, since the performance (what we actually measure) of
an animal in a learning task is dependent upon many
variables (e.g., the motivational state of the animal).
Consequently, the performance of animals on a learning
task could vary for reasons other than the degree of
"plasticity" in the circuitry that will store the critical
information. Nevertheless, it can be assumed that at
least some of the differences between successful and
unsuccessful retention will be due to success or failure of
the mechanism of engram formation itself. If this is true,
there should be some correlation between measures of
retention and measures of LTP, so long as the same neuronal
and synaptic elements are involved.

An obvious question is whether structures shown to be
involved in learning will support LTP. Unfortunately, we
do not really know with any certainty where memories are
stored. Not only is it difficult to identify the elements
involved in memory storage, it is difficult to identify
which brain structures are involved. A lesion might result
in the loss of ability to recall specific information, but
it is always possible that the information is still
present, but can no longer be retrieved. Nevertheless, it
is assumed that forebrain tissue has a greater capacity for
storage than brainstem or spinal cord tissue, and that
cortical structures are heavily involved in the storage
process. It is reassuring, then, that LTP is readily
induced in the forebrain, and that it is reliably found in
neocortical, paleocortical and archicortical tissue
(Racine, Milgram and Hafner, 1983; Wilson and Racine, 1983).
Non-hippocampal limbic system structures, which have also
been implicated in learning, also generally show good LTP
effects (Racine et al., 1983).

Many neuroscientists would make the further assumption
that plasticity should relate to the distance from the
"periphery". Motor and sensory systems should, to some
extent, be hardwired, at least in the adult (Goddard, 1980).
Consequently, the ability to support LTP might be expected
to increase as more "central" pathways are tested. Again,
this appears to be true. Racine et al. (1983) were unable
to produce LTP in the lateral olfactory tract projections
to the pyriform cortex. Also, D. Wilson (personal

communication) was unable to produce LTP by activation of the optic radiations.

Although brainstem sites may be less heavily involved in engram formation than forebrain structures, there is evidence that new information can be stored at these levels. For example, the plasticity evident in the readjustment of the vertibulo-ocular reflex, in response to distorting lenses, appears to involve the vestibular nucleus (Galliana, Flohr and Melville Jones, 1984). The conditioning of the nictating membrane reflex appears to involve the deep cerebellar nuclei (e.g., the interpositus). Racine, Wilson, Gingell and Sunderland (1985) have found that both the vestibular and interpositus nuclei will support LTP.

So, LTP can be induced in structures that we presume to be involved in some aspect of the storage process, but does it otherwise have the right characteristics? Without knowing more about the nature of engram formation, it is impossible to specify in any detail what characteristics a model phenomenon should have. One feature that is generally accepted as promising is the degree of specificity in the effects of the LTP-inducing treatments. Most forebrain cells receive inputs from many different sources. It does not seem reasonable that an inactive line should be strengthened by any process that underlies memory formation. It is even more difficult to imagine a system where information is stored by a totally nonspecific increase in the sensitivity of a cell to all of its inputs. So, the question is raised: Is LTP specific to the activated inputs? The answer is not an unqualified 'yes' (see Misgeld, Sarvey and Klee, 1979; Yamamoto and Chujo, 1978), but it does appear to be true for most systems (e.g., Andersen, Sundberg, Sveen and Wigstrom, 1977; Lynch, Dunwiddie and Gribkoff, 1977; McNaughton and Barnes, 1977; Robinson and Racine, 1982).

Although this restriction of the effects to the activated inputs seems to be a desirable feature, there should be some way of modulating the level of the effect according to the spatial pattern of input. In other words, there should be some form of heterosynaptic interaction between active lines. This would allow us to account for associative memory mechanisms. It is not clear where this interaction should occur. Although it logically follows that there must be some point of interaction at the cellular

level between associated inputs, this does not necessarily
mean that there must be such an interaction at the point
of modification (Racine and Zaide, 1978). Nevertheless, it
is easier to model a system that involves changes at the
sites of neuronal interaction, and LTP satisfies this
criterion rather well. Coactivation of the medial and
lateral components of the perforant path results in a
greater magnitude of potentiation of the component pathways
than if they were activated independently (McNaughton,
Douglas and Goddard, 1978). Similar forms of cooperative
interaction have been demonstrated between the contralateral
and ipsilateral entorhinal projections to the dentate gyrus
(Levy and Steward, 1983), the adjacent components of
s. radiatum pathways projecting to area CA1 (Lee, 1983;
Barrionuevo and Brown, 1983), and between the septal and
entorhinal inputs to the dentate gyrus (Robinson and Racine,
1982; Robinson, 1985; Robinson and Racine, 1985).

Another approach aimed at establishing links between
LTP and engram formation involves direct comparison of the
retention of a memory with "retention" of LTP. The memory
test typically utilizes a task (e.g., spatial learning)
that is presumed to require the involvement of a certain
structure (e.g., the hippocampus). Measures of memory for
the task are then compared with measures of LTP induced in
the same structure. Barnes (1979) compared the acquisition
and decay of LTP in the perforant path-dentate system with
acquisition and retention of a spatial maze task that is
presumed to require hippocampal processing. In addition,
she looked at old as well as young animals, because old
animals were known to show poor performance on these tasks.
She found that the old animals exhibited a more rapid
forgetting of the task and a more rapid decay of LTP. Even
more impressive, she found a correlation between the LTP
and memory measures within the groups, as well.

If we assume that information is stored as a set of
synaptic weighting that determines the pattern of
transmission, it would be expected that LTP, which appears
to produce an increase in efficacy at all activated synapses,
should interfere with the subsequent storage capacity of the
circuitry — much of the 'plasticity' will have been used up.
McNaughton, Barnes, Rao, Baldwin and Rasmussen (1986) have
shown that the induction of LTP in the hippocampus can
interfere with subsequent acquisition of a spatial task.
Since the LTP did not disrupt access to previously stored

information, the possibility arises that the hippocampus functions as a temporary storage system.

Berger (1984) reported an apparent exception to this disruption of acquisition by prior induction of LTP. He found that induction of LTP in the hippocampus resulted in a subsequent facilitation of classical conditioning of the nictitating membrane response. This may have been due to an increase in the saliency of the auditory CS. In the spatial task used by McNaughton et al., the hippocampus was presumably involved in the processing of highly complex patterned input. In the conditioning task used by Berger, the CS was a relatively simple discrete auditory stimulus, and the hippocampus may have been involved in the relaying, rather than the processing, of information. If this was the case, then potentiation of transmission over the relaying pathways could have increased the saliency of the cue and facilitated conditioning.

Another prediction is that any manipulation which blocks LTP should also block engram formation. The reverse, of course, is not necessarily true. Learning can be disrupted in many ways, by interference with motor, perceptual, motivational, attentional and arousal mechanisms. The techniques for induction of LTP probably bypass most of these correlative processes. The most effective way of blocking LTP appears to be with the pharmacological agent D-2-amino-5-phosphonovalerate (APV). Morris, Anderson, Lynch and Baudry (1986) have found that the same dose of APV that blocks LTP in the hippocampus also blocks acquisition of a spatial task. The importance of this finding depends upon the specificity of the effects of APV. Unfortunately, APV can produce effects on background activity (Hablitz and Langmoen, 1986). In fact, the doses that are used to produce the LTP-blocking effects can often lead to some ataxia and other behavioral abnormalities suggesting that APV may be interfering with more than just storage processes.

It is not logically imperative that LTP follows all the same rules as behavioral learning but the confidence that we have in the model will depend to some extent upon the correlates that are established. One such set of correlates is the conditioning-like temporal patterns that appear to be a requirement for the induction of the cooperativity effect. Barrionuevo and Brown (1983) adjusted

the intensities of pulses applied to two separate electrodes
in s. radiatum. This resulted in a "weak" and a "strong"
input to CA1, which were intended to model the CS and UCS
of classical conditioning. LTP could be induced in the weak
pathway only if its activation was paired with activation
of the strong pathway. Kelso and Brown (1985) used two
"weak" inputs and one "strong" one. In order to produce
LTP in a weak pathway, it was necessary that its activation
be followed by activation in a strong pathway. Other
combinations were ineffective. Levy and Steward (1983)
obtained similar results using the strong ipsilateral and
weak contralateral entorhinal inputs to the dentate gyrus.
Again, it was necessary to activate the weak input prior to,
or simultaneous with, the strong input.

Other demonstrations of correlates with learning
phenomena include those reported by Laroche and Bloch (1982).
They found that stimulation of the mesencephalic reticular
formation could facilitate both learning and the induction
of LTP.

PROBLEMS WITH THE MODEL

Although these results are encouraging, there are a
number of problems with the LTP model. A major one is that
all of the LTP effects so far described require a highly
synchronous activation of a large number of input fibres to
produce an effect. It seems unlikely that these levels of
synchronization are achieved under normal physiological
conditions.

Also, if LTP is the basis for memory storage, then
using the activation of a pathway as a cue in a learning
task should result in some potentiation in that pathway.
We have attempted to use stimulation pulses applied to the
perforant path as the cue for various types of learning
(de Jonge and Racine, unpublished observations). We were
unable to effect changes in the response evoked by these
pulses, even though the animals were able to learn the
tasks. The tasks included a go no-go task and a spatial
task (in which the pulses were part of an overall stimulus
set associated with place).

Staubli, Roman and Lynch (1985) have found the reverse,
a learning-induced potentiation-like effect in a pathway

that does not appear to show LTP. They found that contingent (water reward) pulses applied to the olfactory bulb would lead to an increase in the response evoked in the pyriform cortex. As pointed out above, however, repetitive stimulation of the olfactory tract does not appear to induce LTP effects at this site. It may be that these effects require cooperative interaction with other pathways. This was suggested by Racine et al. (1983) who found that kindling (epileptogenic) stimulation, which leads to the activation of multiple sets of pathways, does produce an LTP-like effect in the LOT-pyriform response.

Another problem in the LTP area is the lack of permanence of the effect. The few experiments that have carefully monitored the duration of the effect in chronic animals have shown it to be relatively short-lived. Racine, Milgram and Hafner (1983) found that LTP rarely lasted for more than a few weeks. de Jonge and Racine (1985) attempted to increase the duration of LTP effects by the application of repeated sets of trains. They measured the threshold for the effect, the asymptotic levels, and the decay rate. None of these measures were affected by repeated induction of LTP. Because of our lack of understanding of how memories are actually maintained, it is not clear how serious this problem is. Memories may be lost (forgotten) by a passive decay-type process or by some active removal or retrieval block (e.g., due to proactive or retroactive interference). Similarly, if a memory is retained for months or years, we do not know if it is a "permanent" store or whether it is continually refreshed. The difficulty arises because the mechanism by which the memory is refreshed could occur at an "unconscious" level. For example, it may be sufficient to read out information that is similar to that in store 'X' in order to maintain the store, even though the activation of store 'X' never reaches the level required for conscious awareness. If this was the case, then it would not be surprising that LTP decays - there is no mechanism by which the store can be refreshed, except by appropriate reactivation of the inputs.

There is, however, an even more fundamental problem. LTP involves rather large changes in synaptic response. If we are to assume that animals are always learning something about their environments (particularly in the novel experimental setting), why do responses in control animals appear to remain stable? Why are responses in mature but young animals as large as those in older animals? It does not seem sufficient to suggest that one memory may pre-empt the storage of another, because we know that the storage capacity is quite large. Perhaps these problems arise because our view of the links between memory and potentiation phenomena is too simplistic. We will get back to this problem at the end of the paper.

In any case, these findings raise concerns about the validity of the LTP phenomenon as a memory model. If the model is eventually shown to be valid, then these seemingly paradoxical findings will have provided us with additional means for determining the rules that the engram formation process itself follows at the unit level.

THE MECHANISMS

The more we learn about events at the cellular level, the more daunting the search for mechanisms becomes. The number of known electrochemical processes that could affect the function of the cell is increasing dramatically. Although most neuroscientists begin their investigations with a search for a unitary mechanism, even this would likely involve alterations in one component of a long sequence of events that controls synaptic function. At this stage, we do not even know whether the mechanisms underlying LTP are presynaptic (e.g., an increase in the output of transmitter), postsynaptic (e.g., an increase in the number of receptors), or both (e.g., an increase in the numbers of synapses).

Several lines of evidence have been presented in support of a presynaptic mechanism for LTP. Sastry and co-workers have reported that the threshold for triggering an antidromic response in a hippocampal pathway, by stimulation via an electrode placed near the synaptic terminations, is increased after induction of LTP in that pathway. Sastry (1982) reported this effect for the perforant path input to the dentate gyrus, and Sastry, Murali Mohan and Goh (1985) reported a similar effect for the Schaffer collateral input to CA1. They have argued that these increases in threshold for the antidromic response are a result of changes in the presynaptic terminals. This argument is reminiscent of those presented by Lloyd (1949) and others (e.g., Wall and Johnson, 1958) that post-tetanic potentiation in the spinal cord is due to hyperpolarizing afterpotentials in the terminals which lead to larger action potentials and increased transmitter release. Those reports gave rise to a large number of studies designed to investigate that hypothesis. Although the issue was never completely resolved, most of the published papers reported a lack of correlation between afterpotentials and LTP (e.g., Eccles and Rall, 1951; Liley and North, 1953; Eccles and Krnjevic, 1959a,b; Martin and Pilar, 1964; Gage and Hubbard, 1966).

In a more convincing series of experiments, an increase in the release of transmitter has been demonstrated after induction of LTP in the hippocampus. Skrede and Maltheson (1981), for example, reported an increase in resting and evoked release of glutamate in area CA1 following induction of LTP by stimulation of the Schaffer collaterals. Dolphin, Errington and Bliss (1982) found an increased glutamate release following the induction of LTP in the dentate gyrus by activation of the perforant path, and Feasey, Lynch and Bliss (1985) and Lynch, Feasey and Bliss (1985) reported an increased output of glutamate and aspartate in area CA3 following induction of LTP by activation of the commissural pathway. They found these increases to be calcium-dependent. In a subsequent study they found that Ruthenium Red, which apparently releases calcium from mitochondrial stores, triggered a significantly greater release of glutamate from potentiated tissue than did caffeine, which triggers release of calcium from the endoplasmic reticulum. The authors concluded that LTP depended upon an increase in the mitochondrial storage of calcium in the activated terminals.

A conclusive demonstration of a presynaptic mechanism may be difficult to obtain for central neurons. Because of the large number of terminations and the distance from the soma, the quantal analysis technique is not easily applied. This technique depends upon the assumption that transmitter is released in packets (quanta) of fixed size, and upon the ability to resolve these unit components of the synaptic response (see Liley, 1956). A presynaptic mechanism is then seen as an increase in number of quanta released, while a postsynaptic mechanism is seen as an increase in the size of the quantal response. Voronin (1983) made an attempt to apply this technique in the hippocampus, and reported an apparent LTP-induced increase in quantal release with no change in quantal size. He conceded, however, that the data were not readily interpretable. An increase in the number of synapses, for example, could also account for the data. Baxter, Bittner and Brown (1985) performed a quantal analysis on a long-lasting potentiation effect induced at the neuromuscular junction of the opener muscle of the crayfish and also found an increase in quantal content. It is not clear, however, whether this form of potentiation is the same as that observed in the mammalian forebrain. Koyano, Kuba and Minota (1985) ran a quantal analysis in potentiated frog sympathetic ganglia and found both an increase in quantal content <u>and</u> an increase in quantal size. It is possible that there is more than one component of LTP (see Raine et al., 1983), and that the early component depends upon an increase in transmitter release, while the second depends upon an increase in the number of receptors.

There appears to be more support for a postsynaptic mechanism for LTP. Part of the reason for this may be the view that a postsynaptic mechanism would allow for a greater storage capacity (see Goddard, 1980). That view rests on the assumption that a presynaptic mechanism would likely involve a nonspecific change at <u>all</u> of the terminals of the activated cell. The case for a postsynaptic mechanism has been reinforced by the previously mentioned demonstrations of various forms of cooperative interaction between activated inputs, together with the lack of any obvious means by which such interactions could occur presynaptically. Even those who support presynaptic mechanisms now concede that the triggering mechanism is likely to be postsynaptic.

Another line of evidence that has been presented in support of a postsynaptic mechanism is the demonstration of postsynaptic structural alterations. Fifkova and co-workers, for example, have reported that dendritic spines are increased in size after the induction of LTP in the hippocampus. They argue that a decreased resistance in the spine will result in a greater delivery of synaptic current to the dendritic shaft (Van Harreveld and Fifkova, 1975; Fifkova and Van Harreveld, 1977). In subsequent experiments, they have presented arguments for a contractile process, located in the spine, which could mediate these effects (Fifkova and Delay, 1982; Fifkova, Markham and Delay, 1983). Other workers reporting LTP-induced alterations in spine morphology include Desmond and Levy (1981), who reported an increase in the size of spine heads, and Lee, Schottler, Oliver and Lynch (1980) who reported a decrease in the

variability of spine morphology. Most of these experiments
were done in the dentate gyrus.

Perhaps the most prolific advocates of postsynaptic
mechanisms are G. Lynch and co-workers at the University of
California at Irvine. They have reported that the induction
of LTP in the hippocampus leads to an increase in glutamate
binding, attributable to an increase in the number of
glutamate receptors (Lynch, Halpain and Baudry, 1982). They
also showed that the increased binding was dependent upon
calcium, and others have shown that LTP is dependent upon
calcium or the activation of calcium binding proteins (e.g.,
Wigstrom, Swann and Andersen, 1979; Dunwiddie, Robertson and
Worth, 1982; Mody, Baimbridge and Miller, 1984). Although
these demonstrations could apply to a presynaptic as well as
a postsynaptic mechanism, Lynch, Kelso, Barrioneuvo and
Schottler (1983) reported that the intracellular injection
of EGTA, a Ca^{++} chelater, blocked LTP in that cell. As the
synaptic response did not appear to be affected by this
treatment, the authors concluded that the mechanisms of LTP
must be postsynaptic. These workers have also presented
evidence that the increase in the number of receptors is due
to the calcium-induced activation of a protease (calpain)
which degrades a spectrin-like protein (fodrin) which, in
turn, leads to the exposure of previously inactive glutamate
receptors (Baudry and Lynch, 1980; Lynch and Baudry, 1984).

It appears that it may be possible to potentiate
inhibitory as well as excitatory systems, and this effect
may also be due to an increase in the number of postsynaptic
receptors. Tuff, Racine and Adamec (1983) and Tuff, Racine
and Mishra (1983) have reported evidence for a kindling-
induced potentiation of inhibition in the dentate gyrus.
Kindling is an epilepsy model in which increased
epileptogenic activity is produced by repeated stimulation.
This treatment results in potentiation effects in several
pathways (Racine, Gardner and Burnham, 1972; Racine,
Newberry and Burnham, 1975; Douglas and Goddard, 1975;
Racine, Milgram and Hafner, 1983). Further evidence that a
potentiation effect can be induced in hippocampal inhibitory
systems has been provided by King, Dingledine, Giacchino and
McNamara (1985) and by Oliver and Miller (1985). These
results show that inhibitory systems can be potentiated, and
the experiments of Tuff, Racine and Mishra (1983) and Valdes,
Dasheiff, Birmingham, Crutcher and McNamara (1982) suggest
that this effect may be due to an increase in the number of

benzodiazepine receptors. These have been identified as a component of the inhibitory GABA receptor complex (Haefely, 1984).

Other workers, however, have failed to find an LTP-induced increase in receptor binding (e.g., Sastry and Goh, 1984; Lynch, Feasey and Bliss, 1985).

Confronted with these apparently conflicting data, several workers have suggested that LTP might involve changes at both pre and postsynaptic sites (e.g., Bliss and Dolphin, 1982). Stimulation-induced synaptogenesis, for example, could account for most of the data thus far presented. This appears to be the opinion of Greenough and co-workers who have found that both experience and LTP induction can lead to an increase in the number of synapses associated with "sessile" (small, stubby) spines (Greenough, 1984; Chang and Greenough, 1984). Because they also found an increase in polyribosomal aggregates associated with spine synapses in animals exposed to complex environments, they suggested that these spines could be an indication of newly forming synapses (Greenough, Hwang and Gorman, 1985).

Another line of research that is consistent with a synaptogenic mechanism is that of Routtenberg and co-workers. They have consistently found an increase in the phosphorylation of the so-called "F1 protein" (47 KD) as a result of either learning or the induction of LTP (Routtenberg, Lovinger, Cain, Akers and Steward, 1983; Routtenberg, Lovinger and Steward, 1985; Routtenberg, 1985). As this protein has been associated with growth cones, the authors have suggested that new synapses may be developing (Nelson, Routtenberg, Hyman and Pfenniger, 1985, Routtenberg, 1985).

A POSSIBLE TRIGGER FOR LTP MECHANISMS: THE NMDA RECEPTOR

Whatever the alteration that actually supports increased synaptic efficacy, it is the trigger for this alteration that is of primary interest. One of the goals of those who work with memory phenomena is the eventual development of a "label" for the engram - some means by which those synapses that have been recently recruited into a memory trace can be identified. A label that is specific for newly formed traces will most likely be associated with

transient triggering events. These will be activated under
appropriate conditions, and, in turn, will activate the
chain of events leading to long-term storage.

The work of Greenough and Routtenberg is directed
towards the identification of recently affected synapses.
The recent work related to the function of the N-methyl-D-
aspartate (NMDA) receptor might also lead to the elusive
label. There are apparently at least 3 types of glutamate
receptor. Two of these, the quisqualate and kainate
receptors (named after the pharmacological agents to which
they are most sensitive), appear to mediate normal baseline
synaptic activity. The third, the NMDA receptor, requires
more than the presence of transmitter to affect membrane
conductance. The ion channels associated with this receptor
are also voltage-dependent. This means that the synaptic
activation of these receptors will have no effect unless
there is a suitable background of depolarization
(Collingridge, 1985; Fagg, 1985; Coan and Collingridge,
1985; Herron, Lester, Coan and Collingridge, 1986). It has
been shown by Collingridge, Kehl and McLennan (1983) and
others (Wigstrom and Gustaffson, 1984; Wigstrom, Gustaffson
and Huang, 1985; Morris, Anderson, Lynch and Baudry, 1986)
that LTP can be reliably blocked by agents which appear to
be selective to the NMDA receptor (e.g., D-2-amino-5-
phosphonovalerate). These agents have been reported to
block LTP without blocking normal baseline synaptic
transmission. A voltage-dependency for LTP has also been
demonstrated. Wigstrom and Gustaffson (1983a,b), for
example, have shown that blockade of GABA inhibition by
picrotoxin, biicuculline or penicillin can enhance LTP.
Malinow and Miller (1986) have shown that direct
hyperpolarizing pulses can block the induction of LTP in
single cells. Wigstrom and Gustaffson (1984) and Wigstrom,
Gustaffson and Huang (1985) found that the late components
that appear in the responses of animals treated with
picrotoxin are associated with the activation of the NMDA
receptor and that these appear to be highly correlated with
the induction of LTP. If a train does not evoke these NMDA
components, it will not induce LTP. These findings provide
an attractive hypothesis about the induction of LTP. The
voltage-dependency accounts reasonably well for various
cooperativity effects that have been reported. If
activation of this receptor is the trigger for the events
that alter synaptic transmission, then it may be possible
to discover a label associated with activation of the

receptor or with one of the stages in the chain of events triggered by this activation.

There are still some problems with the NMDA receptor theory. One is that the evidence for voltage-dependency for LTP is not as clear as it should be. Douglas, Goddard and Riives (1982) found that a level of inhibition which was sufficient to block cell discharge (including the cell discharge triggered during the potentiation train) would not block LTP. It was necessary to co-activate the inhibitory pathway with a high frequency train before LTP could be affected. Also, Wigstrom, McNaughton and Barnes (1982) were unable to affect LTP with direct 1 nAmp hyperpolarizing pulses applied to a cell. While Malinow and Miller (1986) were able to block LTP with hyperpolarizing pulses, it was necessary to use at least 3 nA and to apply the potentiating stimulation to inputs that terminated close to the soma (where the hyperpolarizing current was applied). They argued that the excitatory inputs were too electrotonically distant to be affected in the Wigstom et al. study. If that is the case, however, it is difficult to see how distant inputs, such as those onto the basal and apical dendrites, could interact cooperatively (e.g., Gustaffson and Wigstrom, 1986).

Other manipulations which should strongly affect voltage-dependent processes have not been found to block LTP. LTP can be readily induced in animals anesthetized with barbiturates which facilitate inhibitory events (e.g., McNaughton, Douglas and Goddard, 1978). The benzodiazepines, another group of pharmacological agents which facilitate activity in GABA systems, also do not appear to block LTP (Stringer and Guyanet, 1983; Racine, unpublished observations).

Perhaps the biggest problem with the proposed NMDA mechanism is that it remains to be seen whether APV or other agents that affect the NMDA receptor are as specific in the effects as has been claimed. Some of the experiments that have used NMDA blocking agents, for example, have reported a depression of the baseline response (i.e., responses presumed by others to be mediated by activation of "non-NMDA" receptors - Hablitz and Langmoen, 1986). Other studies have shown rather strong behavioral effects of NMDA blockers (Croucher, Collins and Meldrum, 1982; Croucher, Meldrum and Collins, 1984; Erez, Frenk, Goldberg,

Cohen and Teichberg, 1985; Peterson, Collins and Bradford, 1983; Peterson, Collins and Bradford, 1984). Even Morris et al., who claimed that APV produced a specific effect that interfered with both LTP and learning, reported that APV-treated animals occasionally fell off the platform in their water maze task.

LTP AND CONTEXT SPECIFICITY

It has been suggested that the quisqualate and NMDA receptors are linked in the mechanisms underlying LTP. Activation of the NMDA receptor somehow leaves the quisqualate-mediated response potentiated. This opens up the possibility of other types of linkages between synapses or receptor pools. These linkages could themselves be plastic and could conceivably provide the basis for a kind of "tuning" of the response of the cell to temporo-spatial patterns of input (see John, 1967). Few people have pursued these ideas, because it has not been clear how the cell could become tuned to specific patterns of input. Most workers have favoured the hypothesis that engrams are based upon simple increases in synaptic connectivity. That various types of linkage might exist between receptor systems, however, raises the possibility that some context specificity might exist at the cellular level. The moment to moment strength of a synapse, or the local consequences of activation of a synapse, might be determined not only by the strength of its connection, but also by the levels of activation of nearby inputs (or in the distribution of activity in the associated receptor systems). Each synapse would be a context sensitive element containing some local information about how it is related to neighboring elements in the set. Imagine, for example, a set of synapses, A, B, C and D, where A and B have been coactive and potentiated, and C and D have been coactive and potentiated. What should happen when B and C or A and D are activated? A simple connectivity hypothesis would predict that all pairings will be equally strong because all synapses have already been potentiated. If the information conveyed over adjacent sets of synapses is sufficiently similar, then this could serve as a basis for various generalization phenomena. If it is not, then some means of distinguishing the patterns is required. If such context-dependence occurred at the cellular level, it could account for the fact that evoked activity does not appear to increase in strength with age, at least not dramatically, even though the animal is presumably storing new information all the time. It would also lead to the prediction that LTP induced by more complex spatio-temporal patterns of input (e.g., with distributed electrodes) should depend upon how closely the original patterns are duplicated by the test stimuli, and not simply by how many of the potentiated component pathways are activated. We are currently testing these hypotheses.

REFERENCES

Andersen P, Sundberg S, Sveen O, Wigstrom H (1977). Special long-lasting potentiation of synaptic transmission in hippocampal slices. Nature 266:736-737.

Barnes CA (1979). Memory deficits associated with senescence: A neurophysiological and behavioral study in the rat. J Comp Physiol Psychol 93:74-104.

Barrionuevo G, Brown TH (1983). Associative long-term potentiation in hippocampal slices. Proc Nat Acad Sci USA 80:7347-7351.

Baudry M, Lynch G (1980). Hypothesis regarding the cellular mechanisms responsible for long-term synaptic potentiation in the hippocampus. Exp Neurol 68:202-204.

Baxter D, Bittner GD, Brown TH (1985). Quantal mechanism of long-term potentiation. Proc Nat Acad Sci USA 82:5978-5982.

Berger TW (1984). Long-term potentiation of hippocampal synaptic transmission affects rate of behavioral learning. Science 224:627-630.

Beswick FB, Conroy RTWL (1965). Optimal tetanic conditioning of heteronymous monosynaptic reflexes. J Physiol 180:134-146.

Bliss TVP, Dolphin AC (1982). What is the mechanism of long-term potentiation in the hippocampus? TINS 5:289-290.

Bliss TVP, Lomo T (1973). Long-lasting potentiation of synaptic transmission in the dentate area of the anaesthetized rabbit following stimulation of the perforant path. J Physiol 232:331-356.

Bliss TVP, Gardner-Medwin AR, Lomo T (1973). Synaptic plasticity in the hippocampus. Ansell GB (ed), "Macromolecules and Behavior." MacMillan London 193-203.

Chang F-L F, Greenough WT (1984). Transient and enduring morphological correlates of synaptic activity and efficacy change in the rat hippocampal slice. Brain Res 309:35-46.

Coan EJ, Collingridge GL. (1985). Magnesium ions block an N-methyl-D-aspartate receptor-mediated component of synaptic transmission in rat. Neurosci Letters 53:21-26.

Collingridge GL (1985). Long-term potentiation in the hippocampus: Mechanisms of initiation and modulation by neurotransmitters. TIPS 407-411.

Collingridge GL, Kehl SJ, McLennan H (1983). Excitatory amino acids in synaptic transmission in the Schaffer collateral-commissural pathway of the rat hippocampus. Exp Brain Res 52:170-178.

Croucher MJ, Collins JF, Meldrum BS (1982). Anticonvulsant action of excitatory amino acid antagonists. Science 216:899-901.

Croucher MJ, Meldrum BS, Collins JF (1984). Anticonvulsant and proconvulsant properties of a series of structural isomers of piperidine dicarboxylic acid. Neuropharmacol 23:467-472.

de Jonge R, Racine RJ (1985). The effects of repeated induction of long-term potentiation in the dentate gyrus. Brain Res 328:181-185.

Desmond NL, Levy WB (1981). Ultrastructural and numerical alteration in dendritic spines as a consequence of long-term potentiation. Anat Rec 199:68A-69A.

Dolphin AC, Errington ML, Bliss TVP (1982). Long-term potentiation of the perforant path in vivo is associated with increased glutamate release. Nature 297:496-498.

Douglas RM, Goddard GV (1975). Long-term potentiation of the perforant path-granule cell synapse in the rat hippocampus. Brain Res 86:205-215.

Douglas RM, Goddard GV, Riives M (1982). Inhibitory modulation of long-term potentiation: Evidence for a postsynaptic locus of control. Brain Res 240:259-272.

Dunwiddie TV, Robertson NL, Worth T (1982). Modulation of long-term potentiation: Effects of adrenergic and neuroleptic drugs. Pharm Biochem & Behavior 17:1257-1264.

Eccles JC, Krnjevic K (1959). Potential changes recorded inside primary afferant fibres with the spinal cord. J Physiol 149:250-273.

Eccles JC, Krnjevic K (1959) Presynaptic changes associated with post-tetanic potentiation in the spinal cord. J Physiol 149:274-287.

Eccles JC, McIntyre AR (1951). Plasticity of mammalian monosynaptic reflexes. Nature 167:466-468.

Eccles JC, Rall W (1951). Effects in a monosynaptic reflex path by its activation. J Neurophysiol 14:353-376.

Erez U, Frenk H, Goldberg O, Cohen A, Teichberg VI. (1985).

Anticonvulsant properties of 3-hydroxy-2-quinoxalinecarboxylic acid, a newly found antagonist of excitatory amino acids. Eur J Pharmacol 110:31-39.

Fagg GE (1985). L-Glutamate, excitatory amino acid receptors and brain function. TINS 8:207-210.

Feasey KJ, Lynch MA, Bliss TVP (1985). Ca++ induced long-term potentiation in CA3 region of the hippocampus is associated with an increased release of aspartate: An in vivo study in the rat. Neurosci Letters Supple 21:S45.

Fifkova E, Delay RJ (1982). Cytoplasmic actin in dendritic spines as a possible mediator of synaptic plasticity. J Cell Biol 95:345-350.

Fifkova E, Van Harreveld A (1977). Long-lasting morphological changes in dendritic spines of the dentate granular cells following stimulation of the entorhinal area. J Neurocytol 6:211-230.

Fifkova E, Markham JA, Delay RJ (1983). Calcium in the spine apparatus of dendritic spines in the dentate molecular layer. Brain Res 266:163-168.

Gage PW, Hubbard JI (1966). An investigation of the post-tetanic potentiation of end-plate potentials at a mammalian neuromuscular junction. J Physiol 184:353-375.

Galliana HL, Flohr R, Melville Jones G (1984). A reevaluation of intervestibular nuclear coupling: Its role in vestibular compensation. J Neurophysiol 51:242-259.

Goddard GV (1980). Component properties of the memory machine: Hebb revisited. Jusczyk PW, Klein RM (eds), "The Nature of Thought: Essays in Honor of DO Hebb." Lawrence Erlbaum Assoc Hillsdale NJ.

Greenough WT (1984). Structural correlates of information in the mammalian brain: A review and hypothesis. TINS 7:229-233.

Greenough WT, Hwang H-MF, Gorman C (1985). Evidence for active synapse formation or altered postsynaptic metabolism in visual cortex of rats reared in complex environments. Proc Nat Acad Sci USA 82:4549-4552.

Gustaffson B, Wigstrom H (1986). Hippocampal long-lasting potentiation produced by pairing single volleys and brief conditioning tetani evoked in separate afferents. Neurosci (in press).

Hablitz JJ, Longmoen IA (1986). N-methyl-D-aspartate receptor antagonists reduce synaptic excitation in the hippocampus. J Neurosci 6:102-106.

Haefely W (1984). Benzodiazepine interactions with GABA receptors. Neurosc Letters 47:201-206.

Herron CE, Lester RAJ, Coan EJ, Collingridge GL (1985). Intracellular demonstration of an N-methyl-D-aspartate receptor mediated component of synaptic transmission in the rat hippocampus. Neurosci Letters 60:19-23.

John ER (1967). "Mechanisms of Learning." Acad Press New York.

Kelso SR, Brown TH (1985). Differential induction of associative LTP. Neurosci Abstr 11:225.14.

King GL, Dingledine R, Giacchino JL, McNamara JO (1985). Abnormal neuronal excitability in hippocampal slices from kindled rats. J Neurophysiol 54:1295-1304.

Koyano K, Kuba K, Monota S (1985). Long-term potentiation of transmitter release induced by repetitive presynaptic activities in bull-frog sympathetic ganglia. J Physiol 359:219-233.

Laroche S, Bloch V (1982). Conditioning of hippocampal cells and long-term potentiation: An approach to mechanisms of partial memory facilitation. Ajmone-Marsan C, Matthies H (eds), "Neuronal Plasticity and Memory Formation." Raven Press New York p.575-578.

Lee KS (1983). Cooperativity among afferents for the induction of long-term potentiation in the CA1 region of the hippocampus. J Neurosci 3:1369-1372.

Lee KS, Schottler F, Oliver M, Lynch G (1980). Brief burst of high-frequency stimulation produces two types of structural changes in rat hippocampus. J Neurophysiol 44: 247-258.

Levy WB, Steward O (1983). Temporal contiguity requirements for long-term associative potentiation/depression in the hippocampus. Neurosci 8:791-797.

Liley AW (1956). The quantal components of the mammalian end-plate potential. J Physiol 133:571-587.

Liley AW, North KAK (1953). An electrical investigation of effects of repetitive stimulation on mammalian neuromuscular junction. J Neurophysiol 16:509-527.

Lloyd DPC (1949). Post-tetanic potentiation of response in monosynaptic reflex pathways of the spinal cord. J Gen Physiol 33:147-170.

Lomo T (1966). Frequency potentiation of excitatory activity in the dentate area of the hippocampal formation. Acta Physiol Scand Supple 277:128.

Lomo T (1971). Patterns of activation in a monosynaptic cortical pathway: The perforant path input to the dentate area of the hippocampal formation. Exp Brain Res 12:18-45.

Lomo T (1971). Potentiation of monosynaptic EPSPs in the

perforant path-dentate granule cell synapse. Expt Brain Res 12:46-63.

Lynch G, Baudry M (1984). The biochemistry of memory: A new and specific hypothesis. Science 224:1057-1063.

Lynch GS, Dunwiddie T, Gribkoff V (1977). Heterosynaptic depression: A postsynaptic correlate of long-term potentiation. Nature 266:737-739.

Lynch G, Halpain S, Baudry M (1982). Effects of high-frequency synaptic stimulation on glutamate receptor binding studied with a modified in vitro hippocampal slice preparation. Brain Res 244:101-111.

Lynch G, Larson J, Kelso S, Barrionuevo G, Schottler F (1983). Intracellular injections of EGTA block induction of hippocampal long-term potentiation. Nature 305:719-721.

Lynch MA, Errington ML, Bliss TVP (1985). Long-term potentiation of synaptic transmission in the dentate gyrus: Increased release of [14C] glutamate without increase in receptor binding. Neuroscience Letters 62: 123-130.

Lynch MA, Feasey K, Bliss TVP (1985). Long-term potentiation in the hippocampus: Increased release of preloaded glutamate and aspartate without increase in glutamate receptor binding. Neurosci Letters Suppl. 22 S48.

McNaughton BL, Douglas RM, Goddard GV (1978). Synaptic enhancement in fascia dentate: Cooperativity among coactive afferents. Brain Res 157:277-293.

McNaughton BL, Barnes CA, Rao G, Baldwin J, Rasmussen M (1986). Long-term enhancement of hippocampal synaptic transmission and the acquisition of spatial information. J. Neurosci 6:563-571.

Magleby KL (1973). The effect of repetitive stimulation on facilitation of transmitter release at the frog neuromuscular junction. J. Physiol 234:327-352.

Magleby KL (1973). The effect of tetanic and post-tetanic potentiation on facilitation of transmitter release at the frog neuromuscular junction. J Physiol 234:353-371.

Magleby KL, Zengel J (1975). A dual effect of repetitive stimulation on post-tetanic potentiation of transmitter release at the frog neuromuscular junction. J Physiol 245:163-182.

Magleby KL, Zengel JE (1975). A quantitative description of tetanic potentiation of transmitter release at the frog neuromuscular junction. J Physiol 245:183-208.

Magleby KL, Zengel JE (1976). Augmentation: A process that

acts to increase transmitter release at the frog
neuromuscular junction. J Physiol 257:449-470.

Malinow R, Miller JP (1986). Postsynaptic hyperpolarization
during conditioning reversibly blocks induction of long-
term potentiation. Nature 320:529-530.

Martin AR, Pilar G (1964). Presynaptic and post-synaptic
events during post-tetanic potentiation and facilitation
in the avian ciliary ganglion. J Physiol 175:17-30.

McNaughton BL, Barnes CA (1977). Physiological stimulation
and analysis of dentate granule cell responses to
stimulation of the medial and lateral perforant pathways
in the rat. J Comp Neurol 175:439-454.

Misgeld U, Sarvey JM, Klee MR (1979). Heterosynaptic
postactivation potentiation in hippocampal CA3 neurons:
Long-term changes of the postsynaptic potentials. Exp
Brain Res 37:217-229.

Mody I, Baimbridge KG, Miller JJ (1984). Blockade of
tetanic and calcium induced long-term potentiation in the
hippocampal slice preparation by neuroleptics. Neuropharm
23:625-631.

Morris RGM, Anderson E, Lynch GS, Baudry M (1986).
Selective impairment of learning and blockade of long-
term potentiation by an N-methyl-D-aspartate receptor
antagonist, AP5. Nature 319:774-776.

Nelson RB, Routtenberg A, Hyman C, Pfenninger KH (1985).
A phosphoprotein in (F1) directly related to neural
plasticity in adult rat brain may be identical to a major
growth cone membrane protein (pp46). Neurosci Abstr 11:
269.4.

Oliver MW, Miller JJ (1985). Alterations of inhibitory
processes in the dentate gyrus following kindling-induced
epilepsy. Exp Brain Res 57:443-447.

Peterson DW, Collins JF, Bradford HF (1983). The kindled
amygdala model of epilepsy: Anticonvulsant action of
amino acid antagonists. Brain Res 311:176-180.

Peterson DW, Collins JF, Bradford HF (1984). Anticonvulsant
action of amino acid antagonists against kindled
hippocampal seizures. Brain Res 311:176-180.

Racine R, Gartner JG, Burnham WM (1972). Epileptiform
activity and neural plasticity in limbic structures.
Brain Res 47:262-268.

Racine R, Newberry F, Burnham W (1975). Post-activation
potentiation and the kindling phenomenon. Electroenceph
clin Neurophysiol 39:261-271.

Racine RJ, Milgram NW, Hafner S (1983). Long-term
potentiation phenomena in the rat limbic forebrain.

Brain Res 260:217-231.

Racine RJ, Wilson DA, Gingell R, Sunderland D (1986). Long-term potentiation in the interpositus and vestibular nuclei in the rat. Exp Brain Res (in press).

Racine R, Zaide J (1978). A further investigation into the mechanisms underlying the kindling phenomenon. In Livingston K, Hornykiewacz O (eds) "Limbic Mechanisms." Plenum Press New York 457-493.

Robinson GB (1986). Enhanced long-term potentiation induced in rat dentate gyrus by coactivation of septal and entorhinal inputs: Temporal constraints. Brain Res (in press).

Robinson GB, Racine RJ (1982). Heterosynaptic interactions between septal and entorhinal inputs to the dentate gyrus: Long-term potentiation effects. Brain Res 249:162-166.

Robinson GB, Racine RJ (1986). Interactions between septal and entorhinal inputs to the rat dentate gyrus: Facilitation effects. Brain Res (in press).

Romanes GJ (1885). "Jelly-fish, Starfish and Sea Urchins Being a Research on Primative Nervous Systems." K Paul Trench & Co London pp 1-323.

Routtenberg A, Lovinger DM, Steward O (1985). Selective increases in phosphorylation of a 47-kDa protein (F1) directly related to long-term potentiation. Behav Neural Biol 43:3-11.

Routtenberg A (1985). Phosphoprotein regulation of memory formation: Enhancement and control of synaptic plasticity by protein kinase C and protein F1. Ann NY Acad Sci 444: 203-211.

Routtenberg A, Lovinger D, Cain S, Akers R, Steward O. (1983). Effects of long-term potentiation of perforant path synapses in the intact hippocampus on in vitro phosphorylation of a 47KD protein (F1). Fed Proc 42:755.

Routtenberg A (1985). Protein kinase C activation leading to protein F1 phosphorylation may regulate synaptic plasticity by presynaptic terminal growth. Behav Neural Biol 44:186-200.

Sastry BR (1982). Presynaptic change associated with long-term potentiation in hippocampus. Life Sci 30:2003-2008.

Sastry BR, Goh JW (1984). Long-lasting potentiation in rat hippocampus is not due to an increase in glutamate receptors. Life Sci 34:1497-1501.

Sastry BR, Murali Mohan P, Goh JW (1985). A transient increase in the activity of CA3 neurons induces a long-lasting reduction in the excitability of Schaffer collateral terminals in rat hippocampus. Neurosci

Letters 53:51-56.

Sechenov I (1863)(1965). "Reflexes of the Brain." US edition/The MIT Press Cambridge Mass. pp 1-49.

Skrede KK, Malthe-Sorensson D (1981). Increased resting and evoked release of transmitter following electrical tetanization in hippocampus: A biochemical correlate to long-lasting synaptic potentiation. Brain Res 208:436-441.

Staubli U, Roman F, Lynch G (1985). Selective changes in synaptic responses elicited in a cortical network by behaviorally relevant electrical stimulation. Neurosci Abstracts 11:245.15

Stringer JL, Guyenet PG (1983). Elimination of long-term potentiation in the hippocampus by phencyclidine and ketamine. Brain Res 258:159-164.

Tuff LP, Racine RJ, Adamec R (1983). The effects of kindling on GABA-mediated inhibition in the dentate gyrus of the rat: I. Paired pulse depression. Brain Res 277:79-90.

Tuff LP, Racine RJ, Mishra RK (1983). The effects of kindling on GABA-mediated inhibition in the dentate gyrus of the rat: II. Receptor binding. Brain Res 277:91-98.

Valdes F, Dasheiff RM, Birmingham F, Crutcher KA, McNamara JO (1982). Benzodiazepine receptor increases after repeated seizures: Evidence for localization to dentate granule cells. Proc Acad Sci USA 79:193-197.

Van Harreveld A, Fifkova E (1985). Swelling of dendritic spines in the fascia dentata after stimulation of the perforant path fibers as a mechanism of post-tetanic potentiation. Exp Neurol 49:736-749.

Voronin LL (1983). Long-term potentiation of a monosynaptic reflex. J Neurosci 10:1051-1069.

Wall PD, Johnson AR (1958). Changes associated with post-tetanic potentiation of a monosynaptic reflex. J Neurosci 21:148-158.

Wigstrom H, Gustafsson B (1983). Facilitated induction of hippocampal long-lasting potentiation during blockade of inhibition. Nature 301:603-604.

Wigstrom H, Gustaffson B (1983). Large long-lasting potentiation in the dentate gyrus in vitro during blockade of inhibition. Brain Res 275:153-158.

Wigstrom H, Gustaffson B (1984). A possible correlate of the postsynaptic condition for long-lasting potentiation in the guinea-pig hippocampus in vitro. Neurosci Letters 44:327-332.

Wigstrom H, Gustaffson B (1985). A synaptic potential

following single volleys in the hippocampal CA1 region possibly involved in the induction of long-lasting potentiation. Acta Physio Scand 124:475-478.

Wigstrom H, McNaughton BL, Barnes CA (1982). Long-term synaptic enhancement in hippocampus is not regulated by postsynaptic membrane potential. Brain Res 233:195-199.

Wigstrom H, Swann JW, Andersen P (1979). Calcium dependency of synaptic long-lasting potentiation in the hippocampal slice. Acta Physiol Scand 105:126-128.

Wilson DA, Racine RJ (1983). The postnatal development of post-activation potentiation in the rat neocortex. Dev Brain Res 7:271-276.

Yamamoto C, Chujo T (1978). Long-term potentiation in thin hippocampal sections studied by intracellular and extracellular recordings. Exp Neurol 58:242-250.

Neuroplasticity, Learning, and Memory, pages 199–229
© **1987 Alan R. Liss, Inc.**

NEURAL CORRELATES OF CONDITIONING ASSESSED BY EXTRACELLULAR
UNIT RECORDING: IMPLICATIONS FOR NEUROPLASTICITY

Earl Thomas and Elna Yadin

Department of Psychology,
Bryn Mawr College
Bryn Mawr, PA 19010

The unique contribution of extracellular recording to
the understanding of brain plasticity in learning is that
it provides for an on-line record of the basic unit of
neuronal information, the action potential of a cell,
throughout the course of learning. Judiciously used,
extracellular recording can be a powerful tool for the
analysis of the brain mechanisms of learning. It is a tool
the use of which is not restricted to any single approach
to the brain mechanisms of learning, but which may be
employed for dealing with a variety of important issues
related to brain plasticity and learning.

The purpose of this paper is to review some of the
approaches to learning based upon the extracellular
recording technique and to present some of the data
obtained in our laboratory that bear upon brain mechanisms
of learning. While the unit-recording technique has been
successfully employed in instrumental learning and cognitive
processing, this paper will deal primarily with unit-
correlates of Pavlovian conditioning. Using the
extracellular recording procedure, plasticity in Pavlovian
conditioning is seen as changes in the rate or pattern of
unit activity as the result of a contingent relationship
between a conditioned stimulus (CS) and an unconditioned
stimulus (US). Many experiments correlate such changes in
unit activity with a particular overt conditioned response
(CR); other studies have not measured overt conditioned
responses, but rather have concentrated on unit activity as
an index of the conditioned state of the animal (such as
conditioned fear).

EARLY STUDIES

Early studies on unit-recording did not bode particularly well for the use of the procedure for examining the plastic properties of the brain that might mediate learning. Indeed, the very first such study, by Jasper, Ricci and Doane (1960), pointed to a complexity of unit responding in conditioning that seemed to preclude any simple relationship of unit responding to conditioning. Jasper et al. attempted to correlate unit activity in the cortex of Rhesus and Cynomolgous monkeys with acquisition of a discriminated avoidance response to a flashing light CS. Sampling unit activity in the frontal, motor, sensory and parietal cortex, they found a number of differences in the pattern of firing in the various cortical regions. The general finding, however, was that, in all of these regions, some cells increased their firing rates to the CS, some decreased their rates and a great many cells were unresponsive. Moreover, the unit responses were inconsistently related either to the significance of the CS (whether it was reinforced or unreinforced) or to the occurrence of the CR.

A second example of the complexities seen in early studies is Olds' attempt to subject single units in the hippocampus to operant conditioning (e.g., Olds, 1965). While the activity of many units throughout the brain could be modified by reinforcement, either food or rewarding brain stimulation, there was no consistent relation to the known function of the particular structure or to its role in operant conditioning. In addition, the cause-effect relationship between changes in unit responding to operant reinforcement and overt behavioral changes was never fully established. Thus, in most brain regions changes in unit responses appeared to result from sensory feedback from the animal's postural adjustments or orientation. In the hippocampus, where the unit responses seemed independent of response-produced feedback, the evidence suggested that the changes in unit activity were not sensitive to the instrumental contingencies, but rather to the simple Pavlovian conditioning components which accompany instrumental learning.

In spite of the complexities raised by these early studies, the pursuit of unit-activity correlates of conditioning began to pay off as a number of specific

paradigms were designed to highlight particular brain
processes correlated with the learning process. Some of
the approaches attempted to use the ability of extracellular
recording to monitor continuously the course of conditioning
as a way to trace information flow through various regions
of the brain as the conditioned response developed. Other
approaches attempted to use the recording procedure as a
way to solve the puzzle of the engram, the locus of the
memory trace. Still other approaches have used the
procedure to determine the role of specific structures in
adaptive behavior related to the conditioning process.

CONDITIONING, INFORMATION PROCESSING AND THE ENGRAM

A perplexing number of areas in the brain show unit
activity changes associated with Pavlovian conditioning.
A representative, but far from exhaustive, sample of such
structures would include the following: 1) sensory systems,
cortical and subcortical (Birt and Olds, 1982; Diamond and
Weinberger, 1986; Disterhoft, Shipley and Kraus, 1976;
Disterhoft and Stuart, 1982; Weinberger, 1982);
2) sensorimotor cortex (Woody and Engel, 1972); 3) limbic
system structures including hippocampus (Berger and Thompson,
1978a; Olds et al., 1972; Segal, 1973; Segal, Disterhoft
and Olds, 1972; Thompson et al., 1980); dentate gyrus
(Segal et al., 1972; Weisz et al., 1982); septum (Berger
and Thompson, 1978b; Segal, 1973; Thomas and Yadin, 1980);
cingulate gyrus and related anteroventral nucleus of the
thalamus (Gabriel et al., 1982) and the amygdala
(Applegate et al., 1982); 4) brainstem, including
hypothalamus (Kopytova, 1981); reticular formation (Vertes
and Miller, 1976); locus coeruleus (Rasmussen and Jacobs,
1986).

The sheer variety of structures showing conditioned
changes implies complex parallel processing of information
in the brain during the course of conditioning. The
question arises as to whether there is any way to establish
a priority among these structures with regard to fundamental
involvement in the conditioning process. Presumably,
establishing a priority among the structures would provide
a clue as to which neurons were actually involved in the
storage of the memory trace, the so-called engram. There
have been a variety of approaches to the question of
priority and the engram, and it will pay to examine some of

these and to assess the degree to which such approaches have been, or could be, successful.

An ingenious approach to the priority question was made by Olds and his colleagues using a latency analysis (Olds et al., 1972; Segal, 1973). Olds et al., argued that neurons ought to exist whose function it is to make the initial determination that a particular stimulus presented to the nervous system is a valid conditioned stimulus. These decision-making neurons would then shunt the information in the appropriate direction to effect a conditioned response. Such neurons would have to meet two conditions: First, they would have to be specifically activated by a CS that had been previously associated with US and not by stimuli that had not been associated with the US. Secondly, the latency of these neurons in response to the CS should be sufficiently short so that it would be implausible that these neurons could have been influenced by cells in other structures. The criterion adopted by Olds et al. was that the latency of these cells should be of the same order as the latencies observed in cells in the sensory pathways related to the particular CS.

The initial experiment of Olds et al. identified neurons in a number of structures which appeared to meet these criteria. The largest number of cells meeting the criteria (3 cells or more) were found in the ventral tegmentum, the pontine reticular formation, the posterior thalamus, and field CA3 of the hippocampus.

While there is a certain plausibility to the argument of Olds et al., Gabriel (1976) has provided a trenchant critique of the concept that short-latency conditioned unit responses rule out influences of remote structures upon these cells and therefore identify "engrams" within the brain. According to Gabriel's analysis, remote influence could derive from a tonic response bias placed upon these cells, by distant structures, such as the cortex. The presumption is that the remote cells might become tonically activated as a result of conditioning to the experimental context. These cells would then prime other cells, via centrifugal pathways, to respond to the appropriate CSs with very short latencies. That such tonic contextual conditioning exists and has profound effects upon conditioning to specific CSs is now well established (e.g., Balsam and Tomie, 1985). Moreover, we have recently obtained evidence of contextual conditioning of cells in the septal region that gives added support to Gabriel's contention (Yadin and Thomas, 1981). The details of our own results will be given in a later section.

Although it seems likely that the latency analysis provided by Olds et al. does not specify the location of engrams, an analysis of relative latencies can give substantial information about input-output relationships among structures during the course of conditioning. Such an analysis was performed on a variety of limbic system structures by Segal (1973).

Conditioned unit activity was found in several of the limbic regions studied, including fields CA3 and CA1 of the ventral hippocampus, the dentate gyrus, the entorhindal area, the cingulate gyrus, and the lateral and medial septum. When examined for several parameters related to conditioning, including latency to respond, rate of acquisition and extinction, persistence of responding beyond the duration of the CS, and amount of pseudoconditioning to unpaired presentations of the CS and US, each region appeared to have a distinctive pattern of responding. The details of all of these patterns need not concern us here (the interested reader is referred to the original publications), but one of the comparisons, between field CA3 of the hippocampus and the dentate gyrus, is instructive.

The dentate gyrus is a major source of input to CA3 and indeed both conditioning and extinction occurred earlier in the dentate gyrus than in the hippocampus. However, while the dentate cells seem to acquire earlier over the course of learning, they do not appear to pass their information on to the hippocampus, since when the hippocampal cells do show learning they respond with considerably shorter latencies than do cells in the dentate gyrus. Since one structure shows earlier conditioning over trials and the other shows shorter latency responses within trials, it seems unlikely that either structure provides input to the other. In fact, the distinctive pattern of responding found in each of these highly interrelated limbic areas makes it unlikely that the conditioned activity can be understood in terms of simple input-output relations between the structures. Instead, it would appear that each structure has something independent to contribute to the

neural architecture of the conditioned response. These
experiments pointedly illustrate that even closely related
structures may contribute to very different aspects of
conditioning. We will return in a later section to a
further discussion of how these two areas may relate to
the conditioned response.

A second approach to establishing priority among
structures has employed the conditioned nictitating membrane
response (NMR) in the rabbit as a model system. Utilizing
this system, Thompson and his group initially localized the
site of the "engram" for the conditioned NM response in the
hippocampus (Berger and Thompson, 1978a; Thompson et al.,
1980). Hippocampal pyramidal cells showed changes in firing
during acquisition of NMR conditioning in the rabbit. The
changes in unit activity were demonstrated to be associative,
to occur earlier in the course of conditioning than the
overt NMR and, within a trial, to precede the occurrence of
the overt NMR. Moreover, time histograms of unit firing
formed an extremely accurate temporal model of the overt
conditioned NMR. The close correspondence between the
temporal pattern of the unit activity and the topography
of the conditioned response suggested that these hippocampal
cells were very specific in function, presumably mediating
the NMR response which the activity of the cells modeled
and not any of the myriad other conditioned responses which
were not measured, but which assuredly were occurring at
the same time. The idea that the hippocampal cells which
so precisely modeled the CR might represent the engram for
this particular CR was appealing but was inconsistent with
considerable data which showed that hippocampal ablation
had no deleterious effect upon conditioning of the NMR
(Solomon and Moore, 1975). It appears, however, an intact
hippocampus is necessary for certain higher order
conditioning phenomena such as trace conditioning (Weisz
et al., 1980), latent inhibition (Solomon and Moore, 1975)
and blocking (Solomon, 1977).

More recently, the cerebellum has been proposed as the
site of the engram for the conditioned NMR (McCormick and
Thompson, 1983; Thompson et al., 1983). Increased unit
activity forming a temporal model of the CR was found in
the cortex and deep nuclei of the cerebellum and associated
circuitry, including pontine nuclei, the red nucleus,
inferior olive and the motor cortex (Thompson et al.,
1984a, 1984b). Moreover, lesions of the dentate-

interpositus complex permanently abolished the conditioned
NMR response (McCormick and Thompson, 1983) as well as the
conditioned leg flexion response (Donegan, Lowry and
Thompson, 1983) without affecting the unconditioned
response.

An interesting feature of these data is that while
discrete phasic somatomotor responses are abolished by
dentate-interpositus lesions, gross motor activity and
autonomic CRs are not affected. A similar circuit analysis
of an autonomic CR has not been undertaken in the mammal,
but Cohen (1974, 1984) using a combination of recording and
lesioning procedures, has defined such a circuit in the
pigeon. The model used by Cohen was cardiac conditioning
to a visual CS and an electric-shock US. Although it is
dangerous to compare across species and somewhat different
paradigms, the circuit described by Cohen (1984) would
appear to have minimal overlap with the circuit for the
conditioned NMR. Recently Pascoe and Kapp (1985), using
rabbits as subjects, have found units in the central nucleus
of the amygdala which appear to mediate the cardiac
conditioned response.

Another approach to determining what cells may underlie
engrams for Pavlovian conditioning is to combine the
recording procedure with microstimulation techniques in
order to assess changes in excitability of the neurons which
respond to CSs. Such an approach was adopted by Woody
(1982) using a conditioned eyeblink and nose-twitch
preparation in the cat. Using these procedures, Woody has
located at least a portion of the engram for eyeblink and
nose-twitch conditioning in the pericruciate sensorimotor
cortex, on the motor neurons themselves. The argument for
the localization of the engram here is as follows: 1) Cells
which can be identified as motor cells, projecting to target
muscles which were conditioned, show increased firing rates
to CSs (Woody, Vassilevsky, and Engel, 1970); 2) When small
groups of motor cells were stimulated extracellularly
(Woody and Engel, 1972) or when single motor cells were
stimulated by intracellular injection of current (Brons
and Woody, 1980; Woody and Black-Cleworth, 1973), the
proportion of cells which upon stimulation activated the
muscle group that was conditioned increased after
conditioning; 3) The excitability of these cells as
assessed by their responsiveness to intracellular current
injection was increased for a relatively long time after

conditioning (Brons and Woody, 1980).

Whether or not excitability changes actually localize engrams is somewhat problematic. In general, such excitability changes are tested either in the presence of the CSs or in the environment where conditioning has occurred and therefore are tapping retrieval mechanisms rather than storage mechanisms. That is, these excitability changes may well reflect the kinds of remotely generated biasing processes due to contextual conditiong as outlined by Gabriel (1976) and discussed in a prior section. Whether or not these excitability changes represent engrams that the animal carries around with it even when not in the conditioning environment remains to be determined.

In general, a number of very important issues are raised by the "model systems" engram hunting approach. Are NMR conditioning, eyeblink, and cardiac conditioning represented by independent reflex arcs that can be traced in a serial fashion from sensory input to the ultimate motor output? Certainly, for those studying the details of conditioning from a behavioral standpoint, the process is considerably more complicated. There is evidence that conditioning involves representations in the brain of many aspects of the reinforcer including its sensory properties and its affective properties (Konorski, 1967; see also Mackintosh, 1984, for a review of representational processes). The richness of response forms seen in conditioning suggests a mechanism for response production with properties considerably more complex than that implied by the "model systems" approaches. Thus CRs need not resemble the UR upon which they are based and often are much more complex than the corresponding UR (see Rescorla and Holland, 1982, for an excellent review of the many variables that determine response form in Pavlovian conditioning).

Thus, the attempts to understand the substrates of conditioning from the model systems approach raises an interesting dilemma. If modern behavior theory is correct and conditioning has a complicated structure, involving elaborate representational processes and complicated performance rules for converting the representations into behavior, then the tracing of simple, linear pathways and circuits is not likely to yield a great deal of information on engrams for conditioning. On the other hand, if the

model systems approach is correct and one can understand
conditioning in terms of fairly straightforward S-R circuits,
then what appear to behavior theorists as representations,
expectancies, contingency learning and other elaborations
of conditioning are somewhat illusory, perhaps due to the
sheer number of S-R circuits that might mediate conditioning
to various properties of the US. We believe here, however,
that the weight of evidence favors the behavior theorists.
We would argue that what is being mapped in most cases are
not engrams but motor plans for non-reflexively initiated
behavior, i.e., performance rules for conditioning. Under
this assumption it is not surprising that some unit
responding closely models CRs but not URs, nor is it
surprising that the system would have extensive involvement
of the pyramidal and extrapyramidal motor systems.

In sum, the very nature of conditioning would suggest
that the crucial element in the much talked about S-R
pathway is the hyphen, and that the hyphen is very complex
indeed, involving many systems for stimulus representation
and performance rules. In order to understand the nature
of the contribution of the various regions involved in
conditioning, it is necessary to look at conditioned unit
responding in the context of what is generally known about
the behavioral function of the given structure, relating
conditioned unit activity to data obtained by other
techniques such as lesioning, stimulation and pharmacological
techniques. Slowly, but surely these functions are being
unraveled and we are gaining a fuller understanding of the
role of specific limbic regions in conditioning.

Our own interest in unit correlates of conditioning has
been in the understanding of some of the performance rules
in conditioning and the role that brain structures might
play in such performance rules. In particular we have been
interested in the central role of the septal region of the
brain in mediating both excitatory, and especially inhibitory
components of Pavlovian conditioning.

SEPTUM: A POSSIBLE INTERFACE BETWEEN THOUGHT AND ACTION

One of us has argued elsewhere (Thomas, 1986) that the
septal region is in a highly strategic position to mediate
affective components of the conditioned response and to
translate the cognitive components of conditioning into

action. It is clear from the studies described above that the CA fields of the hippocampus participate in the conditioning process at a very early and intimate level. These data are consistent with the notion that the hippocampus is largely concerned with the cognitive components of conditioning. The lateral septum is an important recipient of efferents from the CA fields of the hippocampus and appears to be the only means of communication between the CA fields and the diencephalon and the rest of the brainstem (Swanson and Cowan, 1979). Therefore, the hippocampal-septal connection seems to be critical for the expression of the emotional components of conditioning.

Several kinds of evidence from our laboratory have suggested that the particular role of the lateral septum in conditioning is the inhibition of aversive emotional states such as fear or anxiety. Such a function of the septum, we believe, is important in providing goal direction for aversively motivated behavior which is reinforced by fear- or anxiety-relief. Support for a fear-relief role for the septum comes from a confluence of evidence based upon electrical stimulation and lesioning experiments. This evidence has been reviewed extensively in another publication (Thomas, 1986) and therefore will not be presented here. Our work on septal unit correlates of Pavlovian conditioning has supported such a role for the lateral septum and suggests that the modulation of affect by the septal region is an important element in the architecture of the conditioned response. Our data are based on both multiple- and single-unit recording from the lateral and medial septum. We will first describe the general methodology of our recording and conditioning experiments, and then outline some of the implications of our data for concepts of neuronal plasticity in conditioning.

Recording Procedure

The electrodes for multiple unit recording were 75 micron wire, insulated to the tip. A single twisted pair was implanted into the septal region and recording was monopolar between the recording electrode and an indifferent electrode wrapped around a stainless steel screw mounted on the surface of the skull. For single unit recording, either 25 or 50 micron wire were twisted and formed into bundles of eight. The end of the bundle was cut on a bias so that there was a displacement of the tips in a dorsal ventral direction of about 1/2 mm. This arrangement emulates a chronically mounted microdrive. In our experience there has been little difference between the 25 and 50 micron wire in ability to discriminate single units. We have found, however, that bipolar, differential recording between two electrodes within the active region greatly facilitates discrimination of single units, as opposed to the monopolar procedure we employed for multiple unit recording.

Electrode wires were connected to JFET operational amplifiers in a voltage follower configuration and then to a differential preamplifier/amplifier combination. Single unit activity was sampled by connecting successive pairs of electrodes to the amplifier. The output of the amplifier was fed to a window discriminator for isolation of single-unit spikes and to a computer for data reduction and analysis and construction of peristimulus time histograms of the unit activity. The raw activity is also recorded on tape for further off-line analysis.

For our purposes the criterion for a single unit was that the unit appear under only one electrode tip and appear as a single spike discriminable from background activity. Using this criterion approximately 70% of the animals had at least one electrode yield a single unit. In many cases different clearly discriminable units could be isolated under two or three electrodes. In these cases each unit was sampled for response to the CS in separate conditioning sessions after the animal's conditioning was asymptotic.

Conditioning Procedure

In all cases the CSs were a light and a tone. For aversive conditioning the US was a 1 ma, 100 pulse per second square wave grid shock with a pulse duration of 1 ms. For appetitive conditioning the US was either condensed milk or chocolate milk delivered by a dipper. The CS-US interval was 10 sec. with the CS overlapping and coterminating with the US. For aversive conditioning the US duration was 1 sec.; for appetitive conditioning the US duration was 3 sec. The intertrial interval averaged approximately 90 sec.

There were 40 trials per session, each session lasting an hour. Half of the trials were CS+ trials with the CS paired with the US. The other half of the trials were CS- trials with the CS presented, but not followed by the US. The order of the trials was quasi-random and the stimuli serving as CS+ and CS- were counterbalanced. In some instances, we utilized a truly random control procedure for conditioning (Rescorla, 1967) as a baseline against which to assess both excitatory and inhibitory conditioning. In this case animals received the tone and light CSs in the same sequence as did the conditioning group but received the USs randomly with respect to the CSs.

Some Principles of Neuronal Plasticity in the Septum as Revealed by Extracellular Recording

1. Unit activity can reflect both excitatory and inhibitory mechanisms in conditioning.

One of the things that Pavlov (1927) emphasized about conditioning was that inhibition and excitation shared equal importance in the structure of the conditioned response. In contemporary terms, conditioned excitation occurs when there is a positive correlation between the presentation of the CS and a US, i.e., when the probability of occurrence of a US is greater in the presence of a CS than in its absence. Conditioned inhibition occurs when there is a negative correlation between the presentation of a CS and a US, i.e., when the probability of occurrence of a US is smaller in the presence of a CS than in its absence (cf. Rescorla, 1967). Conditioned inhibition appears to be an independent process in its own right from conditioned excitation. Conditioned inhibition also appears to be an active process involving the activation of structures which are inhibitory to the expression of the conditioned excitatory response (Konorski, 1967; Thomas, 1972). Finally, conditioned inhibition is hedonically and motivationally the opposite of conditioned excitation. Thus, for instance, if the US is aversive and a CS paired with the US produces conditioned fear, then a CS unpaired with the US acquires the property of inhibiting fear and providing for conditioned relief from fear (e.g., Rescorla, 1969).

All of these properties of both conditioned excitation

and inhibition are reflected in extracellular unit recording. That cells will fire in the presence of a conditioned inhibitor of fear was found independently by de Toledo-Morrell, Hoeppner, and Morrell (1979) and in our laboratory (Thomas and Yadin, 1980; Yadin and Thomas, 1981). de Toledo et al. found specific cells in the parastriate cortex in cats which were activated by a conditioned inhibitor of fear. In the initial studies in our laboratory, using multiple unit activity, we found that cells in the lateral septal region increased their firing rates in the presence of a conditioned inhibitor of fear. Multiple-unit activity was suppressed in the presence of a conditioned excitor of fear. Increased unit activity was also seen at the termination of a shock US and at the termination of a tail-pinch (Thomas and Yadin, 1980). Evidence from the learning literature indicates that the termination of an aversive stimulus is associated with the relief of fear (e.g., Denny, 1971; Konorski, 1972). Thus, in these experiments, we had a variety of stimuli known to be associated with fear-relief, the presentation of a conditioned inhibitor and the termination of two kinds of aversive stimulus, footshock and a tail-pinch. Increased multiple-unit activity was seen in the lateral septum in all these cases. This effect was quite specific and was not seen in other brain regions nor in the septum to a CS- when the US was appetitive rather than aversive (Thomas and Yadin, 1980). Moreover, the effect was consistent with considerable evidence based upon lesioning and electrical stimulation data (Thomas, 1986) that the inhibition of aversive states such as fear or anxiety is an important function of the lateral septum.

Fig. 1 depicts the opposite multiple unit responding to CS+ and CS- over several days of conditioning compared to a truly random control group. The ordinate for this graph is a measure we refer to as the unit activity ratio. This ratio is expressed as (B-A)/(B+A) where B is the total number of spikes during the CS-US interval and A is the number of spikes during an equivalent pre-CS period. With this measure, values may range from -1.00 (representing complete suppression) to +1.00 (maximum facilitation) with 0 representing no change. One nice feature of the ratio is that it symmetrically depicts excitation and inhibition around a zero baseline. As may be seen in the figure, there is no conditioning in the control group, an acquired increase in multiple-unit activity in the presence of CS-,

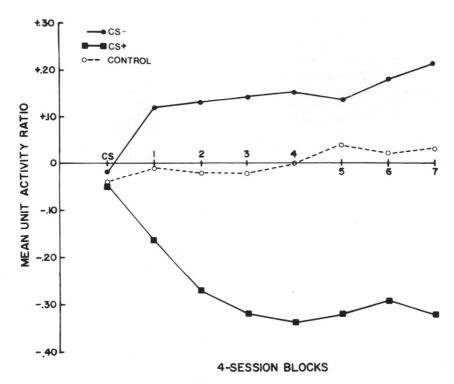

Figure 1. Mean unit activity ratio for the CS+ and CS-
over four-session blocks. The point marked "CS" refers to
the mean unit activity ratio to the conditioned stimuli
alone during the session prior to conditioning. From Yadin
and Thomas (1981).

and an acquired suppression of multiple-unit activity in
the presence of CS+.

Multiple unit recording yields a kind of average of
the activity of a particular structure and therefore it
would be useful to determine if the activity of single units
reflects this average activity. When we examined single-
unit activity we found that single cells did not always
show the entire spectrum of responses seen in the multiple-
unit activity, but individual cells appeared to contribute
components of what is observed with multiple-unit recording.
For instance, in the lateral septum, we have found some
single cells which do seem to represent the spectrum of

multiple unit activity, i.e., which fire in the presence of
a conditioned inhibitor of fear and which are inhibited in
the presence of a conditioned excitor of fear. An example
of such a cell may be seen in Fig. 2. This figure depicts
a peristimulus time histogram of unit responding summed for
20 trials for each of CS+ and CS-. It can be seen that
this cell is suppressed in the presence of CS+ and
increases its rate in the presence of CS-. Note also, an
appreciable increase in unit responding post-US.

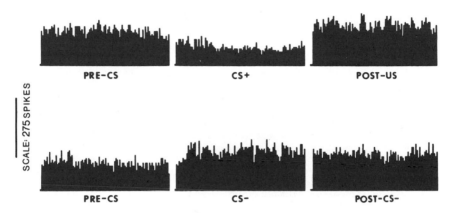

Figure 2. Peristimulus time histograms for unit responding
in a conditioning session. The histograms are summed over
20 trials. Each of the Pre-CS, CS and Post-US intervals
are 10 seconds in duration and are divided into 100 ms time
bins.

We also have seen units which show only one of these
characteristics, i.e., units which fire to a conditioned
inhibitor of fear but which do not respond to a conditioned
excitor of fear, or units which inhibit to a conditioned
excitor of fear but do not respond to a conditioned
inhibitor of fear. Fig. 3 shows an example of a unit which
fires in the presence of CS-, but which is relatively
unaffected by CS+. Similarly, Fig. 4 is an example of
suppression in the presence of CS+ with relatively little
effect of CS-. In general, however, there is great
consistency in the manner in which units in the lateral
septum respond to the CSs. Of the considerable number of

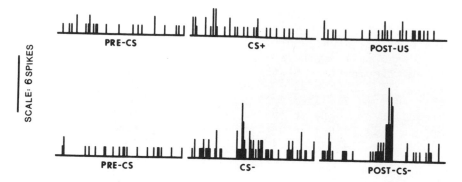

Figure 3. Peristimulus time histograms for a cell in the lateral septum excited by CS-. The parameters are the same as in Fig. 2.

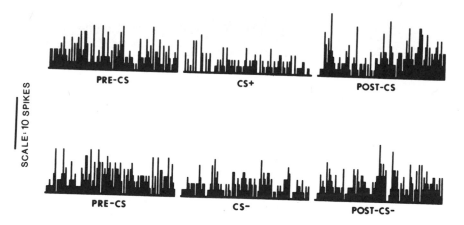

Figure 4. Peristimulus time histogram for a cell in the lateral septum inhibited by CS+. The parameters are the same as in Fig. 2.

units assessed to date, none has shown a response that is inconsistent with the notion that lateral septal activity is enhanced by stimuli which reduce fear and is suppressed by stimuli which signal fear.

The picture in the medial septum is somewhat more complicated, with cells showing a variety of response patterns including 1) "non-plastic cells" which show no response to any stimulus during conditioning, 2) cells which show theta bursting in the presence of a conditioned inhibitor of fear, and 3) cells which respond to conditioned stimuli in a manner directly opposite to those in the lateral septum (i.e., which increase activity in the presence of a conditioned fear stimulus and suppress in the presence of a conditioned inhibitor of fear). An example of a medial-septal cell which shows increased responding to CS+ may be seen in Fig. 5. As can be seen this cell is relatively unreactive to CS-. In a similar manner we have also observed medial septal cells which inhibit responding in the presence of a CS- but which are unreactive to CS+.

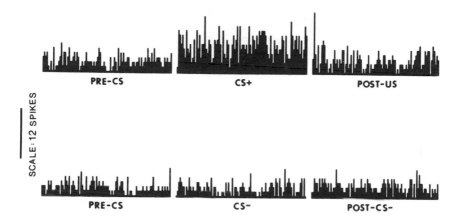

Figure 5. Peristimulus time histogram for a cell in the medial septum excited by CS+. The parameters are the same as in Fig. 2.

Obviously, in the case of the medial septum, the individual units reflect a variety of different functions, some of which are unrelated to learning, and others of which may relate to different aspects of conditioning. Theta driving cells in the medial septum bear a particularly interesting relation to conditioned inhibition. We have noticed that as a CS- becomes established as a conditioned inhibitor of fear a variety of response patterns emerge

de novo. These response patterns include postural
adjustments, changes in body orientation and exploratory
behavior. The emergence of new behavior to CS- is another
example of conditioned inhibition as an active brain process.
These kinds of behavior have been directly linked to
hippocampal theta activity (Vanderwolf et al., 1975). We
have found recently that theta bursting in medial septal
cells is greatly increased in the presence of CS-, precisely
tied to the emergence of CS- specific behavior patterns.
We are presently exploring this phenomenon in greater
detail. Category three cells, which are the most common
cells we have seen in the medial septum, seem to reflect
the hedonic aspects of the CS, but in a manner directly
opposite to that seen in the lateral septum. This last
category of cell has suggested to us that there may be,
at least in part, a reciprocal relationship between the
lateral and medial septum.

     The fact that cells which respond to a conditioned
inhibitor of fear are seen in structures as diverse as the
parastriate cortex and the lateral septum suggests that
cells mediating conditioned inhibition probably occur at
several levels of processing. It is tempting to speculate
that cells in the visual association area may be involved
in making the decision that there is indeed a negative
contingency between the CS and the US, whereas cells in the
septal region may be involved considerably later along the
line, and by mediating the motivational consequences of the
negative contingency.

2.   Unit activity recorded in a given structure during
conditioning should relate to known functions of that
structure and should be consistent with well established
behavioral principles.

     Given the large number of structures, cited above,
whose cells show plasticity in conditioning, it should be
obvious that the role of any given structure in conditioning
cannot be understood on the basis of unit recording alone.
Rather the data from the recording experiments must be
related to what is known about the general functioning of
the structure based upon information derived from a variety
of techniques. This is essentially the kind of analysis we
have applied to the septum. Here, the kinds of plastic
changes seen during conditioning seem consistent with the
role of the septum as a general inhibitor of behavior,

especially aversively motivated behavior. To the extent that the lateral septum is involved in the inhibition of aversion, external stimuli that have such a property should activate cells in the lateral septum. There is considerable evidence from the behavioral literature to suggest that a CS- in an aversive conditioning situation actively acquires the ability to inhibit fear. If so, then the finding that such a CS also activates cells in the lateral septum fits well onto this proposed function of the lateral septum. Moreover, the observation that a conditioned excitor of fear suppresses firing of cells in the lateral septum fits well with the behavioral principle that conditioned inhibitors are hedonically the opposite of conditioned excitors.

Our findings with appetitive Pavlovian conditioning are also consistent with the behavioral concept that there is a hedonic equivalence between appetitive excitatory CSs and aversive inhibitory CSs (Dickinson and Pearce, 1976; Dickinson and Dearing, 1979). Yadin and Thomas (1981) have shown that with an appetitive US, the effects of CSs on lateral septal firing are the mirror image of what is seen for conditioning with an aversive US. That is, in appetitive conditioning, cells in the lateral septum increase their firing to CS+ and are inhibited by CS-. Finally, our recent data (Thomas and Yadin, 1984, 1986) suggest at least a partial reciprocal relationship between the medial and lateral septum. In the medial septum there is nearly an inverse relationship between conditioned unit activity and the hedonic properties of the US to that seen in the lateral septum. Lest the reader be somewhat confused (as indeed at times we are) by double, and sometimes triple negatives, the following table provides a summary of our findings to date.

3. Some cells which show plasticity in conditioning reflect hedonic processes in conditioning; others may reflect associative processes.

In 1972 Segal, Disterhoft and Olds reported an important experiment on unit correlates of conditioning in the hippocampal formation that anticipated our own in the septal region. They recorded from units in fields CA3 and CA1 in the hippocampus and from granule cells in the dentate gyrus. On alternate days of conditioning they used either food or shock as the US. Different response patterns emerged from cells in the CA fields and the dentate gyrus. In the

TABLE 1. Direction of conditioned unit changes in the
lateral and medial septum with appetitive and aversive USs.

	AVERSIVE US		APPETITIVE US	
	CS+	CS−	CS+	CS−
LATERAL SEPTUM	↓	↑	↑	↓
MEDIAL SEPTUM	↑*	↓*	↓	↑

The asterisked arrows for the medial septum indicate a
preponderant response where other responses are seen as
well, as discussed in the text.

dentate gyrus the cells were differentially responsive to
the hedonic properties of the US. These cells increased
their rate of firing in the presence of the CS for food
and decreased their rate in the presence of the CS for
shock. In this respect these cells are very much like the
cells we have observed in the lateral septum. Cells in the
hippocampus did not differentiate between the aversive and
appetitive USs but responded in a like manner, increasing
their rate, to both. Adequate controls for conditioning
suggested that unit responses in both regions were true
conditioned responses.

The pattern of data obtained by Segal et al. suggests
that unit activity in these two highly related structures
subserve quite different functions in the conditioning
process. It is of considerable importance to determine
specifically what the different functions might be.
Lacking further data, however, one might speculate. It
is not unreasonable, and consistent with much of the data
cited earlier, that the hippocampal unit activity may

reflect basic associative functions that are in common with all CSs, perhaps even representing some global contingency-detecting mechanism. The dentate gyrus on the other hand, much like the septal region, reflects the hedonic content of the conditioned stimuli. The mechanism by which one function, the "cognitive", gets transformed into the other, the "hedonic", remains unresolved. Also awaiting further clarification is the manner in which the dentate gyrus and other limbic structures are organized to mediate the hedonic components of conditioning.

4. Extracellular recording can reflect both tonic and phasic properties of conditioning.

Konorski (1967) distinguished between two types of CR, which he termed preparatory and consummatory. In general, consummatory CRs are reflexive and phasic in nature and typically a close copy of the UR. Preparatory CRs are generally tonic and may consist of general motor arousal and autonomic discharge. The best examples of phasic forms of conditioning are seen where the responses that are measured during conditioning are discrete skeletal reflexes such as leg flexion or eyelid closure. The chief characteristics of the conditioned response with these kinds of reflex are that they are rapid and relatively short lasting. With these kinds of response close temporal contiguity between the CS and the US seems to be a prerequisite. The optimal CS-US interval (the time between the onset of the CS and the US) appears to be about 0.5 sec or less (e.g., Smith, 1968; Smith, Coleman and Gormezano, 1969; see also Gormezano, 1983), and the strength of conditioning falls off quite rapidly as the CS-US interval is varied from the optimal.

The best examples of tonic forms of conditioning are emotional responses, especially the CER. Tonic conditioned responses can extend over several seconds and even minutes. The CER, for example, shows substantial conditioning with CSs as long as 3 min (e.g., Kamin, 1965). Not only do these kinds of responses condition well with long duration CSs but the CRs themselves are tonic in that they are manifest through the entire duration of the CS and can even be shown to be chronically manifest to the contextual cues of the conditioning environment throughout the entire conditioning session (Balsam, 1984; Rescorla, Durlach and Grau, 1985).

Most investigators have chosen phasic CRs to derive their models of conditioning based upon unit recording (e.g., Olds et al., 1972; Segal, 1973; Thompson et al., 1983; Woody, 1986). The rationale seems to be that, since for phasic CRs temporal contiguity is extremely important, such a CR provides the best model for the associative process. Woody (1986) has recently suggested that tracing the circuitry of the CR requires very short duration CSs and short latency CRs otherwise it cannot be determined which portion of the CS was actually effective in eliciting the CR. The problem with this approach is that, for any US, a wide variety of CRs may be elicited, some of which have tonic properties and some of which have phasic properties. We still do not know whether or not all of the CRs that might be elicited by the CS are the result of a single associative engram under which there are a number of response production rules or whether there are multiple, independently laid down engrams.

While numerous studies have shown good correlations of unit responding to rapid phasic responses it is also clear that unit recording can reflect the tonic aspects of conditioning that are particularly characteristic of emotional responses. A perusal of the peristimulus time histograms for conditioning illustrates the tonic properties of conditioned unit responding in the septal region. For instance, in Fig. 5 it can be seen that the facilitatory effect of CS+ upon medial septal units is relatively constant throughout duration of the 10 sec. CS. This reflects very well the kinds of processes seen in the conditioned emotional response. This tonic effect can also be seen in the lateral septum both for the suppressive effect of CS+ and for the facilitatory effect of CS- (Figs. 2, 3 and 4). This tonic effect is most characteristic of the units that we have conditioned and is seen both early and late in conditioning even after as many as 20 sessions.

Perhaps a more dramatic example of tonic conditioning of unit responding can be seen in changes in baseline unit activity as a result of conditioning to the contextual cues of the conditioning environment. Certainly the most powerful current model of Pavlovian conditioning is the Rescorla-Wagner (1972) model. The model asserts that there is a competition among CSs for association with a US. Among the stimuli that may be associated with the US are the environmental cues. To the extent that there are

specific CSs associated with the US these can overshadow
conditioning to background cues and perhaps even prevent
substantial conditioning to contextual cues.

Unit activity in the pre-CS period reflects spontaneous
activity of the cells in the conditioning context and may be
used to reflect conditioning of unit activity to the context.
An example of this may be seen in Fig. 6. This figure
depicts changes in lateral septal multiple-unit responding
in the pre-CS period over sessions. Changes in spontaneous
unit activity were calculated according to the ratio (A-B)/
(A+B), where A represents the mean spontaneous activity
during a 10 sec. pre-CS period of each session and B
represents the mean spontaneous activity in a 10-sec. period
recorded during the initial habituation session.

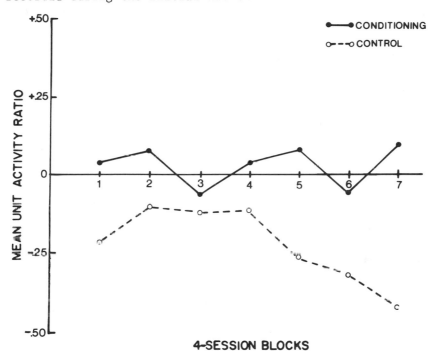

Figure 6. Mean spontaneous activity ratio for cells in the
lateral septum during the pre-CS period over four-session
blocks of conditioning. From Yadin and Thomas (1981).

Positive scores represent baseline increases relative to
preconditioning levels and negative scores reflect baseline
suppression. The solid line represents pre-CS activity for
animals subjected to Pavlovian discrimination and the dashed
line represents pre-CS activity for "truly random" control
animals. As can be seen, animals for which the CSs are
random with regard to the US show considerable depression
of baseline unit activity. When there are CSs which
adequately predict the occurrence of the US, then there is
no baseline change in unit activity.

Two significant conclusions may be derived from this
observation. First, unit activity can reflect conditioning
to contextual cues as well as to specific CSs. Such
conditioning occurs under conditions that are predicted by
current conditioning theories, such as the Rescorla-Wagner
model. Secondly, unit activity correlates of such
conditioning show that, at least in some structures, cells
can alter their responding persistently and tonically and
can therefore reflect long term changes in conditioning that
might be important in theories of memory. Wagner (1979),
for instance, has argued that the conditioning context
might serve as a trigger for priming short term memory.
Cells which are tonically affected by environmental cues
would be well suited to perform such a function. In fact
this kind of memory-triggering mechanism is not very
different from the context-primed biasing mechanism described
by Gabriel (1976) in his critique of the use of response
latencies for determining engrams. Again, cells which can
respond tonically to contextual cues might serve such a
biasing function.

CONCLUSION

The technique of recording unit activity during the
course of conditioning is by its very nature a retrieval-
time technique and as such is much more well suited to
provide information about retrieval processes in conditioning
than about storage processes. Therefore, the procedure is
not well suited per se for the characterization of engrams.
It can be, however, a useful adjunct in combination with
other procedures for localization of the fundamental changes
associated with the learning process. At the outset of the
paper we said that the chief value of the technique is that
it can monitor on a continuous basis the fundamental

means of communication between regions of the nervous system. The procedure's chief value, then, is in determining the paths of communication that distinguish the conditioning process. Ultimately what unit-recording can do very well is provide us with a functional architecture of the conditioned response and allow us to understand the manner in which the many structures involved contribute to the organization of conditioning. In this respect we believe that the unit correlates of conditioning in the septum provide a good example of the participation of at least one region in conditioning.

The precise manner in which unit activity in the septal region appears to reflect the affective aspects of conditioning suggests an important role for this region in mediating the affective components of conditioning. It is particularly reassuring that this model fits so well with the bulk of the evidence in the contemporary learning literature concerning the conditioning of affect. This is particularly true in the ability of the septal region to mirror the symmetry in hedonic states, as, for instance, in mirroring the hedonic equivalence of a conditioned inhibitor of fear and a conditioned appetitive excitor. The reciprocal effects seen in the lateral and medial septum suggest that the interaction of these two regions plays an important role in modulating affective tone in conditioning. The recent work of Applegate et al. (1982) on unit correlates of cardiac conditioning in the rabbit, when compared with our own work, supports a reciprocal relationship between the amygdala and the septum in modulating affective tone. These relations need to be worked out in considerably more detail.

Finally, one of the great problems in understanding the neural basis of conditioning is how the brain transforms the cognitive and other higher order aspects of conditioning into action. It has always seemed to us that the critical link between thought and action is the affective system and that the communicative pathways between "cognitive" structures such as the hippocampus and "emotional" structures such as the septum and amygdala provides such a link. Needless to say this is all much too simple a concept and, undoubtedly, there is no such neat parceling of function anywhere in the nervous system. But it does represent a way of understanding the pathways of communication in the limbic system as they pertain to plastic functions associated with conditioning.

ACKNOWLEDGEMENTS

    A portion of the data reported here was collected
while the authors were visiting scientists and the Weizmann
Institute of Science. We gratefully acknowledge the
generosity of the Institute and of Dr. Menahem Segal.
This research was also supported by a faculty grant from
Bryn Mawr College.

REFERENCES

Applegate CD, Frysinger RC, Kapp BS, Gallagher M (1982).
  Multiple unit activity recorded from the amygdala central
  nucleus during Pavlovian heart rate conditioning in the
  rabbit. Brain Res 238:457.
Balsam PD (1985). The functions of context in learning and
  performance. In Balsam PD, Tomie A (eds): "Context and
  Learning," Hillsdale: Erlbaum, p 1.
Balsam PD, Tomie A (1985) (eds). "Context and Learning,"
  Hillsdale: Erlbaum.
Berger WT, Thompson RF (1978a). Neuronal plasticity in the
  limbic system during classical conditioning of the rabbit
  nictitating membrane response. I. The hippocampus. Brain
  Res 145:323.
Berger WT, Thompson RF (1978b). Neuronal plasticity in the
  limbic system during classical conditioning of the rabbit
  nictitating membrane response. II. Septum and mammillary
  bodies. Brain Res 156:293.
Birt D, Olds ME (1982). Auditory response enhancement
  during differential conditioning in behaving rats. In
  Woody CD (ed): "Conditioning: Representation of Involved
  Neural Structures," New York: Plenum, p 483.
Brons J, Woody CD (1980). Long-term changes in excitability
  of cortical neurons after Pavlovian conditioning and
  extinction. J Neurophysiol 44:605.
Cohen DH (1974). The neural pathways and informational flow
  mediating a conditioned autonomic response. In DiCara LV
  (ed): "Limbic and Autonomic Nervous Systems Research,"
  New York: Plenum, p 223.
Cohen DH (1984). Identification of vertebrate neurons
  modified during learning: Analysis of sensory pathways.
  In Alkon DL, Farley J (eds): "Primary Neural Substrates

of Learning and Behavioral Change," Cambridge: Cambridge University Press, p 129.

Denny MR (1971). Relaxation theory and experiments. In Brush FR (ed): "Aversive Conditioning and Learning," New York: Academic Press, p 235.

Diamond DM, Weinberger NM (1986). Classical conditioning rapidly induces specific changes in frequency receptive fields of single neurons in secondary and ventral ectosylvian auditory cortical fields. Brain Res 372:357.

Dickinson A, Dearing MF (1979). Appetitive-aversive interactions and inhibitory processes. In Dickinson A, Boakes RA (eds): "Mechanisms of Learning and Motivation," Hillsdale: Erlbaum, p 203.

Dickinson A, Pearce JM (1976). Inhibitory interactions between appetitive and aversive stimuli. Psychol Rev 84: 690.

Disterhoft JF, Stuart DK (1976). The trial sequence of changed unit activity in auditory system of alert rat during conditioned response acquisition and extinction. J Neurophysiol 39:266.

Disterhoft JF, Shipley MT, Kraus N (1982). Analyzing the rabbit NM conditioned reflex arc. In Woody CD (ed): "Conditioning: Representation of Involved Neural Structures," New York: Plenum, p 433.

Donegan NH, Lowry RW, Thompson RF (1983). Effects of lesioning cerebellar nuclei on conditioned leg-flexion responses. Neuroscience Abstr 9:331

Gabriel M (1976). Short-latency unit discriminative response: Engram or bias? Physiol Psychol 4:275

Gabriel M, Orona E, Foster K, Lambert RW (1982). Mechanisms and generality of stimulus significance coding in a mammalian model system. In Woody CD (ed): "Conditioning: Representation of Involved Neural Structures," New York: Plenum, p 535.

Gormezano I, Kehoe EJ, Marshall BS (1983). Twenty years of classical conditioning research with the rabbit. Prog Psychobiol Physiol Psychol 10:198.

Grauer E, Thomas E (1982). Conditioned suppression of medial forebrain bundle and septal intracranial self-stimulation in the rat: Evidence for a fear relief mechanism of the septum. J Comp Physiol Psychol 96:61.

Jasper HH, Ricci G, Doane BK (1960). Microelectrode analysis of cortical cell discharge during avoidance conditioning in the monkey. In Jasper HH, Smirnov GD (eds): "The Moscow Colloquium of Electroencephalography of Higher Nervous Activity," Electroencephalography and

clinical neurophysiology 13 suppl. p 137.
Kamin, LJ (1965). Temporal and intensity characteristic of
  the conditioned stimulus. In Prokasy WF (ed): "Classical
  Conditioning: A Symposium," New York: Appleton-Century-
  Crofts, p 118.
Konorski J (1967). "Integrative Activity of the Brain,"
  Chicago: University of Chicago Press.
Konorski J (1972). Some ideas concerning physiological
  mechanisms of so-called internal inhibition. In Boakes
  RA, Halliday MS (eds): "Inhibition and Learning," New York:
  Academic Press, p 341.
Kopytova FV (1981). Hypothalamic unit activity during
  defensive conditioning. Neurosci Behav Physiol 10:452.
Lashley K (1950). In search of the engram. Soc Exp Biol
  symposium 4:454.
Mackintosh NJ (1984). "Conditioning and Associative
  Learning," New York: Oxford University Press.
Olds J (1965). Operant conditioning of single unit
  responses. Excerpta medica international congress 87:372.
Olds J (1969). The central nervous system and reinforcement
  of behavior. Amer Psychol 24:114.
Olds J, Disterhoft JF, Segal M, Kornblith CL, Hirsh R (1972).
  Learning centers of rat brain mapped by measuring latencies
  of conditioned unit responses. J. Neurophysiol 35:202.
Pascoe JP, Kapp BS (1985). Electrophysiological
  characteristics of amygdaloid central nucleus neurons
  during Pavlovian fear conditioning in the rabbit. Behav
  Brain Res 16:117.
Pavlov IP (1927). "Conditioned Reflexes." Oxford: Oxford
  University Press.
Rasmussen K, Jacobs BL (1986). Single unit activity of
  locus coeruleus neurons in the freely moving cat. II.
  Conditioning and pharmacologic studies. Brain Res 371:
  335.
Rescorla RA (1967). Pavlovian conditioning and its proper
  control procedures. Psychol Rev 74:71.
Rescorla RA (1969). Pavlovian conditioned inhibition.
  Psychol Bull 72:77.
Rescorla RA, Durlach PJ, Grau JW (1985). Contextual
  learning in Pavlovian conditioning. In Balsam PD, Tomie
  A (eds): "Context and Learning," Hillsdale: Erlbaum, p 23.
Rescorla RA, Holland PC (1982). Behavioral studies of
  associative learning in animals. Ann Rev Psychol 33:265.
Rescorla RA, Wagner AR (1972). A theory of Pavlovian
  conditioning: Variations in the effectiveness of
  reinforcement and non-reinforcement. In Black AH,

Prokasy WF (eds): "Classical Conditioning II: Current Research and Theory," New York: Appleton-Century-Crofts, p 64.

Segal M (1973). Flow of conditioned responses in limbic telencephalic system of the rat. J Neurophysiol 36:840.

Segal M, Disterhoft JF, Olds J (1972). Hippocampal unit activity during classical aversive and appetitive conditioning. Science 175:792.

Smith MC (1968). CS-US interval and US intensity in classical conditioning of the rabbit's nictitating membrane response. J Comp Physiol Psychol 66:679.

Smith MC, Coleman SR, Gormezano I (1969). Classical conditioning of the rabbit's nictitating membrane response at backward, simultaneous, and forward CS-US intervals. J Comp Physiol Psychol 69:226.

Solomon PR (1977). Role of the hippocampus in blocking and conditioned inhibition of the rabbit's nictitating membrane response. J Comp Physiol Psychol 91:407.

Solomon PR, Moore JW (1975). Latent inhibition and stimulus generalization of the classically conditioned nictitating membrane response in rabbits (Oryctolagus cuniculus) following dorsal hippocampal ablations. J Comp Physiol Psychol 89:1192.

Swanson LW, Cowan WM (1979). The connections of the septal region of the rat. J Comp Neurol 186:621.

de Toledo-Morrell L, Hoeppner TJ, Morrell F (1979). Conditioned inhibition: Selective response of single units. Science 204:528.

Thomas E (1972). Excitatory and inhibitory processes in hypothalamic conditioning. In Boakes RA, Halliday MS (eds): "Inhibition and Learning," New York: Academic Press, p 359.

Thomas E (1986). Forebrain mechanisms in the relief of fear. Submitted.

Thomas E, Evans GJ (1983). Septal inhibition of aversive emotional states. Physiol and Behav 31:673.

Thomas E, Yadin E (1980). Multiple unit activity in the septum during Pavlovian aversive conditioning: Evidence for an inhibitory role of the septum. Exper Neurol 69:50.

Thomas E, Yadin E (1983). Septal unit activity in Pavlovian conditioning: A regional comparison. Neurosci Abstr 9:518.

Thomas E, Yadin E (1986). Single unit response in the lateral and medial septal area to conditioned emotional stimuli. Neurosci Abstr In press.

Thompson RF, McCormick DA, Lavond DG, Clark GC, Kettner RE,

Mauk MK (1983). The engram found? Initial localization of the memory trace for a basic form of associative learning. Prog Psychobiol Physiol Psychol 10:167.

Thompson RF, Barchas JD, Clark GA, Donegan N, Kettner RE, Lavond DG, Madden J IV, Mauk MD, McCormick DA (1984). Neuronal substrates of associative learning in the mammalian brain. In Alkon DL, Farley J (eds): "Primary Neural Substrates of Learning and Behavioral Change," Cambridge: Cambridge University Press, p 71.

Vanderwolf CH, Kramis R, Gillespie LA, Bland BH (1975). Hippocampal rhythmic slow activity and neocortical low-voltage fast activity: Relations to behavior. In Isaacson RL, Pribram, KH (eds): "The Hippocampus: Vol. 2: Neurophysiology and Behavior," New York: Plenum Press, p. 101.

Vertes R, Miller NE (1976). Brain stem neurons that fire selectively to a conditioned stimulus for shock. Brain Res 103:229.

Wagner AR (1979). Habituation and memory. In Dickinson A, Boakes RA (eds): "Mechanisms of Learning and Motivation," Hillsdale: Erlbaum, p 53.

Weinberger NM (1982). Sensory plasticity and learning: The magnocellular medial geniculate nucleus of the auditory system. In Woody CD (ed): "Conditioning: Representation of Involved Neural Structures," New York: Plenum, p 697.

Weisz DJ, Solomon PR, Thompson, RF (1980). The hippocampus appears necessary for trace conditioning. Bull Psychon Soc Abstr 193:244.

Weisz DJ (1982). Activity of dentate gyrus during NM conditioning in rabbit. In Woody CD (ed): "Conditioning: Representation of Involved Neural Structures," New York: Plenum, p 131.

Woody CD (1984). The electrical excitability of nerve cells as an index of learned behavior. In Alkon DL, Farley J (eds): "Primary Neural Substrates of Learning and Behavioral Change," Cambridge: Cambridge University Press, p 101.

Woody CD (1986). Understanding the cellular basis of memory and learning. Ann Rev Psychol 37:433.

Woody CD, Black-Cleworth P (1973). Differences in excitability of cortical neurons as a function of motor projection in conditioned cats. J Neurophysiol 36:1104.

Woody CD, Engel J Jr (1972). Changes in unit activity and thresholds to electrical microstimulation at coronal-pericruciate cortex of cat with classical conditioning of different facial movements. J Neurophysiol 35:230.

Woody CD, Vassilevsky NN, Engel J (1970). Conditioned eye-blink: Unit activity at coronal-precruciate cortex of the cat. J Neurophysiol 33:851.

Yadin E, Thomas E (1981). Septal correlates of conditioned inhibition and excitation in rats. J Comp Physiol Psychol 95:331

Neuroplasticity, Learning, and Memory, pages 231–263

THE NEUROANATOMY OF LEARNING AND MEMORY IN THE RAT

Robert Thompson and Jen Yu

State Developmental Research Institutes, Costa
Mesa, California 92626 and University of California Irvine Medical Center, Orange, California
92668

INTRODUCTION

Through the eyes of a neuroanatomist, the brain lit-
erally consists of thousands of distinct cortical areas,
subcortical nuclei and fiber pathways. Given such a complex organ, it is only natural that one of the goals of
the neurosciences has been to discover the functions of
these different parts of the brain. Since the turn of the
century, enormous strides have been made along the lines
of cerebral localization, ranging from the parcellation of
the cerebral cortex into visual, auditory, somatosensory,
motor and speech areas to the fractionation of subcortical
formations into mechanisms concerned with hunger and
thirst, sex, fear, pain, pleasure, arousal, attention,
posture and the like.

Similar strides in cerebral localization have been
made in the domains of learning and memory to the extent
that specific neuroanatomical mechanisms have been identified which are engaged in the performance of certain
classes of learned responses, but not others. In the rat,
for example, some specific mechanisms would include the
occipital cortex, lateral geniculate nuclei and zona incerta for the execution of visual discrimination habits,
the cingulate cortex, hippocampus, septal area and mammillary bodies for spatial learning and memory, the amygdala
and mediodorsal thalamic nucleus for the performance of
active and passive avoidance responses and the motor cortex and cerebellum for the preservation of skilled movement learning (Thompson 1982a; 1983a).

However, a second and equally important goal of the brain sciences (though not enunciated as frequently nor pursued as assiduously as cerebral localization) is to determine how the functionally differentiated mechanisms of the brain interact to produce unity and flexibility evident in a wide variety of goal-seeking behaviors. Progress along these lines of "cerebral integration" has lagged far behind that associated with cerebral localization. Even the broadest outlines of the neural circuitry underlying the organization of behavior in general and the elaboration of learning and memory in particular remain obscure.

Most investigators, like Lashley (1929; 1950), have assumed or at least have taken for granted that the multiplicity of pathways within the cerebral cortex is sufficient to mediate the complexities of learned behaviors. Others, like Penfield (1954; 1958), have proposed the existence of a "centrencephalic" (nonspecific) system within the upper brainstem that coordinates the activities of the specialized cortical and subcortical learning and memory mechanisms.

One of us has been persuaded for a number of years (Thompson, 1965) that subcortical mechanisms take precedence over cortical mechanisms in the final integration of behavior, at least with respect to the rat. Other scientists who have also posited at one time or another the existence of a subcortical nonspecific mechanism concerned with higher cognitive functions include Fessard (1954), MacKay (1966), Kilmer, McCulloch and Blum (1968), Knoll (1969), Reader (1974) and Klopf (1982). However, no concordance prevails as to the particular neuroanatomical make-up of this hypothetical nonspecific mechanism. The main reason for this is that different authors have developed different criteria for the determination of those brain sites that should be incorporated into a central integrating mechanism. Penfield, for example, claimed that a given brain region was a component of the centrencephalic system if (1) interference with the function of that region by vascular insufficiency, lesions or electrical stimulation abolished consciousness and (2) bilateral reciprocal connections existed between that region and the cerebral hemispheres. Our principal working hypothesis is that those brain sites implicated in the learning and retention of a diversity of laboratory tasks are the very

same sites that compose a central integrating mechanism.
Thus, this chapter will deal with those brain structures
that appear to play a nonspecific role in learning and
memory. More specifically, it focuses on a series of lesion studies on albino rats which have yielded findings
suggesting that destruction of certain brain sites is associated with a global learning and memory impairment--an
impairment that is not limited to one sense modality, to
one class of laboratory tasks or to one motivational state.

Use of the lesion method to investigate nonspecific
(or specific) mechanisms underlying learning and memory
requires no explanation. Lesion studies continue to con-
stitute one of the most reliable and straightforward approaches to acquire clues concerning the identity of (and
the role played by) those nuclei and pathways implicated
in the acquisition and retention of simple and complex
learned activities. Admittedly, a number of authors have
been critical of the lesion method in its application to
the study of learning and memory (see, for example, John
1972; Lynch 1976; and Schoenfield and Hamilton 1977), but
it should be emphasized that many of the charges against
the method are either exaggerated, ill-conceived or hardly
serious enough to discredit the technique (Thompson
1983a).

Limiting the empirical findings largely to investigations using laboratory rats as subjects likewise needs no
apology. In the United States, the rat has become the
most popular laboratory animal used in neurobehavioral
research. In fact, much of what is already appreciated
about the neural substrates of learning and memory is
based upon, or at least supplemented by, studies on the
rat. Virtually every part of the brain of this animal has
been subjected to examination by the lesion method and the
variety of learning situations in which the brain-damaged
rat has been observed provides a richness to the literature that has yet to be matched with the use of any other
laboratory animal. Besides, probably more is known about
the cytoarchitecture, chemoarchitecture and connectivity
of the different regions of the rat brain than of any
other laboratory animal (Paxinos 1985a; 1985b).

The feature about this chapter that is unusual, and
therefore requires a comment, concerns the topic of nonspecific learning and memory mechanisms. Most of the ex-

tensive literature dealing with the neuroanatomical basis
of learning and memory focuses on specific mechanisms;
that is, mechanisms which are engaged in the performance
of certain classes of learned responses, but not others.
While identification of (and the role played by) specific
learning and memory mechanisms is undeniably important,
this knowledge alone will not deepen our understanding
about how the relevant specific mechanisms are recruited
and the irrelevant ones inhibited in the acquisition or
retention (expression) of a given learned response. Conceivably, a nonspecific mechanism, through which attentional influences can operate within the context of an
"anticipatory set" (Sperry 1955), could exert an organizing effect on the brain (activate the appropriate specific
mechanisms) for the task at hand. In other words, acquisition and retention of most learned responses (excluding
possibly taste aversions, eyelid conditioning and other
tasks that place minimal demands upon cognitive functioning) can be viewed as the mobilization of one or more specific mechanisms by a nonspecific mechanism. This view
is vague and incomplete, but it does provide a conceptual
framework against which the findings derived from a long
series of lesion studies (Thompson 1984) can be interpreted. Furthermore, the foregoing conceptualization of
learning and memory bears a remarkable resemblance to one
of the more popular and enduring theories of intelligence;
namely, Spearman's (1927) two-factor theory. According to
this theory, performance on any given cognitive task is a
function of both a general intelligence factor or "g" and
one or more specific ability factors or "s". If overall
learning and memory abilities can be equated with intelligence, then it is not unreasonable to envisage a nonspecific learning and memory mechanism as the neural substrate of g and the specific learning and memory mechanisms as neural substrates of corresponding s'. Thus, the
study of nonspecific learning and memory mechanisms may
conceivably interface not only with findings on the neurology of intelligence, but with findings on the neuropathology of mental retardation as well (see Thompson,
Huestis, Crinella and Yu 1986). Such a rapprochement is
long overdue, considering the fact that the hallmark of
mental retardation is a nonspecific learning (and to a
lesser extent memory) deficiency (Campione & Brown 1984;
Denny 1964).

MAPPING THE BRAIN FOR NONSPECIFIC MECHANISMS IN LEARNING
AND MEMORY

Since the cognitive demands during the formation of a
habit (learning) may be quite different from those during
the performance of an already acquired habit (memory), it
is reasonable to assume that the nonspecific neural mechanism underlying learning will not exactly coincide with
that underlying memory. Thus, the quest for these nonspecific mechanisms necessarily requires two separate research
projects.

The lesion method is ideally suited to carry out each
project. With respect to learning, different groups of
laboratory animals would first be subjected to bilateral
cortical or subcortical lesions and subsequently would be
trained on a wide variety of tasks. Those lesion placements producing significant acquisition deficits on all
tasks investigated could be viewed as defining those sites
within the brain having a nonspecific function in learning. In the case of memory, normal laboratory animals
would first be trained on a wide variety of tasks and then
would be subjected to bilateral lesions of different cortical or subcortical regions. Following an appropriate
recovery period, the animals would be tested for retention
of each of the tasks learned preoperatively. Those lesion
placements producing significant retention deficits on all
tasks investigated could similarly be viewed as defining
those sites within the brain having a nonspecific function
in memory. For convenience, those structures found to
play a nonspecific role in learning will be termed the
"general learning system" (GLS) and those found to play a
nonspecific role in retention will be termed the "general
memory system" (GMS).

Like most neurobehavioral research projects, the approach outlined above is not devoid of weaknesses nor free
from pitfalls. It is obvious, for example, that the inclusion of a given brain structure within the GLS or GMS
will depend upon such variables as the size and locus of
the lesions investigated, the length of the recovery period, the composition of the test battery and the age and
previous experience of the subjects. Furthermore, since
the foregoing research projects will utilize electrolytic
and aspirative methods to inflict localized brain inju-
ries, it will not be known to what extent any lesion-

induced nonspecific learning or memory deficit is due to
cell damage within the brain structure as opposed to the
destruction of fibers of passage. How, then, does one interpret data in relation to the GLS and GMS in the absence
of studies assessing the importance of the foregoing variables? Consider the following hypothetical pattern of
results: Of the 25 different brain sites convassed with
lesions, only eight were associated with a nonspecific
memory impairment. On the strength of these results, it
may be inferred that these eight brain regions, which are
included within the GMS, are potentially more involved in
the general memory process than the remaining 17 brain regions that were excluded from the GMS.

About two decades ago, one of us (RT) began using the
lesion method for the purpose of identifying the GMS of
the rat brain. The results of this early effort will be
described first, followed by a description of more recent
data related to the identification of the GLS of the rat
brain.

GENERAL MEMORY SYSTEM

The initial evidence favoring the existence of a GMS
within the rat brain arose from a series of studies on the
comparative effects of various cortical and subcortical
lesions on retention of visual and nonvisual (vestibular-
proprioceptive-kinesthetic) discrimination tasks (Thompson 1976; Thompson, Arabie and Sisk 1976). Both tasks
were based upon the motive of escape-avoidance of mild
foot shock. With respect to the visual habit, the animals
were required to approach a white (or horizontally black
and white striped) card and to avoid an adjacent black (or
vertically black and white striped) card in order to gain
access to the goal box (area of safety). In the case of
the nonvisual (inclined plane discrimination) habit,
blinded animals were required to approach the upward sloping arm of a single unit T-maze and to avoid the adjacent
downward sloping arm in order to reach the goal box.

As might be expected, three functionally separate
groups of brain structures emerged. One group was concerned with retention of the visual habit only (components of the specific visual discrimination mechanism),
the second group was concerned with retention of the nonvisual habit only (components of the specific vestibular-

proprioceptive-kinesthetic discrimination mechanism) and
the third group was concerned with retention of both the
visual and nonvisual habits (possibly components of the
GMS). Figure 1 summarizes some of these results. (There
was a fourth group of brain structures; those that were
found not to be concerned with retention of either discrimination habit.)

Since both habits described above involved the task
of approaching a positive nonspatial stimulus "object" and
avoiding an adjacent negative nonspatial stimulus object,
this third group of brain structures could, in fact, be
components of a specific nonspatial sensory discrimination
mechanism rather than being components of the GMS. To
test this possibility, different subjects were trained on
a 3-cul maze habit under the motive of escape-avoidance of
mild foot shock and subsequently underwent bilateral lesions to those structures composing the third group.
Postoperative retention scores revealed that those lesion
placements impairing retention of the visual and nonvisual
discrimination problems also impaired retention of the
maze problem (Thompson 1974). On the strength of these
results, the function of this third group was not specialized for the maintenance of nonspatial sensory discrimination tasks.

It will be noted that all three laboratory problems
discussed so far were performed under the motive of
escape-avoidance of foot shock. The possibility exists,
therefore, that the lesion placements producing deficits
in retention of the discrimination and maze tasks actually
define those brain sites having a specific function in the
retention of aversively motivated habits rather than defining those brain sites having a nonspecific function in
retention. That this is not the case is suggested by the
findings that the brain mechanisms underlying retention of
an appetitively (thirst) motivated white-black discrimination are not remarkably different from those underlying
retention of an aversively motivated white-black discrimination (Thompson and Spiliotis 1981). Consistent with
the foregoing findings are the reports that retention of
latch box habits acquired under thirst motivation is impaired by the same lesions that disrupt both discrimination and maze habits (Spiliotis and Thompson 1973; Thompson, Gates and Gross 1979). Thus, even the retention of
learned skilled movements in the rat is susceptible to in-

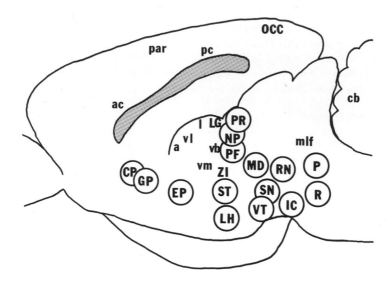

Figure 1. Schematic drawing of a parasagittal section of the rat brain, showing the relative positions of lesion placements producing retention deficits on the inclined plane discrimination only (lowercase letters), visual discrimination only (capital letters), and both discriminations (encircled capital letters). (From Thompson 1984).

terference by the same lesions that impair retention of discrimination and maze habits.

Summary

Based upon currently available data, rats with focal bilateral lesions to either the caudoputamen (intermediate division), globus pallidus, entopeduncular nucleus, subthalamus, posterolateral hypothalamus, parafascicular nucleus, nucleus posterior thalami, pretectal area, ventral tegmental area, substantia nigra, red nucleus, interpeduncular-central tegmental area (posterior division), median raphe or brainstem reticular formation (medial portion at the dimesencephalic juncture and paramedial portions at both pontomesencephalic and pontine levels) exhibit retention deficits on visual and nonvisual discriminations, a 3-cul maze and latch box problems. By virtue of the general nature of this series of problems, it seems reasonable to assume that selective damage to the aforementioned brain structures produces a generalized memory impairment and that these structures compose the GMS of the rat brain. Obviously, rats with these lesions will have to be assessed in retention of other kinds of laboratory tasks before this assumption can go unchallenged. While these lesion placements would more than likely disturb retention of more complex laboratory tasks, such as radial maze performance, delayed alternation and oddity learning, they could conceivably leave intact retention of simple associative learning (e.g., eyelid conditioning, taste aversions, and certain passive avoidance problems) which invokes minimal cognitive intervention. It has already been reported that retention of a particular passive avoidance response (refraining from entering a small dark compartment from a large illuminated compartment) is unaffected by lesions to certain elements of the GMS (Thompson 1978).

Before discussing the anatomical and functional interrelationships among the structures composing the GMS, it is necessary to present some relatively recent data gathered on the composition of the GLS of the rat brain.

GENERAL LEARNING SYSTEM

The first hint that a GLS exists within the rat brain came from a series of studies comparing the effects of various cortical and subcortical lesions in adult rats on original and reversal learning of both a simple spatial (nonvisual) discrimination habit formed in a single unit T-maze and a nonspatial white-black (visual) discrimination habit formed in a Thompson-Bryant box. Of the 38 different cortical and subcortical sites canvassed with lesions, 29 were found to be associated with deficits in original and reversal learning of the spatial discrimination (Thompson 1983b). Of these 29 brain sites, only 12 were subsequently found to be critical for the acquisition and reversal of the visual discrimination habit (Thompson 1982b; 1982c; Thompson, Gallardo and Yu 1983). Those 12 regions implicated in both nonvisual and visual discrimination learning included the occipital cortex, globus pallidus, ventrolateral thalamus, lateral thalamus, parafascicular nucleus, posterolateral hypothalamus, substantia nigra, red nucleus, central gray, interpeduncular-central

tegmental area, median raphe and pontine reticular formation (see Figure 2).

Despite the use of only a visual and a spatial discrimination problem, these results are remarkable to the
extent that most of the structures appearing to have a
nonspecific function in learning have already been demonstrated to have a nonspecific function in memory. On the
other hand, it was clear that this initial estimate of the
composition of the GLS was not entirely satisfactory since
one of the components (occipital cortex) has not been
found to be essential for normal acquisition of other
types of sensory discrimination problems (Finger and
Frommer 1968; Thompson 1982b).

As a consequence, the decision was made to develop a
battery of laboratory problems that would sample a broad

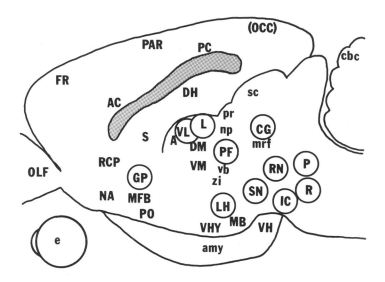

Figure 2. Schematic drawing of a parasagittal section of
the rat brain, showing the relative positions of lesion
placements producing no deficits in spatial discrimination
learning (lowercase letters), deficits in spatial discrimination learning (capital letters) and deficits in both
spatial and visual discrimination learning (encircled capital letters). (From Thompson 1984).

range of learning activities in the rat. This test battery was composed of six separate learning tasks and our
criterion of a nonspecific learning impairment arising
from a focal brain lesion was defective acquisition of all
six tasks. The individual tasks included a visual (white-
black) discrimination, a nonvisual vestibular-proprio-
ceptive-kinesthetic (inclined plane) discrimination, an
enclosed 3-cul maze and three distinct detour problems
(mounting a raised platform, entering an elevated cylinder
and climbing a ladder in order to gain access to the goal
box). The first three tasks utilized the motive of
escape-avoidance of mild foot shock, while the last three
utilized the motive of thirst.

Although this test battery may be criticized for
omitting certain problems, such as radial maze learning,
olfactory discriminations and delayed alternation, it is a
reasonably rigorous test of a nonspecific learning impairment, that is, an impairment that is not limited either to
one sense modality, to one class of laboratory problems
or to one motivational state. Furthermore, it contains
tasks (detour problems) that are sensitive to the presence
of a deficit in "response flexibility" (Thompson, Harmon
and Yu 1984a; 1984b). Response flexibility, which may be
defined in the context of a problem situation as "the
ability rapidly to discard unsuccessful responses and to
attempt new ones, until the correct one is found" (Riopelle 1967, p 253) is one of the more important features
of adaptive (intelligent) behavior. In addition, it
should be noted that these problems do not impose undue
demands on the sensory or motor capacities of the rat and,
as a consequence, the presence of subtle sensory or motor
disturbances arising from any given brain lesion can
largely be ruled out as a possible explanation for defective acquisition of all six problems.

Well over 500 rats receiving lesions to different
parts of the brain have been tested for acquisition of
either the three discrimination and maze habits, the three
detour problems or all six problems. Because of an interest in developing a brain-injured animal model of mental
retardation, these subjects sustained their brain lesions
(or sham operations in the case of the controls) at 21-24
days of age and began training on the test battery three
weeks later. A major portion of the findings of this
study has recently been published (Thompson et al. 1986).

TABLE 1. Brain regions critical for acquisition of various laboratory tasks in the white rat*

Brain Region	Visual Problem	Maze	Inclined Plane Problem	Detour Problem 1	2	3
Frontal (motor) cortex				X	X	X
Parietal cortex	X	X	X	X	X	X
Occipitotemporal cortex	X	X			X	
Frontocingulate cortex		X	X	X	X	
Posterior cingulate cortex		X	X	X		X
Hippocampus (dorsal)		X		X	X	X
Amygdala		X				
Caudoputamen (rostral)		X		X		X
Globus pallidus	X	X	X	X	X	X
Entopeduncular nucleus	X	X		X	X	X
Subthalamus	X	X		X	X	X
Anterior thalamus		X	X	X	X	X
Lateral thalamus		X	X			X
Ventrolateral thalamus	X	X	X	X	X	X
Mediodorsal thalamus		X	X	X		X

Parafascicular thalamus		X		X	X
Ventral thalamus	X	X			X
Hypothalamus (lateral)	X	X		X	X
Substantia nigra	X	X		X	X
Central gray (midbrain)	X	X		X	X
Red nucleus		X		X	
Median raphe	X	X		X	X
Lateral midbrain area					
Midbrain reticular formation	X	X		X	X
Pontine reticular formation	X	X		X	X

*A critical brain region is indicated by the letter "X" within a cell.

Table 1 summarizes the main findings of this research effort. Of the 25 different cortical and subcortical areas of the brain canvassed with focal lesions, only six were associated with significant learning deficits on all six problems of the test battery and therefore met the criterion for inclusion within the GLS. These areas consisted of the parietal cortex, globus pallidus, ventrolateral thalamus, substantia nigra, median raphe and pontine reticular formation.

It is important to note that this pattern of results is not readily explicable in terms of either the nonspecific debilitating effects arising from brain damage in the weanling rat or the magnitude of the lesions. In the first place, selective damage to 19 other brain sites (see Table 1) did not lead to a learning impairment on all six problems of the test battery. Furthermore, some of the brain-damaged groups that did not exhibit a nonspecific learning impairment, such as those with rostral caudoputamenal or lateral midbrain lesions, suffered greater damage to brain tissue than those groups with lesions to the globus pallidus, ventrolateral thalamus, substantia nigra, median raphe or pontine reticular formation.

It is also important to note that the nature of the test battery makes it unlikely that a specific sensory or motor defect underlies the nonspecific learning impairment. Attributing this impairment to general malaise or to an arousal-motivational-emotional defect also seems unlikely since the animals with selective lesions to the parietal cortex, globus pallidus, ventrolateral thalamus, substantia nigra, median raphe and pontine reticular formation were alert, healthy and active at the time of the first learning test, responded with what appeared to be normal vigor in pursuit (and in the presence) of the goal object and failed to evidence any emotional lability.

As might be expected, the essential findings of the foregoing study, which utilized young rats as subjects, have led to a different estimate of the composition of the GLS from that suggested by the findings of the initial study, which utilized adult rats as subjects. Both studies concurred in including the globus pallidus, ventrolateral thalamus, substantia nigra, median raphe and pontine reticular formation within the GLS, but differed with respect to the inclusion of the parietal cortex, occipitotemporal cortex, lateral thalamus, parafascicular nucleus, lateral hypothalamus, red nucleus and midbrain central gray. In view of the possibility that these discrepancies could have arisen either from the age difference (weanlings versus adults) at the time of surgical brain damage or from lesion differences in topography and magnitude, it seemed reasonable to avoid choosing the results of one study over the other in determining the constituents of the GLS. Instead, those lesion placements that were associated with either deficits in original and reversal learning of both visual and spatial discrimination problems (adult rat study) or deficits in learning all six problems of the test battery (weanling rat study) were considered to provide the best estimate of the composition of the GLS.

If the aforesaid structures are indeed components of the GLS, then it would be expected that selective damage to these structures would significantly impair skilled (manipulative) movement learning. It should be noted that none of the laboratory tasks used in the two preceding studies has tapped this kind of learning ability.

We have recently been examining the effects of focal cortical and subcortical lesions in adult rats on the learning of various latch box tasks, such as rotating a button latch in a clockwise direction, sliding a barrel bolt to the right or elevating a hook in order to open a door leading to a reward. The studies pertaining to certain cortical and subcortical structures have already been published (Thompson, Gallardo and Yu 1984a; 1984b), while those pertaining to other brain structures are either in progress or have just been completed.

Table 2 presents the main findings of these experiments with respect to acquisition of the bolt latch. (The button latch was used preoperatively to identify and discard those rats that were reluctant to manipulate latches or open doors under conditions of thirst, while the hook latch was omitted in some experiments because it proved to be too difficult to learn for some sham-operated control animals.) First of all, it should be noted that this latch box problem seems to be sensitive to those lesions invading structures traditionally associated with motor function (frontal cortex, globus pallidus and substantia nigra), while being insensitive to those lesions invading

structures not traditionally associated with motor function (occipitotemporal cortex, anterior thalamus and midbrain central gray). Of most importance, however, are the
findings relative to those brain structures which were
identified by the two earlier studies to be possible components of the GLS. While damage to the globus pallidus,
substantia nigra, ventrolateral thalamus, parafascicular
thalamus, lateral hypothalamus, median raphe or pontine
reticular formation impaired acquisition of the bolt latch
problem, damage to the parietal cortex, occipitotemporal
cortex, lateral thalamus, or midbrain central gray did
not. (No comparable data are available for the red nucleus or interpeduncular-central tegmental area.)

Summary

Adult rats with focal lesions to either the globus
pallidus, ventrolateral thalamus, parafascicular thalamus,
lateral hypothalamic area, substantia nigra, median raphe
or pontine reticular formation have been found to be retarded in original and reversal learning of both visual
and spatial discrimination habits and in the acquisition
of a latch box task. In most cases, weanling rats sus-
taining similar lesion placements exhibit acquisition deficits on visual and nonvisual discriminations, mazes and
detour problems. On the strength of these findings, it is
speculated that selective damage to the foregoing brain
structures produces a generalized learning impairment and
that these structures compose the GLS of the rat brain.
(The regions of the intermediate division of the caudoputamen, ventral tegmental area, red nucleus and interpeduncular-central tegmental area may also be components
of the GLS, but have yet to be fully evaluated.) Again, it
must be emphasized that although described as manifesting
a generalized learning impairment, rats with lesions to
any one of the proposed components of the GLS may learn
certain "simple" problems as fast as controls. It has already been reported that damage to the globus pallidus,
median raphe or pontine reticular formation, while impairing acquisition of a white-black discrimination (Thompson,
Ramsay and Yu 1984; Thompson and Yu 1983), fails to impair acquisition of an easier light-dark discrimination
(Thompson, Harmon and Yu 1985). This pattern of results
may be understood by assuming that simple problems do not
place as much demand upon cognitive functioning as more
difficult problems and, as a consequence, would be less

TABLE 2. Performance of the brain-damaged groups (relative to that of the sham-operated control groups) on the acquisition of a latch box task.

Brain Region	Sliding Bolt Latch
Cortex	
Frontal (motor)	loss
Parietal*	normal
Occipitotemporal*	normal
Frontocingulate	loss
Posterior cingulate	normal
Basal Ganglia	
Globus pallidus*	loss
Substantia nigra*	loss
Thalamus	
Anterior	normal
Mediodorsal	loss
Ventromedial	loss
Lateral*	normal
Ventrolateral*	loss
Midline	normal
Parafascicular*	loss
Hypothalamus	
Lateral*	loss
Brainstem	
Red nucleus*	not tested
Central gray*	normal
Interpeduncular-central tegmentum*	not tested
Median raphe*	loss
Pontine reticular formation*	loss

*Possible component of the GLS, based upon earlier studies.

sensitive to the presence of <u>small</u> lesions to brain regions concerned with the general learning process.

GENERAL MEMORY SYSTEM VERSUS GENERAL LEARNING SYSTEM

Comparing the current composition of the GMS with
that of the GLS reveals some striking similarities as well
as differences (see Table 3). Both embrace the globus
pallidus, parafascicular nucleus, lateral hypothalamus,
substantia nigra, median raphe and pontine reticular formation, but the GLS additionally contains the ventrolateral thalamus, while the GMS exclusively contains the caudoputamen (intermediate division), entopeduncular nucleus,
pretectal area, nucleus posterior, subthalamus and midbrain reticular formation. These differences are of considerable interest and could bear upon a number of issues
related to learning and memory. However, it would be
treacherous to speculate at this time about the functional
significance of the dissimilarities between the GMS and
GLS because of the possibility that the locus and size of
the lesions examined in the GLS experiments may not have
been totally comparable to those examined in the GMS experiments. Furthermore, the strain of subjects used in
the GMS studies (Wistar albino rats) was different from
that used in the GLS studies (Sprague-Dawley albino rats).
(This switch in the strain of rats occurred when the
senior author moved from Louisiana where all of the GMS
studies were performed to California where all of the GLS
studies were performed.) This methodological difference
may be significant when it is considered that Wistar rats
appear to require almost three times the number of errors
to learn the inclined plane discrimination as Sprague-Dawley rats (compare Thompson et al. 1976 with Thompson et
al. 1986). (Differences in the speed of learning the visual discrimination and maze habits were also present, but
fell considerably short of that existing for the inclined
plane problem.) What this difference means is that the
inclined plane problem used in the GMS studies was considerably more difficult to master than that used in the GLS
studies. This factor alone could account for the greater
number of components comprising the GMS relative to the
GLS since difficult problems are more sensitive to the
presence of brain damage than easy problems of the same
class.

Despite the difference in the strain of rats used and

TABLE 3. The composition of the GMS and GLS of the rat brain*

Brain Region	GMS	GLS
Basal Ganglia		
Caudoputamen (intermediate division)	X	?
Globus pallidus	X	X
Entopeduncular nucleus	X	
Subthalamus	X	
Substantia nigra	X	X
Red nucleus	X	?
Limbic Midbrain Area		
Ventral tegmental area	X	?
Interpeduncular-central tegmental area	X	?
Median raphe	X	X
Brainstem Reticular Formation		
Pretectum	X	
Nucleus posterior thalami	X	
Parafascicular nucleus	X	X
Lateral hypothalamus	X	X
Midbrain reticular formation (paramedial area)	X	
Pontine reticular formation (paramedial area)	X	X
Other		
Ventrolateral thalamus		X

*A given component is indicated by the letter "X" within a cell.

the probable variations in lesion topography and magnitude, the results of the two sets of experiments still led to a number of common elements composing the GMS and GLS. The extent of this correspondence may even be more striking than that indicated in Table 3. It is not inconceivable, for example, that the caudoputamenal (intermediate division), ventral tegmental, rubral and interpeduncular-central tegmental areas may turn out to be components of the GLS once all of the data on these structures have been collected. It is also noteworthy to mention that the entopeduncular nucleus and subthalamus (components of the

GMS) were excluded from the GLS largely because lesions to
these sites failed to induce a significant learning deficit on the "easy" inclined plane discrimination problem
(see Table 1). Similarly, the only reason that the ventrolateral thalamus (a component of the GLS) was excluded
from the GMS is that lesions to this nucleus fail to impair retention of a white-black discrimination problem
(see Thompson 1982a).

ANATOMICAL ANALYSIS

According to earlier analyses (Thompson 1982a;
1983a), the nonspecific system (GMS) pertaining to the retention of a wide range of laboratory tasks in the rat involves structures which neatly distribute themselves within the basal ganglia (BG), Nauta's (1960) "limbic midbrain
area" (LMA) and the ventral portions of the brainstem reticular formation (BSRF), including the extension of the
latter into the posterolateral hypothalamus ventrally and
parafascicular nucleus, nucleus posterior thalami and pretectum dorsally (Table 3). It was also pointed out that
although customarily viewed as being anatomically and
functionally independent, the degree of interconnectivity
existing among the BG, LMA and BSRF (see Figure 3) allows
for the possibility that these three morphological ensembles form a unit which serves a highly complex function in
memory.

Interestingly, except for the ventrolateral thalamus,
the nonspecific system (GLS) pertaining to the acquisition
of a diversity of laboratory tasks in the rat also involves structures which distribute themselves within the
BG, LMA and BSRF (Table 3). Although the GLS is not as
strongly represented within these three ensembles as the
GMS, there is sufficient overlap to suggest the hypothesis
that the BG, LMA and BSRF are the most likely candidates
among all other recognized anatomical aggregates to underlie nonspecific learning and memory processes. Parenthe-
tically, the involvement of the ventrolateral thalamus
does not detract from this hypothesis nor does it diminish
the possibility that the BG, LMA and BSRF function as a
unit in the cognitive mediation of learning and memory.
First of all, it should be recalled that this thalamic
region was excluded from the GMS only because of earlier
findings suggesting that ventrolateral thalamic lesions
fail to impair retention of a white-black discrimination--

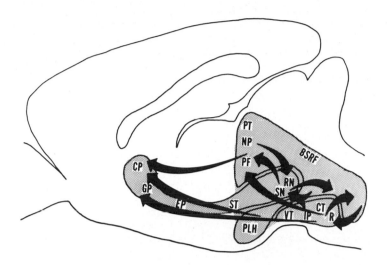

Figure 3. Schematic drawing of a parasagittal section of
the rat brain showing some of the interconnecting pathways
of the GMS. (From Thompson 1982a).

rats with these lesions are impaired in retention of
mazes, nonvisual discriminations, active avoidance responses and latch box habits (Thompson 1982a). Secondly,
this thalamic region is the recipient of projections from
the entopeduncular nucleus and substantia nigra and is
generally considered to be an integral part of any functional circuit diagram involving the BG (Heimer, Alheid
and Zaborszky 1984). Finally, besides being anatomically
related to the BG, this thalamic complex appears to be one
of the targets of projections from both the LMA (Peschanski and Besson, 1984) and BSRF (Purpura, McMurtry and
Maekawa 1966; Steriade, Ropert, Kitsikis and Oakson 1980).

    Perhaps the most disturbing feature about the fore-
going analysis concerns the exclusion of those brain
structures from the GLS and GMS that are most frequently
cited in connection with learning and memory; namely, the
cerebral cortex and hippocampus. This, of course, does
not imply that these (or any other) excluded structures
are devoid of any significant role in learning and memory.
Rather it means that neocortical and hippocampal regions

may be critical for acquisition and retention of certain laboratory tasks, but not for acquisition and retention of other laboratory tasks. In other words, these telencephalic structures have specific functions in learning and memory that are to be contrasted with the seemingly non-specific functions served by the deep structures of the BG, LMA and BSRF (see, for example, Table 1). In the final analysis, the key to the understanding of the neuroanatomy of learning and memory may lie in the identification of those pathways linking cortical and hippocampal structures with the BG, LMA and BSRF that provide the matrix within which the superordinate abilities of the nonspecific systems can set the functions of the specific systems.

FUNCTIONAL CONSIDERATIONS

Granting that the BG, LMA and BSRF largely compose the nonspecific mechanisms involved in learning and memory, the question arises concerning the extent to which each of these anatomical ensembles contributes in a specialized and independent way to the learning and memory process. Conceivably, the BG could be implicated in learning and memory by virtue of its role in motor control, the LMA by virtue of its role in reinforcement processes and the BSRF by virtue of its role in arousal and selective attention. Alternatively, the activities of this anatomical triad could combine to serve a much broader role in learning and memory, whose fulfillment would depend upon elements of motor control, reinforcement processes, arousal and selective attention.

It was suggested previously (Thompson 1982c; 1984) that Sperry's (1955) conceptualization of learning and memory as the establishment and reinstatement of an "expectancy" or "anticipatory set" incorporates those psychological processes that could be mediated by the consortium of the BG, LMA and BSRF. For Sperry, an anticipatory set intermediates between sensory and motor events in a learning situation by exerting an organizing effect on the brain --through the mobilization of both inhibitory and excitatory influences--that facilitates both the reception of the relevant signals and the execution of the appropriate response sequence. The overall readiness to respond, as evidenced by fine motor adjustments in receptor orientation and body posture, constitutes one of the more obvious behavioural expressions of this organizing effect.

Linking anticipatory sets to the BG, LMA and BSRF is plausible for a number of reasons. First of all, this triad features a superabundance of anatomical connections throughout the neuraxis that could arouse particular patterns of central excitation and inhibition in the service of establishing a given behavioral state of readiness. Second, anticipatory sets are reflected electrophysiologically in the phonemenon of "assimilation of rhythms"--the appearance during the intertrial interval of brain activity normally evoked by the conditioned stimulus--and other "endogenous" processes (John 1967; 1972). Of considerable interest is the fact that these assimilated rhythms seem to appear most reliably within the "nonsensory-specific" systems of the brain (see also Olds, Mink and Best 1969 and Ray, Mirsky and Pragay 1982). Similarly, the mapping of those units within the rat brain that exhibit "conditioned responses" (Disterhoft and Olds 1972; Linseman and Olds 1973; Olds, Disterhoft, Segal, Kornblith and Hirsh 1972) has revealed that these learning units are found in several regions of the brain, including those affiliated with the BG (globus pallidus), LMA (ventral tegmental area) and BSRF (nucleus reticularis pontis oralis). Finally, since the cardinal feature of an anticipatory set is a predisposition to respond in a certain way to a given stimulus event, it would follow that such a predisposition would largely be achieved by brain structures having an intermediary role in motor function. It must be more than coincidence that the BG have long been known to be associated with postural mechanisms (Denny-Brown 1962) and that the LMA (Asin and Fibiger 1983; Lorens, Kohler and Guldberg 1975; Montaron, Bouyer, Rougeul and Buser 1982) and BSRF (Siegel 1979) may also function in the modulation of motor output.

The notion that the BG may be implicated in the formation of anticipatory sets is not new. Buchwald, Hull, Levine and Villablanca (1975), for example, concluded that the pattern of learning deficits arising from damage to the BG in cats can be explained in terms of a disturbance in the ability "to adopt and to maintain appropriate cognitive sets." The BSRF has likewise been suggested to be significant for the mediation of "mental sets" (Lindsley 1958). As far as can be determined, the LMA has not been previously proposed as a candidate for the mediation of

anticipatory sets, but the lateral hypothalamus, the posterior part of which is considered to be a component of
the LMA (Nauta 1960), has been speculated to function in
generating various aspects of anticipatory behaviors
(Panksepp 1981).

FINAL REMARKS

One of the pressing questions arising from this research program on the laboratory rat concerns whether or
not nonspecific learning and memory mechanisms exist within the human brain and, if so, whether these mechanisms
also reside, at least in part, within the BG, LMA and
BSRF. Assuming that such mechanisms do exist (see Fodor
1983), it is unlikely that they would involve any discrete
areas of the cerebral cortex since focal neocortical lesions in the adult human are rarely, if ever, accompanied
by a nonspecific learning or memory impairment (Russell
1981). It is also unlikely that the hippocampus, mammillary bodies or mediodorsal thalamus (structures implicated
in the "amnesic syndrome") are involved in these mechanisms inasmuch as patients with pathology to these subcortical regions evidence no serious deficits in the learning
or retention of certain motor, perceptual and cognitive
skills (Cohen 1984; Squire and Cohen 1984).

If the BG, LMA and BSRF of the human brain do indeed
play a significant nonspecific role in learning and memory
processes, then it would be expected that patients with
pathology largely restricted to these anatomical areas
should present with global learning, memory and intellectual disorders. Unfortunately, the clinical literature
lacks a sufficient number of cases in which elements of
this morphological triad sustained histologically verified
lesions that were large, bilaterally symmetrical and un-
attended by pathology to other brain areas. However, the
clinical material that is available, although requiring
further validation, is suggestive that a generalized cognitive disorder may be one of the products of pathology to
the BG, LMA and BSRF. Perhaps the most persuasive clinical material relates to what workers in the field of dementia now refer to as "subcortical dementia", a condition
characterized by such cognitive disorders as the slowing
of thought processes, forgetfulness and reduced drive
(Benson 1983; Huber and Paulson 1985). The location of
the primary neuropathology (and the associated disease

entity) in cases of subcortical dementia include the pars
compacta of the substantia nigra (parkinsonism), caudate
nucleus (Huntington's disease), lenticular nuclei (Wilson's disease), thalamus (thalamic dementia), globus
pallidus and pars reticulata of the substantia nigra
(Hallervorden-Spatz disease) and midbrain (progressive
supranuclear palsy). Since cortical systems responsible
for language functions and for perceiving sensory input
are usually intact, it has been proposed that the cognitive abnormalities associated with subcortical dementia
are due to "disturbances of timing and activation" (Albert, Feldman and Willis 1974). Interestingly, these disturbances could conceivably reflect an impairment in the
establishment, reinstatement or maintenance of anticipatory sets as well.

Other clinical reports suggesting the involvement of
the BG, LMA and BSRF in general cognitive functions include the dementias following brainstem encephalitis (Ueno
and Takahata 1978), the dense retrograde amnesia following
pathology to the ventral tegmental area (Goldberg et al.
1981), the severe intellectual impairments arising from
nonhaemorrhagic thalamic infarction of the ventrolateral
nucleus (Graff-Radford et al. 1985) and cases of mental
retardation associated with pathological changes roughly
restricted to various subcortical sites (Malamud, 1964).

Another issue relevant to the topic of the neuroanatomy of learning and memory concerns the locus of the engrams of experience. It is becoming increasingly apparent
from the recent clinical (Cohen 1984; Warrington 1981) and
experimental (Mishkin and Petri 1984; Oakley 1983) literature on the effects of brain lesions on memory that multiple engram systems rather than a unitary engram system
inhabit the mammalian brain. Richard Thompson et al.
(1984), for example, have presented compelling evidence
for the distinctions among what they term "nonspecific
trace systems" (related to learned motivation), "specific
trace systems" (related to the acquisition of adaptive responses) and "cognitive trace systems" (related to procedural and declarative learning). A different lesion experiment on rats (Thompson 1979) has similarly demonstrated that the performance of a simple white-black discrimination task can be dissociated into an "incentive
habit" (based upon engrams related to the initiation of
the behavioral act leading to the reward), a "location

habit" (based upon engrams related to the location of the reward or correct pathway to the reward) and a "response habit" (based upon engrams related to the nature of the response necessary to gain access to the reward). While lesion data of this sort can be interpreted as being compatible with the notion that different anatomical loci exist for different classes of engram systems, they do not rule out the possibility that these different anatomical loci are, in fact, different specific neural mechanisms and that all engrams systems are established within a nonspecific neural mechanism (GMS).

As discussed earlier, different classes of learned responses can be conceived as being mediated by different specific mechanisms couple with a (common) nonspecific mechanism. Although this conceptualization opens the way for the argument that all engram systems are traceable to the nonspecific mechanism, it also allows for the possibility that the acquisition of any given habit generates two (or more) subsets of engrams. One might convey coarse (rudimentary) information about the habit and be located within the nonspecific mechanism, whereas the other might fill in the details about the habit and be located within the specific mechanism(s).

Finally, the data presented in this chapter on the identification of the GMS and GLS of the rat brain provide remarkable support for Penfield's (1954; 1958) "centrencephalic theory" which acknowledges the presence of a localized collection of subcortical nuclei and fiber pathways responsible not only for conscious awareness and voluntary action, but for the cognitive mediation of diverse problem-solving activities. Although it can be argued that serious conceptual difficulties attend any theory positing the existence of a circumscribed integrating mechanism within the brain (Walshe 1957), any alternate theory that views the brain as an assemblage of specific "informationally encapsulated" mechanisms is no less vulnerable to criticism (see Fodor 1983). Perhaps the difficulties facing a centrencephalic-type theory in the domains of learning and memory will fade away as more is learned about the functional linkage between the upper brainstem and cortical and hippocampal formations. According to our results on the rat, particular attention should be paid to the BG, LMA and BSRF in tracing such functional links.

LIST OF ABBREVIATIONS USED IN FIGURES

a(A), anterior thalamus; ac(AC), anterior cingulate
cortex; amy, amygdaloid complex; cb, cerebellum; cbc,
cerebellar cortex; CG, mesencephalic central gray; CP,
intermediate caudoputamen; DH, dorsal hippocampus; DM,
mediodorsal thalamus; e, eye; EP, entopeduncular nucleus;
FR, frontolateral cortex; GP, globus pallidus; IC,
interpeduncular-central tegmental area; l(L), lateral
thalamic complex; LG, lateral geniculate bodies; LH,
posterolateral hypothalamus; MB, mammillary bodies; MD,
mesodiencephalic reticular formation; MFB, rostral medial
forebrain bundle; mlf, medial longitudinal fasciculus;
mrf, dorsomedial mesencephalic reticular formation; NA,
nucleus accumbens; NP(np), nucleus posterior thalami; OCC,
occipital cortex; OLF, olfactory bulb; P, pontine
reticular formation; par(PAR), parietal cortex; pc(PC),
posterior cingulate cortex; PF, parafascicular nucleus;
PO, preoptic-supraoptic hypothalamus; PR(pr), pretectum;
R, median raphe; RCP, rostral caudoputamen; RN, red
nucleus; S, septal area; sc, superior colliculus; SN,
substantia nigra; ST, subthalamic nucleus; vb, ventrobasal
thalamus; VH, ventral hippocampus; VHY, ventromedial
hypothalamus; vl(VL), ventrolateral thalamus; vm(VM),
ventromedial thalamus; VT, ventral tegmental area; ZI(zi),
zona incerta.

ACKNOWLEDGEMENT

The authors wish to thank Phyllis Wood for her assistance
in preparing this manuscript.

REFERENCES

Albert ML, Feldman RG, Willis NL (1974). The "subcortical
    dementia" of progressive supranuclear palsy. J Neurol
    Neurosurg Psychiat 37:121.
Asin KE, Fibiger HC (1983). An analysis of neuronal ele-
    ments within the median nucleus of the raphe that medi-
    ate lesion-induced increases in locomotor activity.
    Brain Res 268:211.
Benson DF (1983). Subcortical dementia: A clinical ap-
    proach. In Mayeux R, Rosen WG (eds.): "The Dementias,"
    New York: Raven Press, p 185.
Buchwald NA, Hull CD, Levine MS, Villablanca J (1975).
    The basal ganglia and the regulation of response and

cognitive sets. In Brazier (ed.): "Growth and Development of the Brain," New York: Raven Press, p 171.

Campione JC, Brown AL (1984). Learning ability and transfer propensity as sources of individual differences in intelligence. In Brooks PH, Sperber R, McCauley C (eds.): "Learning and Cognition in the Mentally Retarded," Hillsdale: Lawrence Erlbaum, p 265.

Cohen NJ (1984). Preserved learning capacity in amnesia: Evidence for multiple memory systems. In Squire LR, Butters N (eds.): "Neuropsychology of Memory," New York: Guilford Press, p 83.

Denny MR (1964). Research in learning and performance. In Stevens HA, Heber R (eds.): "Mental Retardation," Chicago: University of Chicago Press, p 100.

Denny-Brown D (1962). "The Basal Ganglia." New York: Oxford University Press.

Disterhoft JF, Olds J (1972). Differential development of conditioned unit changes in thalamus and cortex of rat. J Neurophysiol 35:665.

Fessard AE (1954). Mechanisms of nervous integration and conscious experience. In Delafresnaye JF (ed.): "Brain Mechanisms and Consciousness," Springfield: Charles C Thomas, p 175.

Finger S, Frommer GP (1968). Effects of cortical lesions on tactile discrimination graded in difficulty. Life Sciences 7:897.

Fodor JA (1983). "The Modularity of Mind." Cambridge: MIT Press.

Goldberg E, Antin SP, Bilder RM, Gerstman LJ, Hughes JEO, Mattis S (1981). Retrograde amnesia: Possible role of mesencephalic reticular activation in long-term memory. Science 213:1392.

Graff-Radford NR, Damasio H, Yamada T, Eslinger PJ, Damasio AR (1985). Nonhaemorrhagic thalamic infarction. Brain 108:485.

Heimer L, Alheid GF, Zaborszky L (1984). Basal ganglia. In Paxinos G (ed.): "The Rat Nervous System," Vol 1, New York: Academic Press, p 37.

Huber SJ, Paulson GW (1985). The concept of subcortical dementia. Am J Psychiat 142:1312.

Kilmer WL, McCulloch WS, Blum J (1968). An embodiment of some vertebrate command and control principles. Curr Mod Biol 2:81.

Klopf AH (1982). "The Hedonistic Neuron." New York: Hemisphere.

Knoll J (1969). "The Theory of Active Reflexes." New

York: Hafner.

John ER (1967). "Mechanisms of Memory." New York: Academic Press.

John ER (1972). Switchboard versus statistical theories of learning and memory. Science, 177:850.

Lashley KS (1929). "Brain Mechanisms and Intelligence." Chicago: University of Chicago Press.

Lashley KS (1950). In search of the engram. Sympos Soc Exp Biol No IV:454.

Lindsley DB (1958). The reticular system and perceptual discrimination. In Jasper (ed.): "Reticular Formation of the Brain," Boston: Little, Brown, p 513.

Linseman, MA, Olds J (1973). Activity changes in rat hypothalamus, preoptic area, and striatum associated with Pavlovian conditioning. J Neurophysiol 36:1038.

Lorens SA, Kohler C, Guldberg HC (1975). Lesions in Gudden's tegmental nuclei produce behavioral and 5-HT effects similar to those after raphe lesions. Pharmacol Biochem Behav 3:653.

Lynch G (1976). Some difficulties associated with the use of lesion techniques in the study of memory. In Rosenzweig MR, Bennett EL (eds.): "Neural Mechanisms of Learning and Memory," Cambridge: MIT Press, p 544.

MacKay DM (1966). Conscious control of action. In Eccles JC (ed.): "Brain and Conscious Experience," New York: Springer-Verlag, p 422.

Malamud N (1964). Neuropathology. In Stevens HA, Heber R (eds.): "Mental Retardation," Chicago: University of Chicago Press, p 429.

Mishkin M, Petri HL (1984). Memories and habits: Some implications for the analysis of learning and retention. In Squire LR, Butters N (eds.): "Neuropsychology of Memory," New York: Guilford Press, p 287.

Montaron M-F, Bouyer J-J, Rougeul A, Buser P (1982). Ventral mesencephalic tegmentum (VMT) controls electrocortical Beta rhythms and associated attentive behavior in the cat. Behav Brain Res 6:129.

Nauta WJH (1960). Some neural pathways related to the limbic system. In Ramey ER, O'Doherty DS (eds.): "Electrical Studies on the Unanesthetized Brain," New York: Paul B Hoeber, p 1.

Oakley DA (1983). The varieties of memory: A phylogenetic approach. In Mayes A (ed.): "Memory in Animals and Humans," Wokingham: Van Nostrand Reinhold, p 20.

Olds J, Mink WD, Best PJ (1969). Single unit patterns during anticipatory behavior. Electroenceph Clin Neurophysiol 26:144.

Olds J, Disterhoft JF, Segal M, Kornblith CL, Hirsh R
(1972). Learning centers of rat brain mapped by measuring latencies of conditioned unit responses. J Neurophysiol 35:202.

Panksepp J (1981). Hypothalamic integration of behavior.
In Morgane PJ, Panksepp J (eds.): "Handbook of the Hypothalamus," Vol 3, New York: Marcel Dekker, p 289.

Paxinos G (1985a). "The Rat Nervous System, Vol 1, Forebrain and Midbrain." New York: Academic Press.

Paxinos G (1985b). "The Rat Nervous System, Vol 2, Hind-
brain and Spinal Cord." New York: Academic Press.

Penfield W (1954). Studies of the cerebral cortex of man:
A review and an interpretation. In Delafresnaye JF
(ed.), "Brain Mechanisms and Consciousness," Springfield: Charles C Thomas, p 284.

Penfield W (1958). "The Excitable Cortex in Conscious
Man." Springfield: Charles C Thomas.

Peschanski M, Besson J-M (1984). Diencephalic connections
of the raphe nuclei of the rat brainstem: An anatomical
study with reference to the somatosensory system. J
Comp Neurol 224:509.

Purpura DP, McMurtry JG, Maekawa K (1966). Synaptic
events in ventrolateral thalamic neurons during suppression of recruiting responses by brain stem reticular
stimulation. Brain Res 1:63.

Ray CL, Mirsky AF, Pragay EB (1982). Functional analysis
of attention-related unit activity in the reticular formation of the monkey. Exp Neurol 77:544.

Reader AV (1974). "Machine, Mind and Brain." Manchester:
AV Reader.

Riopelle AJ (1967). "Animal Problem Solving." Baltimore:
Penguin.

Russell EW (1981). The pathology and clinical examination
of memory. In Filskov SB, Boll TJ (eds.), "Handbook of
Clinical Neuropsychology," New York: Wiley, p 287.

Shoenfeld TA, Hamilton LW (1977). Secondary brain changes
following lesions: A new paradigm for lesion experiments. Physiol Behav 18:951.

Siegel JM (1979). Behavioral functions of the reticular
formation. Brain Res Rev 1:69.

Spearman C (1927). "The Abilities of Man." New York:
Macmillan.

Sperry RW (1955). On the neural basis of the conditioned
response. Brit J Anim Behav 3:41.

Spiliotis PH, Thompson R (1973). The "manipulative response memory system" in the white rat. Physiol Psychol 1:101.

Squire LR, Cohen NJ (1984). Human memory and amnesia. In Lynch G, McGaugh JL, Weinberger NM (eds.): "Neurobiology of Learning and Memory," New York: Guilford Press, p 3.

Steriade M, Ropert N, Kitsikis A, Oakson G (1980). Ascending activating neuronal networks in midbrain reticular core and related rostral systems. In Hobson JA, Brazier MAB (eds.): "The Reticular Formation Revisited," New York: Raven Press, p 125.

Thompson Richard F, Clark GA, Donegan NH, Larond DG, Lincoln JS, Madden J, Mamounas LA, Mauk MD, McCormick DA, Thompson JK (1984). Neuronal substrates of learning and memory: A "multiple-trace" view. In Lynch G, McGaugh JL, Weinberger NM (eds.): "Neurobiology of Learning and Memory," New York: Guilford Press, p 137.

Thompson R (1965). Centrencephalic theory and interhemispheric transfer of visual habits. Psychol Rev 72:385.

Thompson R (1974). Localization of the "maze memory system" in the white rat. Physiol Psychol 2:1.

Thompson R (1976). Sterotaxic mapping of brainstem areas critical for memory of visual discrimination habits in the rat. Physiol Psychol 4:1.

Thompson R (1978). Localization of a "passive avoidance memory system" in the white rat. Physiol Psychol 6:263.

Thompson R (1979). Dissociation of a visual discrimination task into incentive, location and response habits. Physiol Behav 23:63.

Thompson R (1982a). Functional organization of the rat brain. In Orbach J (ed.): "Neuropsychology after Lashley," Hillsdale: Lawrence Erlbaum, p 207.

Thompson R (1982b). Brain lesions impairing visual and spatial reversal learning in rats: Components of the "general learning system" of the rodent brain. Physiol Psychol 10:186.

Thompson R (1982c). Impaired visual and spatial reversal learning in brain-damaged rats: Additional components of the "general learning system" of the rodent brain. Physiol Psychol 10:293.

Thompson R (1983a). Brain systems and long-term memory. Behav Neur Biol 37:1.

Thompson R (1983b). Abnormal learning and forgetting of individual spatial reversal problems in brain-damaged rats. Physiol Psychol 11:35.

Thompson R (1984). Nonspecific neural mechanisms involved

in learning and memory in the rat. In Squire LR, Butters N (eds.): "Neuropsychology of Memory," New York: Guilford Press, p 408.

Thompson R, Arabie GJ, Sisk GB (1976). Localization of the "incline plane discrimination memory system" in the white rat. Physiol Psychol 4:311.

Thompson R, Gallardo K, Yu J (1983). Posterolateral hypothalamic and midbrain central gray lesions impair visual and spatial reversal learning: Further additions to the "general learning system" of the rodent brain. Physiol Psychol 11:93.

Thompson R, Gallardo K, Yu J (1984a). Cortical mechanisms underlying acquisition of latch-box problems in the white rat. Physiol Behav 32:809.

Thompson R. Gallardo K, Yu J (1984b). Thalamic mechanisms underlying acquisition of latch-box problems in the white rat. Acta Neurobiol Exp 44:105.

Thompson R, Gates CE, Gross SA (1979). Thalamic regions critical for retention of skilled movements in the rat. Physiol Psychol 7:7.

Thompson R, Harmon D, Yu J (1984a). Detour problem-solving behavior in rats with neocortical and hippocampal lesions: A study of response flexibility. Physiol Psychol 12:116.

Thompson R, Harmon D, Yu J (1984b). Detour problem-solving behavior in rats with early lesions to the "general learning system." Physiol Psychol 12:193.

Thompson R, Harmon D, Yu J (1985). Deficits in response inhibition and attention in rats rendered mentally retarded by early subcortical brain damage. Develop Psychobiol 18:483.

Thompson R, Huestis PW, Crinella FM, Yu J (1986). The neuroanatomy of mental retardation in the white rat. Neuroscience Biobehav Rev (in press).

Thompson R, Ramsay A, Yu J (1984). A generalized learning deficit in albino rats with early median raphe or pontine reticular formation lesions. Physiol Behav 32:107.

Thompson R, Spiliotis PH (1981). Subcortical lesions and retention of a brightness discrimination in the rat: Appetitive vs. aversive motivation. Physiol Psychol 9:63.

Thompson R, Yu J (1983). Specific brain lesions producing nonspecific (generalized) learning impairments in weanling rats. Physiol Psychol 11:225.

Ueno T, Takahata N (1978). Chronic brainstem encephalitis with mental symptoms and ataxia. J Neurol Neurosurg

Psychiat 41:516.

Walshe FMR (1957). The brain-stem conceived as the "highest level" of function in the nervous system; with particular reference to the "automatic apparatus" of Carpenter (1850) and to the "centrencephalic integrating system" of Penfield. Brain 80:510.

Warrington EK (1981). Neuropsychological evidence for multiple memory systems. Acta Neurol Scand 64:13.

Neuroplasticity, Learning, and Memory, pages 265–278
© **1987 Alan R. Liss, Inc.**

NEURAL GRAFTS IN THE STUDY OF BRAIN PLASTICITY

Menahem Segal

Center for Neurosciences
The Weizmann Institute of Science
Rehovot, Israel

Mammalian brain transplantation has been in the realm of science fiction for many years. The possibility of changing behavior by grafts of neural tissue was not conceived by scientists as a viable approach to studying brain functions because it was assumed that neural circuits in mammalian brain are rigid. Thus, very few reports on mammalian brain grafting were published in the first 70 years of this century. This contrasts with a larger volume of studies in lower vertebrates, known to have a more plastic brain.

It was not until the late seventies that brain grafts began to gain momentum and to be used in several fields of research. Two major developments have encouraged research into brain grafting. The first was the realization that central neurons possess greater plastic abilities than had been thought previously. Thus, mature central neurons can extend axons into denervated regions not seen by them normally, and cut axons can grow across bridges to reach their normal target organs (Raisman, 1969; Zimmer, 1971; Lynch et al., 1972). Furthermore, certain neuron groups, particularly those containing biogenic amines, have more pronounced plastic properties than other cell types (Stenevi et al., 1976). The other major impetus for brain graftology is the accumulated evidence relating behavioral, neural or hormonal deficits to damage to specific cell groups in the brain. Thus, parkinsonism is associated with degeneration of dopaminergic neurons of the substantia nigra (SN), Alzheimer's disease with loss of cholinergic neurons in the nucleus basalis and perhaps of noradrenergic neurons of the nucleus locus coeruleus (LC) (Corkin et al., 1982). In Brattleboro rats, specific cells in the hypothalamus do not produce vasopressin which results in diabetes insipidus. These two main groups of observations culminated in the late seventies with the pioneering discovery that one can cure diabetes in Brattleboro rats by injecting normal hypothalamus into their third ventricle (Gash et al., 1980) and parkinsonian symptoms in rat model by injecting SN cells into the striatum (Perlow et al., 1979).

Not surprisingly, these observations were followed by numerous animal experiments on grafting of central and peripheral tissue in various disease models. The nearly unanimous success has prompted some premature human experiments where pieces of adrenal medula were dumped into the basal ganglia of parkinsonian patients, thus far without therapeutic effect (Backlund et al., 1985).

There is an obvious intuitive appeal to using brain grafts for the study of brain functions. The traditional assignment of functions to structure demands that the function be impaired by damage to the structure. While this has been studied in nearly every brain region, this classical approach has an inherent limitation -- there is no easy means of distinguishing cellular damage from damage to fibers of passage or secondary damage inflicted on remote neurons. If one is able to regain a function impaired by damage to a brain nucleus by substituting a grafted nucleus for the damaged nucleus, one can then positively associate the function with that structure. Nonetheless, such conclusions require great caution and the use of proper controls en route to such an association.

Studies of brain grafts can be described along several dimensions: (1) the source of the grafted neural tissue and the site of grafting, (2) the scientific objectives of the research, and (3) the expected effects exerted by the graft. Let us consider each of these in turn.

The Source of the Grafted Tissue

For nearly every brain region, tissue has been taken out of the embryo and grafted into an adult host. The grafted tissue can be either a neurochemically specified nucleus or a piece of highly organized brain region. The former group includes the dopamine-containing substantia nigra (Perlow et al., 1979), the noradrenaline-containing nucleus locus coeruleus (McRae-Degueurce et al., 1985), the serotonin-containing raphe nuclei (Segal and Azmitia, 1986), the acetylcholine-containing septal area (Bjorklund and Stenevi, 1977; Segal et al., 1985), the acetylcholine-containing nucleus basalis (Arendash et al., 1985; Fine et al., 1985), and the peptide-containing hypothalamus (Gash and Scott, 1980).

It must be noted, however, that in none of these cases are the target neurons the only ones to be grafted. The graft most certainly contains much more than the neurochemically specific neurons. In most of the studies where recovery of function is suggested, there is no clear pharmacological evidence that this recovery is due to action of the selected neuron population.

Of the laminated structures of the brain, the cerebellum (Alvarado, Mallart and Sotelo, 1982), neocortex (Labbe et al., 1983), and hippocampus (Raisman et al., 1985) have been implanted into adult rat brain. The rationale for doing these experiments is different from that underlying the chemically specific neural grafting (see below).

The Scientific Objectives

Although research objectives can change in the course of a study, they usually determine the tools and the brain region selected for study. There are two main objectives for using brain grafts: (a) in the analysis of determinants of growth and maturation of neurons and their interconnections, and (b) in the study of recovery of function following specific brain lesions.

Studies aimed at the first objective have been conducted with embryonic hippocampus implanted into a cavity produced in another hippocampus (Raisman et al., 1985; Frotscher and Zimmer, 1986). These studies illustrate the rules governing the connections made by certain hippocampal cell types with one another. Experiments with the serotonergic innervation of the hippocampus (Zhou et al., 1987) have described a factor that is produced in the target

organ and selectively promotes growth of serotonergic fibers
there. While experiments are still being conducted to
identify the factor, it is likely that such a factor might
be effective in guiding serotonergic fibers into the
hippocampus of the developing brain.

A more well known factor, the nerve growth factor (NGF)
associated for many years with the peripheral nervous
system, has been found to have a specific affect on the
cholinergic medial septal neurons which innervate the
hippocampus. Experiments using NGF indicate that it may
support survival of grafted cholinergic neurons in a host
hippocampus. Another structure which has been studied is
the cerebellum. Grafts from embryonic cerebellum have been
used as a model systems for studying the principles of
organization of cerebellar development (Alvarado-Mallart
and Sotelo, 1982).

There have also been studies on the
electrophysiological properties of grafted cells which were
aimed at clarifying the developmental factors responsible
for cellular specificity. The results have been surprising,
but consistant. These studies indicate that the properties
of embryonic hippocampal cells grown in the cerebellum,
cerebellar cells grown in the hippocampus (Hounsgaard and
Yarom, 1985), and dorsal raphe cells grown in the
hippocampus (Segal and Azmitia, 1986) develop normal-like
properties even when they are exposed to an alien
environment in an adult brain. This indicates that ionic
conductances of given cells are determined at a very early
age and are not affected to a significant degree by
changing growth conditions.

The second main objective for using brain graft
methodology is to study recovery of functions following
specific brain lesions. The ultimate objective of such
studies is to use the graft as a means of treatment of
neurodegenerative diseases. Thus, the nigral graft in the
rat striatum is being used to study a model of parkinsonism,
and the cholinergic graft in rat neocortex is being used to
study a model of Alzheimer's disease. Both types of studies
have provided positive results so far. Parkinson-like
symptoms in rats are reduced by nigral transplants, while
cognitive deficits are reduced by grafting cholinergic
tissue. Studies were extended to using grafts in aged rats,
again with reported success (Gage et al., 1984).

One major criticism that can be raised against most studies involving behavioral recovery following grafting of neural tissue into the brain is the lack of knowledge concerning the possible incorporation of the grafted tissue into the host neural circuits. While every grafter likes to believe that the grafted tissue replaces the lost tissue and that is why functions recover, the evidence for this is far from being satisfactory. The following possibilities should be considered:

1. The mechanical effect -- The cavity produced by the lesion or by the preparatory operation for the grafting can be harmful and cause a collapse of adjacent tissue, degeneration of fiber tract, and other indirect effects. The mechanical support provided by the grafted tissue can facilitate restoration of functions of adjacent tissue. Perhaps, then, the actual transplant is not the causal factor.

2. The humoral effect -- The grafted tissue might secrete transiently a factor (some hormone or other substance) that would prevent retrograde degeneration of neurons projecting through the damaged area. This is indicated in studies using gelforam soaked in brain extracts, a procedure that appeared to be beneficial in restoring functions associated with the neocortex (Nieto-Sampedro, personal communication). In such a case, a transient action is sufficient and the grafted tissue can then degenerate and be absorbed by the host. A possibly similar case was illustrated in the septohippocampal system; injection of NGF into the lateral ventricle of fornix-transected rats protected cholinergic septal neurons from undergoing retrograde degeneration (Toniolo et al., 1985; Varon et al., 1987).

3. The neurotransmitter/modulator/hormone effect -- The grafted tissue might be accepted by the host brain, receive a blood supply and be alive. Nevertheless, the behavioral improvement may not be a result of the innervation of host neurons. It is possible that the grafted neurons release their neurotransmitter substance in a non-controlled manner and that the substances diffuse and activate remote receptor sites. This action is different from the more precise, synaptic action of a neurotransmitter. Such a case can be easily distinguished from the normal or completely reinnervated brain where the graft is totally

incorporated in the host. In the latter case, the functional recovery will depend on formation of extensive connections between the graft and the host, which will require at least several months to develop. In the former case, the recovery should be almost immediate, as soon as the cells recover from the grafting trauma and start releasing their neurotransmitter substances.

A confusion between these two cases is exemplified in the nigral graft in the striatum; the original studies demonstrated that the graft develops an extensive, dopaminergic fiber network in the host striatum over a period of several months (Stenevi et al., 1976; Perlow et al., 1979) and that a behavioral recovery is correlated with this. A more recent study on a primate model of parkinsonism (Sladek et al., 1987) demonstrated an immediate recovery of behavioral functions following grafting, indicating that the extensive fiber outgrowth is not relevant to the behavioral recovery. In cortical grafts, recovery can be detected several days to several months after grafting (Labbe et al., 1983; Arendash et al., 1985).

4. The full incorporation of the graft into the host-- To justify a claim for incorporation of a graft in the host circuit, one has to satisfy strict anatomical and physiological criteria. Anatomically, it should be shown that the grafted neurons are innervated by extrinsic afferent and that they innervate the host neurons in about the same locations normally innervated by these neurons. Also, it has to be shown at the ultrastructural level that these neurons make synapses on host neurons. When an intrinsic organization is expected, such as in laminated structures, it should be maintained in a graft. This can be seen both with cerebellar and hippocampal grafts (Raisman and Ebner, 1983; Alvarado-Mallart and Sotelo, 1982). Thus, these criteria have been met in at least some instances.

Physiologically, it must be shown that the grafted neurons receive input from the host brain akin to the normal input seen by the neurons, such that stimulation of host neurons will produce characteristic Ca_2 dependent post synaptic potentials in the grafted neurons. It has to be shown that the grafted neurons share same biophysical properties with their homotypic counterparts and have the same family of ionic conductances typical of normal cells. When stimulated, they produce postsynpatic responses to host neurons similar to those seen in the normal innervation of host neurons. A correlation between the anatomical, physiological and behavioral levels of recovery should be established. To the best of my knowledge, these criteria have not been met fully in any test system studied thus far.

Undoubtedly, several series of experiments using grafts for behavioral analysis of brain functions may have important theoretical implications if replicated and extended to include the necessary controls and graft criteria listed above. Examples include the description of self stimulation in nigral grafts (Fray et al., 1983). Self brain stimulation has been studied for over 30 years, yet the mechanisms underlying this phenomenon (as well as the brain regions involved) are far from being understood. If this observation is indeed replicated and strengthened, it will contribute enormously to the understanding of the phenomenon of self stimulation, as it can help to isolate the brain substrate for self stimulation. Likewise, if indeed grafts of cholinergic or cortical tissue into cortex produces behavioral recovery of function by incorporating into cortical circuitry, it will provide an extremely potent tool for the study of cortical plasticity. Unfortunately, the evidence for this is far from satisfactory. The fact that one can get fairly rapid recovery of functions along with the lack of convincing anatomical and physiological evidence for interconnections between the graft and the host make it unlikely that the recovery is due to the incorporation of the graft into the host networks.

Our attempts to correlate physiological and behavioral recovery subsequent to grafting of neural tissue involved the septohippocampal (Segal et al., 1985) and the raphe-hippocampal systems (Segal and Azmitia, 1986). Initially, we transected the fimbria-fornix where the cholinergic fibers travel into the hippocampus. Alternately, we lesioned the septal area, where these fibers originate. Several days later we dissected the septal area out of Day 16 embryos, minced them, and injected them into the denervated hippocampus. At various times after the injection, we tested the behavior of the rats in tasks including an open field and a water maze. Some of the rats were sacrificed and slices of their hippocampus were used for assessment of graft host interactions. Rats were implanted with recording electrodes for a quantitative assessment of their hippocampal EEG (Segal et al., 1987).

The results thus far indicate that within 4-6 months there is a nearly complete restoration of cholinergic innervation of the hippocampus as measured by intensity of acetylcholinesterase (AChE) staining of the host hippocampus (Fig. 1). This cannot originate from the regrowth of intrinsic cholinergic fibers as one could detect a gradient of intensity of AChE staining that centers in the graft area and diminishes away from the graft.

The studies with the slices indicated that grafted cells possessed some of the same properties as normal medial septal cells. Septal neurons characteristically show a high rate of spontaneous firing, even when they are disconnected from other neurons in the brain or slice. We have found similar spontaneously active cells while recording from grafted tissue. Further, electrical stimulation of the graft cells produces the same effect as topical application of ACH. Both produce voltage-dependent depolarization of target neurons in CA1. Moreover, the effect of electrical stimulation was enhanced by the cholinergic agonist, physostigmine, and blocked by atropine.

In studies with intact organisms, however, the electrophysiological findings were more difficult to interpret. Both septal and fornix lesions abolished the normal movement related pattern of hippocampal activity (theta rhythm). Despite a nearly normal-looking AChE staining in the hippocampus, we could not detect a restoration of normal hippocampal EEG in any of the grafted rats (Fig. 2). In fact, in some of them, an abnormal type of rhythm associated with arrest of motion was recorded. Such an effect has been seen by others (Bussaki et al., submitted). The absence of normal electrical activity in the presence of an apparently normal cholinergic reinnervation of the hippocampus indicates that acetylcholine might be necessary but certainly not sufficient to evoke the rhythmic activity, and that the entire circuitry responsible for generation of this rhythm has not recovered.

The behavioral deficits seen after a hippocampal lesion, fornix transection, or septal lesion involve inability to perform well in spatial memory tasks, as measured in a water maze (Morris, 1985). We found a differential effect of the graft on recovery from the deficit depending on the initial lesion; the graft

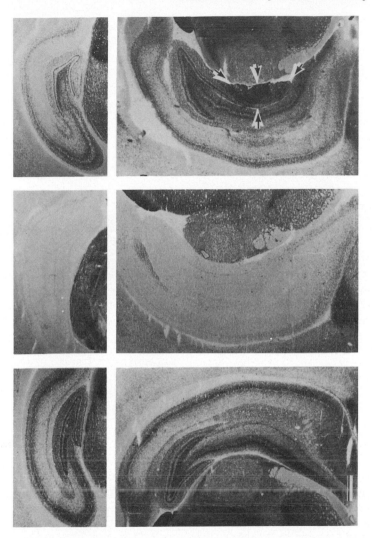

Figure 1. Acetylcholine-esterase (AChE) staining of normal
control hippocampus (bottom), fornix fimbria (FF) transected
(middle), and FF transected with septum-grafted hippocampus
(top). The animals were sacrificed three months after the
transplantation. The left row is of the dorsal hippocampus
and the right row of the main body of the hippocampus. The
transplant is marked with arrowheads at the level of the
main body of the hippocampus. Calibration bar 0.5 mm. Note
that the AChE staining did not reach the entire extent of
the dorsal hippocampus in the rat with the transplanted
tissue.

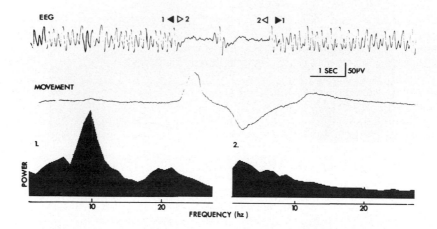

Figure 2. EEG recording from awake rat hippocampus. Top
record is a continuous chart record of the EEG. The rat
movement is depicted below the EEG record. Power spectra
of the EEG recorded during arrest (left) and movement
(right) are seen below. The rat was fornix-lesioned and
septum-grafted 4 months before recording. Unlike normal
rats, where hippocampal theta is associated with locomotion,
theta is associated with arrest in this rat (From Segal et
al., 1987).

ameliorated the initial deficit after a septal lesion but
not after a fornix transection, regardless of the magnitude
of AChE reinnervation. It appears that when the initial
damage is large enough to include efferent and afferents
fibre bundles that are not replaced by the grafted neurons,
the graft might be ineffective. If, on the other hand, the
lesion is restricted to the nucleus where the cholinergic
fibers arise, there is a good chance of recovery.

Prospects for Neural Grafting

    The initial wave of studies on brain grafts and neural
plasticity is over. These studies are encouraging in that
they illustrate that grafting can correct behavioral

deficits. It is not generally clear whether the recovery
results from incorporation of the grafted tissue into the
host brain circuits or whether the graft somehow facilitates
restoration of functions of the remaining host brain tissue.
Parametric studies are still needed to determine the
relevance of the age of the graft, the source of the tissue
and its placement, and the roles of facilitating factors on
behavioral recovery. More information is needed to confirm
that the graft is integrated into the host tissue
morphologically and physiologically. It should ultimately
prove possible to use an analysis of behavioral recovery
following grafting to further our understanding of the role
of neural structures and circuits in behavior.

REFERENCES

Alvarado-Mallart RM, Sotelo C (1982). Differentiation of
cerebellar anlage heterotopically transplanted to adult
rat brain: a light and electron microscopic study. J
Comp Neurol 212:247-267.
Arendash GW, Strong PN, Mouton PR (1985). Intracerebral
transplantation of cholinergic neurons in a new animal
model for alzheimer's disease. In "Senile Dementia of the
Alzheimer's Type," New York: Alan R. Liss, pp 351-376.
Backlund EO, Granberg PO, Hamberger B, Sedvall G, Seiger A,
Olson L (1985). Transplantation of adrenal medullary
tissue to striatum in parkinsonism. In Bjorklund A,
Stenevi U (eds): "Neural Grafting in the Mammalian CNS,"
New York: Elsevier, pp 551-558.
Bjorklund A, Stenevi U (1977). Reformation of the severed
septohippocampal cholinergic pathway in the adult rat by
transplanted septal neurons. Cell Tiss Res 185:289-302.
Bjorklund A, Stenevi U, Svendgaard NA (1976). Growth of
transplanted monoaminergic neurons into the adult
hippocampus along the perforant path. Nature 262:787-790.
Buzsaki G, Gage FH, Czopt J, Bjorklund A (submitted).
Restoration of rhythmic slow activity (theta) in the
subcortically denervated hippocampus by fetal CNS
transplants.
Corkin S, Davis KL, Growdon JH, Usdin E, Wurtman RJ (1982).
Alzheimer's disease: a report of progress in research.
New York: Raven Press.
Deckel WA, Robinson RG, Coyle JT, Sandberg PR (1983).
Reversal of long term locomotor abnormalities in the kainic

acid model of huntington's disease by day 18 fetal
striatal implants. Eur J Pharmacol 93:287-288.

Dunnett SB, Low CW, Iversen SD, Stenevi U, Bjorklund A
(1982). Septal transplants restore maze learning in rats
with fornix fimbria lesions. Brain Res 251:335-348.

Dunnett SB, Toniolo G, Fine A, Ryan CN, Bjorklund A,
Iversen SD (1985). Transplantation of embryonic ventral
forebrain neurons to the neocortex of rats with lesions
of nucleus basalis magnocellularis II sensorimotor and
learning impairments. Neuroscience 16:787-797.

Fine A, Dunnett SB, Bjorklund A, Clarke D, Iversen SD
(1985). Transplantation of embryonic ventral forebrain
neurons to the neocortex of rats with lesions of nucleus
basalis magnocellularis 1. biochemical and anatomical
observations. Neuroscience 16:769-786.

Fray PJ, Dunnett SB, Iversen SD, Bjorklund A, Stenevi U
(1983). Nigral transplants reinnervating the dopamine-
depleted neostriatum can sustain intracranial self
stimulation. Science 219:416-419.

Freed WJ (1983). Functional brain tissue transplantation:
Reversal of lesion-induced rotation by intraventricular
substantia nigra and adrenal medulla grafts, with a note
on intracranial retinal grafts. Biological Psychiatry
18:1205-1267.

Frotscher M, Zimmer J (1986). Intracerebral transplants of
the rat fascia dentata: a golgi/electron microscope study
of dentate granular cells. J Comp Neurol 246:181-190.

Gage FH, Bjorklund A, Stenevi U, Dunnett SB, Kelly PTA
(1984). Intrahippocampal septal grafts ameliorate
learning impairments in aged rats. Science 225:533-636.

Gash DM, Scott DE (1980). Fetal hypothalamic transplants
in the third ventricle of the adult rat brain.
Correlative scanning and transmission electron microscopy.
Cell Tissue Res 211:191-206.

Gash DM, Sladek JR, Sladek CD (1980). Functional development
of grafted vasopressin neurons. Science 210:1367-1369.

Hounsgaard J, Yarom Y (1985). Cellular physiology of
transplanted neurons. In Bjorklund A, Stenevi U (eds):
"Neural Grafting in the Mammalian CNS," New York:
Elsevier, pp 401-408.

Kimble DP, Bremiller R, Stickrod G (1986). Fetal brain
implants improve maze performance in hippocampal lesioned
rats. Brain Res 363:358-363.

Labbe R, Firl A, Mufson EJ, Stein DG (1983). Fetal rat
brain transplants: reduction of cognitive deficits in rats
with frontal cortex lesions. Science 221:470-472.

Low WC, Lewis RP, Terri-Bunch S, Dunnett SB, Thomas SR, Iversen SD, Bjorklund A, Stenevi U (1982). Function recovery following neural transplantation of embryonic septal nuclei in adult rats with septohippocampal lesions. Nature 300:260-262.

Lynch G, Matthews DA, Mosco S, Parks T, Cotman C (1972). Induced acetylcholinesterase-rich layer in the rat dentate gyrus following entohinal lesions. Brain Res 42:311-318.

McRae-Degueurce A, Bellin SI, Serrano A, Landas SK, Wilkin LD, Scatton B, Johnson AK (1985). Behavioral and neurochemical models to investigate functional recovery with transplants. In Bjorklund A, Stenevi U (eds): "Neural Grafting in the Mammalian CNS," New York: Elsevier, pp 431-436.

Morris R (1984). Developments of a water maze procedure for studying spatial learning in the rat. J Neurosci Methods 11:47-60.

Nieto-Sampedro M, Lewis ER, Cotman CW, Manthorpe M, Skaper SD, Barbin G, Longo FM, Varon S (1982). Brain injury causes a time-dependent increase in neuronotrophic activity at the lesion site. Science 217:860-861.

Perlow MF, Freed WF, Hoffer BJ, Seiger A, Olson L, Wyatt RJ (1979). Brain grafts reduced motor abnormalities produced by destruction of nigrostriatal dopamine system. Science 204:643-647.

Raisman G (1969). Neuronal plasticity in the septal nuclei of the adult rat. Brain Res 14:25-48.

Raisman G, Ebner FF (1983). Mossy fibre projections into and out of hippocampal transplants. Neuroscience 9: 783-801.

Raisman G, Lawrence JM, Zhou CF, Lindsay RM (1985). Some neuronal, glial and vascular interactions which occur when developing hippocampal primordia are incorporated into adult host hippocampi. In Bjorklund A, Stenevi U (eds): "Neural Grafting in the Mammalian CNS," New York: Elsevier, pp 125-150.

Segal M, Azmitia EC (1986). Fetal raphe neurons grafted into the hippocampus develop normal adult physiological properties. Brain Res 364:162-166.

Segal M, Bjorklund A, Gage FH (1985). Transplanted septal neurons make viable cholinergic synapses with a host hippocampus. Brain Res 336:302-307.

Segal M, Greenberger V, Milgram NW (1987). A functional analysis of connections between grafted septal neurons and a host hippocampus. Progress in Brain Res (in press).

Sladek JR Jr, Redmond E, Roth RH, Collier TJ, Elsworth JD,

Deutch A, Haber SN (1987). Fetal nigral grafts can
reverse parkinsonian symptoms in MPTP lesioned monkeys.
Proc NY Acad Sci (in press).

Stein D (1987). Behavioral effects of intracortical grafts
in rats with lesion-induced cognitive deficits. Proc NY
Acad Sci (in press).

Stenevi U, Bjorklund A, Svendgaard NA (1976).
Transplantation of central and peripheral monoamine
neurons to the adult rat brain: Techniques and conditions
for survival. Brain Res 114:1-20.

Toniolo G, Dunnett SB, Hefti F, Will B (1985).
Acetylcholine-rich transplants in the hippocampus:
influence of intrinsic growth factors and application of
nerve growth factor on choline acetyltransferase activity.
Brain Res 345:141-146.

Varon S, Williams LR, Gage FH (1987). Exogenous
administration of neurotrophic factors in vivo projects
CNS neurons against axotomy-induced degeneration. In
Seil FJ (eds): "Neural Regeneration. Progress in Brain
Research," New York: Elsevier (in press).

Zimmer J (1971). Ipsilateral afferents to the commissural
zone of the fascia dentata, demonstrated in decomissurated
rats by silver impregnation. J Comp Neural 142:393-409.

Zhou F, Auerbach S, Azmitia E (1987). Prior 5,7-DHT lesions
in fornix enhances growth of raphe 5-HT transplants but
not locus coeruleus NE transplants. Proc NY Acad Sci (in
press).

Neuroplasticity, Learning, and Memory, pages 279–300
© 1987 Alan R. Liss, Inc.

DISSOCIABLE FORMS OF MEMORY IN COLLEGE STUDENTS, ELDERLY
INDIVIDUALS, AND PATIENTS WITH ANTEROGRADE AMNESIA:
IMPLICATIONS FROM RESEARCH ON DIRECT PRIMING

Peter Graf

Department of Psychology,
University of Toronto,
Toronto, Ontario, M5S 1A1

In recent years, a growing number of studies of normal
human memory, aging and memory, and memory dysfunction in
patients with anterograde amnesia have converged on a
distinction between two forms of memory. We have labeled
these explicit and implicit memory, respectively (Graf and
Schacter, 1985). Explicit memory refers to performance on
standard memory tests, such as free recall, cued recall, and
recognition. On these tests, subjects are explicitly
instructed to retrieve items from a specific prior episode
and performance thus reflects an intentional or explicit use
of memory. In contrast, implicit memory refers to
performance on priming tests, such as word completion, word
identification, and lexical decision. On these tests, the
instructions make no reference to a specific study episode
and performance thus reflects an unintentional or implicit
use of memory. Performance effects on the latter tests are
generally known as direct or repetition priming effects.

The importance of a distinction between explicit and
implicit memory is underlined by a growing amount of evidence
that performance on explicit memory tests can become
dissociated from performance on implicit memory tests. To
illustrate, experiments with college students have shown
that in contrast to the well-known finding that "levels of
processing" manipulations affect performance on explicit
memory tests (for review see Cermak and Craik, 1979), these
manipulations have a minimal effect or no effect on implicit
memory tests (e.g., Graf and Mandler, 1984; Graf, Mandler,
and Haden, 1982; Jacoby and Dallas, 1981). Studies on
memory and aging have shown that whereas performance on

explicit memory tests declines with increasing age of
subjects, implicit memory shows no age effects (e.g., Graf
and Schacter, 1985; Light and Anderson, 1983; Rabinowitz,
1986; for review see Craik, 1983). It has also been
demonstrated that patients with anterograde amnesia can show
entirely normal performance on implicit memory tests (e.g.,
Cohen and Squire, 1980; Graf, Squire, and Mandler, 1984;
Squire, Shimamura, and Graf, 1985; Warrington and
Weiskrantz, 1968, 1970), despite having severe deficits on
explicit memory tests that have long been viewed as the
hallmark of their condition (Cermak, 1982; Rozin, 1976;
Talland, 1968; Wechsler, 1917). Together, these and similar
findings highlight important differences between explicit
and implicit memory that must be considered by general
theories of "normal" human memory, by theories about aging
and memory, and by theories of memory dysfunction in amnesic
patients.

Several interpretations that have been offered for
performance dissociations have postulated a difference in
the nature of the representations that underlie explicit and
implicit memory. One widespread interpretation known as the
activation view holds that priming effects are mediated by
the activation of pre-existing representations in long-term
memory, whereas explicit memory effects are mediated by
representations that are newly acquired during the study
trial (e.g., Graf and Mandler, 1984; Graf et al., 1982;
Mandler, 1980; Rozin, 1976). In most previous experiments,
subjects studied familiar items, such as individual words,
that were represented in long-term memory prior to their
appearance in the study list. It was assumed that these
pre-existing representations are activated automatically in
the course of processing the study list items, and that this
activation occurs independently of other processes that are
necessary for explicit remembering. By this view, what
underlies the intact implicit memory test performance of
elderly individuals and of amnesic patients is the process
by which pre-existing representations are activated in
long-term memory (e.g., Graf et al., 1984; Rozin, 1976;
Warrington and Weiskrantz, 1982).

Direct support for an activation view comes from the
finding that even severely amnesic patients can show normal
priming for familiar words and related word pairs (e.g.,
TABLE - CHAIR), but show no priming for new items, such as
the unfamiliar pseudoword NUMDY (e.g., Diamond and Rozin,

1984). The latter finding is expected by an activation view because in contrast to words and related pairs, pseudowords have no pre-existing representations in long-term memory that can be activated during the study trial. Indirect support for this view comes from the common observation that it is primarily the ability for new learning that is impaired in elderly individuals and in amnesic patients (see Craik, 1977; Rozin, 1976; Talland, 1968). Nevertheless, the literature does contain scattered reports of implicit memory for new items, such as pairs of unrelated words, that have no pre-existing long-term memory representations (e.g., McKoon and Ratcliff, 1979; Moscovitch, 1984; Salasoo, Shiffrin, and Feustel, 1985; Schacter, Harbluk, and McLachlan, 1984). Because there is no pre-existing representation that can be activated during the study trial, priming for new items must be mediated by other processes. What is the nature of these processes? What is the relation between the processes that mediate priming for old items and priming for new items? Are the processes that mediate priming for new items spared in elderly individuals and in patients with anterograde amnesia?

In an attempt to answer these and related questions, this chapter reviews a series of experiments that examined priming for new items. In these experiments, subjects studied pairs of normatively unrelated words, such as DRYER – BLOCK, that do not have pre-existing representations as pairs in long-term memory. Implicit memory was tested with a completion test that presented word stems (e.g., BLO_____) and required subjects to complete each stem with the first word that came to mind. On this test, priming is revealed by the finding that recently presented words are more likely to be written as completions than nonpresented words. Of primary interest was whether completion test performance would be affected by memory for newly acquired associations between words that were paired on a single study trial. Two normatively unrelated words do not have a pre-existing representation as a pair that can be activated; any associations between them must be established during the study trial. By an activation view, performance on a word completion test should not be affected by these newly acquired associations. To the extent that completion performance is affected, it would suggest that priming is mediated, at least in part, by processes other than activation of pre-existing representations.

IMPLICIT MEMORY FOR NEW ASSOCIATIONS

Demonstration Experiments. The aim of the first
experiment was twofold: first, to examine whether
completion test performance is sensitive to memory for newly
acquired associations between unrelated words and, second,
to examine whether this type of memory occurs automatically.
College students were presented with pairs of normatively
unrelated words (e.g., DRYER - BLOCK) and were then given a
completion test, followed by a cued recall test. For the
completion test, subjects were presented the initial three
letters -- the stems -- of the right-hand or target words
from the study list pairs and instructed to complete the
stems with the first words that came to mind. To assess
whether completion performance is affected by memory for new
associations, some stems appeared on the test together with
the same left-hand or cue words as in the study list (e.g.,
DRYER - BLO_____) [same context test-items], and some stems
appeared together with other cue words (e.g., FLAG -
BLO_____) or alone (e.g., BLO_____) [different context
test-items]. The completion test also included the stems of
non-presented or new words; these stems were used to obtain
an index of chance or baseline performance. It was expected
that the proportion of studied words that subjects write as
completions would be higher than baseline on both same and
different context test-items; this finding would provide
evidence for a word priming effect. To the extent that
completion performance is facilitated primarily by word
priming, a similar level of performance was expected on same
and different context test-items. However, to the extent
that completion performance is also affected by memory for
newly acquired associations, a higher level of performance
was expected on same context test-items than on different
context items.

Thirty-two college students were assigned to two groups
of 16 each. The groups were given different study tasks
that involved either constructing sentences for paired words
or comparing the vowels of paired words. For the sentence
construction task, subjects were presented with cue-target
pairs (e.g., DRYER - BLOCK) and required to construct a
simple sentence that related the two words from each pair in
a meaningful manner (e.g., The clothes DRYER was standing on
a wooden BLOCK). For the vowel comparison task, subjects
were required to decide (Yes/No) whether the two words from
each pair had the same number of vowels. Each subject

studied a list of 32 unrelated cue-target pairs and, then,
following a brief (5 min) filler task, implicit memory was
assessed with a word completion test. Immediately
afterwards, a cued recall test was given in which the cue
words from the study list pairs were provided (e.g., DRYER)
and subjects were required to recollect the words that were
paired with them in the study list. Consistent with
previous reports, a higher level of cued recall was expected
following the sentence construction task than the vowel
comparison task (Graf, 1982).

The mean levels of completion test performance are
shown in Table 1. Three aspects of the results are
noteworthy. First, priming occurred for all test-items, as
revealed by the finding that studied words were produced as
completions more often than baseline words. Second, for the
different context test-items, similar proportions of studied
words were produced as completions after the sentence
construction task (.23) and vowel comparison task (.21).
This finding, which reflects a word priming effect, is
consistent with previous reports that word priming is
comparable across study tasks that engage different levels
of processing (e.g., Graf and Mandler, 1984; Jacoby and
Dallas, 1981). Third, and most important, completion
performance was substantially higher on same context text-
items than on different context items, but this occurred
only following the sentence construction task. The finding
of an associative influence on performance which provides
evidence of memory for newly acquired associations is not
consistent with an activation view of priming. The finding
that this associative influence occurred only following the
sentence construction task and not following the vowel
comparison task suggests that implicit memory for new

TABLE 1. Completion Test Performance as a Function of Study
Task and Test Context (from Graf and Schacter, 1985,
Experiment 1)

Study Task	Type of Completion Test Items	
	Same Context	Different Context
Sentence Construction	.50	.23
Vowel Comparison	.22	.21
Baseline	.12	

associations does not occur automatically, but depends on some form of elaborative processing during the study trial.

Recall test performance was higher following the sentence construction task (.35) than following the vowel comparison task (.02). This finding is consistent with previous demonstrations that explicit memory is dependent on tasks, such as sentence construction, that involve some form of elaborative processing of to-be-remembered materials (for review see Cermak and Craik, 1979).

The main observation from these findings concerns the relation between implicit and explicit memory for new associations. An abundance of previous experiments have shown that explicit memory increases directly with degree of elaborative processing during study (for review see Cermak and Craik, 1979). Consequently, the present finding that implicit memory for new associations occurred only following an elaborative study task raises the possibility that implicit and explicit memory for new associations depend on new representations that are established as a result of engaging the same elaborative processes during the study trial.

Additional evidence that suggests a dependence between the processes that establish the representations that underlie explicit and implicit memory for new associations comes from two further experiments with college students. These experiments were designed to examine what types of elaborative processing are required to obtain implicit memory for new associations. In the first experiment (Schacter and Graf, 1986), subjects were presented with unrelated word pairs, and they either performed the sentence construction task as in the previous experiment, or they rated the pleasantness of the individual words in each pair. The latter task was used to determine whether semantic/elaborative processing of the individual words from the study list pairs would be sufficient to produce implicit memory for new associations. The results were similar to those from the preceding experiment: Completion test performance showed an associative influence following the sentence construction task, but not following the word pleasantness rating task. The latter task produced a comparable amount of priming on the same and different context test-items. Explicit memory also replicated the results from the preceding experiment by showing a significantly higher level of cued recall after the sentence construction task than after the word pleasantness rating task. The second experiment examined whether implicit memory for new associations depends on processing paired words in a meaningful relation to each other. For this purpose, subjects were presented sentences in which two unrelated words were linked either in a meaningful manner (e.g., the clothes DRYER was standing on a wooden BLOCK) or in an anomalous manner (e.g., the grazing DRYER read the BLOCK). During study, subjects read each sentence aloud and rated the extent to which the two capitalized words were related to each other by the sentence in which they occurred. Subsequent cued recall was significantly higher for the pairs from the meaningful sentences than for the pairs from the anomalous sentences. On the word completion test, there was an associative influence on performance for the pairs from the meaningful sentences but not for the pairs from the anomalous sentences. Therefore, based on the findings from the studies described this far, it appears that implicit memory for new associations occurs only with study tasks that involve some form of elaborative processing in which paired words are related to each other in a meaningful manner. Previous work has revealed that this type of processing also determines performance on tests of explicit memory.

Age and Amnesia. The finding that implicit memory for new associations depends on some form of elaborative processing during the study trial has implications for understanding memory dysfunctions in elderly individuals and in patients with anterograde amnesia. An impairment in the ability to perform tests that depend on prior elaborative processing (i.e., explicit memory tests) has long been viewed as the hallmark of memory in elderly individuals and in amnesic patients (e.g., Rozin, 1976; Talland, 1968). Thus, in view of the finding that implicit memory for new associations depends on prior elaborative processing, one might expect that this type of memory would also be impaired in elderly individuals and in amnesic patients. This possibility was examined in the next experiment.

Three types of subjects participated in this experiment: a group of 12 patients with organic anterograde amnesia, a group of 12 age-matched control subjects, and a group of 24 college students. These groups, which have been described in detail elsewhere (Graf and Schacter, 1985), averaged 42, 47, and 22 years of age, respectively. The amnesic patients were of mixed etiologies and their only notable cognitive deficit was on tests of explicit memory. In the study phase of the experiment, all subjects were presented with 12 pairs of unrelated words and required to construct a meaningful sentence for each pair. After a brief (5 min) filler task, a word completion test was given, followed by a cued recall test.

The mean levels of performance on the completion test are presented in Table 2. First, the proportion of words that was produced in the baseline condition was comparable across all subject groups. Second, there was evidence of priming in all subject groups and experimental conditions as indicated by the finding that the completion rate was higher for studied words than for words in the baseline condition. Third, a higher proportion of studied words was produced as completions on same context test-items (.33) than on different context items (.20); this finding provides evidence for an associative influence on performance. Fourth, and most important, the size of this associative influence on performance was comparable across subject groups (.14, .11, and .12 for the amnesic, age-matched, and student subjects, respectively). These findings stand in sharp contrast to the results from the cued recall test, where performance averaged .02, .35, and .64 for the amnesic, age-matched, and student groups, respectively. The latter findings replicate the severe memory performance deficit that has long been viewed as the hallmark of amnesia (Rozin, 1976; Wechsler, 1917), and they show the decrease in performance that is characteristic of memory in elderly individuals (see Craik, 1977; Talland, 1968).

TABLE 2. Completion Test Performance across Subject Groups (from Graf and Schacter, 1985, Experiment 2)

Subject Group	Type of Test Item	
	Same Context	Different Context
Amnesic	.32	.18
Age-matched	.32	.21
Student	.34	.22
Baseline	.13	

The combined pattern of findings from this and the preceding experiments present a challenging interpretive puzzle. On the one hand, it appears that both implicit and explicit memory for new associations depend on elaborative processing during the study trial. This is implied by the finding that performance on both word completion and cued recall tests showed evidence of an associative effect only following study tasks that required subjects to process paired words by relating them in a meaningful manner. On the other hand, the findings from amnesic patients and elderly subjects, whose performance on explicit memory tests was impaired relative to college students, revealed a normal level of performance on a test of implicit memory. The puzzle is this: If elaborative processing is necessary to establish the representations that underlie both explicit and implicit memory for new associations, and if elderly individuals and amnesic patients have an impaired ability to benefit from elaborative processing on tests of explicit memory, what enables them to show normal implicit memory for new associations?

Types of Elaboration. We do not yet have a solution for this puzzle. However, one possibility was suggested by the findings from several related experiments that are described in the following two sections. One experiment examined the relation between different types or degrees of elaborative processing during the study trial and its effects on implicit and explicit memory for new associations. For this purpose, normal college students studied pairs of unrelated words in two different conditions: sentence construction and sentence rating. As in the preceding experiments, the first of these tasks required subjects to construct a meaningful sentence for each study list pair. For the sentence rating task, each word pair was embedded in a meaningful sentence (e.g., The clothes DRYER was standing on a wooden BLOCK). The critical words were printed in capital letters and subjects were required to rate how well the sentence related these words. After a brief (5 min) filler task, memory was assessed with either a completion test or a cued recall test. Previously, it has been suggested that a task such as sentence construction involves a higher degree of elaboration of study materials than a task such as sentence rating (e.g., Graf, 1982) and, thus, a higher level of explicit memory was expected with the sentence construction task. The critical question is whether this manipulation of type or degree of elaboration has a similar effect on implicit memory.

For this and subsequent experiments, we used exactly
the same test form to assess explicit and implicit memory.
This test form showed word-stems, either paired with the
same words as in the study list (e.g., DRYER - BLO_____)
[same context test-items] or paired with different words
(e.g., WINDOW - BLO_____) [different context test-items].
When it was used for completion testing, this form was given
with the instructions simply to complete the stems with the
first words that come to mind; when it was used for cued
recall, subjects were told about the composition of the
test-items and instructed to use these items as aids for
remembering words from the study list. The main advantage
of using the same form for both tests is that it is possible
to compare directly the extent to which newly acquired
associations affect explicit and implicit memory.

Table 3 shows the main findings for each test. For
implicit memory, the overall completion rate was higher for
studied words (.25) than for baseline words (.11). A higher
proportion of studied words was produced as completions on
the same context test-items (.33) than on the different
(.18) context items; this indicates that performance was
affected by memory for newly acquired associations between
unrelated words. More important, the size of this
associative influence on performance was similar for the
sentence construction task (.16) and for the sentence rating
task (.15). This finding suggests that the type or degree
of elaborative processing that is required by different
study tasks has no effect on implicit memory for newly
acquired associations.

The main recall test results are shown at the bottom of
Table 3. Overall recall was higher after the sentence
construction task (.48) than after the sentence rating task
(.33). This finding replicates the results of previous
studies (e.g., Graf, 1982) and, thus, attests to the
effectiveness of the task manipulation. Recall was also
affected by the test context manipulation, as revealed by
the overall higher performance on same (.47) than different
(.34) context test-items. However, as indicated by the
tabled means, recall showed an associative influence on
performance only following the sentence construction task
(.60 and .35, respectively, for same and different context
test-items) and not following the sentence rating task (.34

and .32, respectively, for same and different context test-items). In combination, therefore, these findings indicate that explicit memory for new associations is affected by different types or degrees of elaboration, but that implicit memory for new associations is not affected by such manipulations.

TABLE 3. Completion and Cued Recall Test Performance as a Function of Study Task and Test Context (from Schacter and Graf, 1986, Experiment 2)

Completion Test Performance:

Study Task	Type of Test Item	
	Same Context	Different Context
Sentence Construction	.35	.19
Sentence Rating	.31	.16
Baseline	.11	

Cued Recall Test Performance:

Study Task	Type of Test Item	
	Same Context	Different Context
Sentence Construction	.60	.35
Sentence Rating	.34	.32

Associative Interference. Related experiments examined the effects of another variable -- associative interference -- that is known to have a pronounced influence on explicit memory for new associations (e.g., Barnes and Underwood, 1959; McGovern, 1964; Postman and Stark, 1969). Interference manipulations are known to decrease performance on explicit memory tests, in contrast to elaboration manipulations which increase explicit remembering. We used a retroactive interference paradigm for one experiment (Graf and Schacter, in press). For this purpose, subjects were shown pairs of unrelated words (e.g., WINDOW - FORMULA) and they generated a meaningful sentence for each pair. In the interference condition, the cue words from each critical pair also occurred in five other pairs (e.g., WINDOW - POCKET, WINDOW - DINNER, WINDOW - FATHER, WINDOW - DRINK, WINDOW - FRIEND). In the control condition, each critical pair appeared only once in the study list and neither of its

words appeared in any other pairs. Memory was tested either
with a word completion test or with a cued recall test,
exactly as described in the preceding experiment.

TABLE 4. Completion and Cued Recall Test Performance as a
Function of Study Task and Test Context (from Graf and
Schacter, in press, Experiment 1)

Completion Test Performance:

Study Task	Type of Test Item	
	Same Context	Different Context
Interference	.35	.21
Control	.32	.18
Baseline	.10	

Cued Recall Test Performance:

Study Task	Type of Test Item	
	Same Context	Different Context
Interference	.45	.26
Control	.67	.31

The mean levels of performance are shown in Table 4.
Two findings are noteworthy. First, performance on both
word completion and cued recall tests was higher on same
context test-items than on different context items; this
indicates that both tests were sensitive to memory for newly
acquired associations. Second, and more important, there
was no evidence of an interference effect on the word
completion test but, as expected, cued recall was
significantly impaired by the interference manipulation.
Similar patterns of results have been found with proactive
interference manipulations, as well as when different tests
(e.g., pair matching, modified-modified free recall) were
used to assess explicit memory (Graf and Schacter, in
press). This combination of findings suggests that standard
interference manipulations affect primarily explicit but not
implicit memory for new associations.

A PRELIMINARY HYPOTHESIS

The preceding experiments provide several clues about
the influence of associative elaboration and interference on
implicit and explicit memory for new associations. To
summarize, the findings revealed, first, that both implicit
and explicit memory for new associations are mediated by
representations that are established as a result of
elaborative processing during the study trial; second, that
implicit memory for new associations can be manipulated
independently of explicit memory for new associations by
means of study tasks that involve different types or degrees
of elaborative processing; third, that these forms of memory
can be dissociated by tasks that produce associative
interference. To account for these observations, and for
the puzzling finding of related performance dissociations in
elderly individuals and in amnesic patients (see Table 2),
we have hypothesized that explicit and implicit memory for
new associations are mediated by different components of the
representations of newly acquired word pairs (Graf and
Schacter, 1986, in press; Schacter and Graf, 1986).

These representational components can be envisaged in
terms of a distributed feature set (cf. Hinton and Anderson,
1981; Knapp and Anderson, 1984). Consider a set of features
that represents all aspects of a word pair that were
processed during the study trial: Some features represent
perceptual and conceptual aspects of the individual words,
some features represent perceptual and conceptual aspects of
the two words as a pair, and some features represent
perceptual and conceptual aspects of the experimental
environment. We have speculated that only a subset of all
of these features -- specifically those that represent the
perceptual and conceptual aspects of the two words as a
pair -- is relevant for implicit memory for new associations.
For convenience, in the remainder of this chapter, the
phrase pair representation will be used to describe this
subset of features that represents two words as a pair; the
entire feature set which includes this subset and also
features related to a specific experimental environment will
be described as the episodic representation of a study list
pair. Similar distinctions between representational
components have been suggested by other investigators (e.g.,
Humphreys, 1978; Mandler, 1980; Wickelgren, 1979).

We have assumed that pair representations are

established as a result of processing two words in a
meaningful relation to each other, and that processing the
same words in relation to other study list pairs and
environmental cues ensures that episodic representations are
larger than and/or different from pair representations.
Based on these assumptions, the episodic representation of a
study list pair may change in terms of distinctiveness
depending on the extensiveness of processing environmental
cues and relations with other pairs in the study list; this
may account for the finding that different types of
elaborative study tasks affected explicit memory for new
associations in the preceding experiments. The
distinctiveness of a pair's episodic representation can
decrease when features related to the same environmental
cues are included in the episodic representations of several
different study list pairs; this might occur, for example,
in an associative interference experiment of the sort
described in the preceding pages (cf. Graf and Schacter, in
press). Previously, it has been argued that the more
distinctive the representation of an item in memory, the
greater the probability of its subsequent retrieval (e.g.,
Eysenck, 1979; Jacoby and Craik, 1979).

The assumption that only a subset of the features of a
pair's episodic representation, that is, its pair
representation, is relevant to implicit memory for new
associations is plausible in view of the performance
requirements of implicit memory tests. Consider, for
example, that a word completion test presents subjects with
test items (e.g., WINDOW – FOR_____) that must be completed
with the first words that come to mind. Under these
conditions, an associative influence on performance is
expected to the extent that the completion for a stem (e.g.,
FOREST) is associated with its cue (e.g., WINDOW). More
specifically, because the test does not require retrieval
from a particular study episode, it is assumed that an
associative influence on performance is mediated primarily
by activation of features that represent perceptual and
conceptual aspects of two words as a pair, and does not
involve activation of features related to a specific study
environment. In contrast, explicit memory tests, such as
cued recall, require subjects to remember items from a
specific prior study episode. It is assumed that under
these conditions, an associative influence on performance is
mediated by activation of both features that represent
aspects of two words as a pair and features that represent

aspects of the study environment. In short, the different performance requirements of implicit and explicit memory tests suggest that implicit memory for new associations is mediated primarily by pair representations, whereas explicit memory is mediated by episodic representations.

A recent experiment tested this hypothesis about memory for newly acquired associations. In this experiment, implicit and explicit memory for new associations were compared across two tasks: One task involved extensive processing of the relation between the pairs in the study list and the other task involved relatively little of this type of processing. For this purpose, subjects were presented with 24 meaningful sentences, each of which contained a pair of unrelated words printed in capital letters. This list of sentences was presented twice. For the first pass through the list, subjects were required to rate each sentence in terms of how well it related the capitalized words; this task was assumed to entail primarily processing of two words as a pair and, thus, result in the construction of pair representations. For the second pass through the list, subjects were required to sort the sentences into 4 groups either on the basis of their semantic content (theme sort) or on the basis of number of words (length sort). These two sorting tasks were assumed to require different degrees of elaborative processing of relations among sentences and, thus, to establish episodic representations for the pairs that have either a high degree of distinctiveness (theme sort) or a low degree of distinctiveness (length sort). Memory was tested with a completion test and a cued recall test.

The main findings are shown in Table 5. Performance on both completion and cued recall tests was higher on same context test-items than on different context test-items; this indicates that both tests were sensitive to memory for newly acquired associations. The critical new finding is that the theme sort task produced a higher level of cued recall performance than the length sort task, but this task manipulation had no effect on completion test performance. This pattern of findings was expected; it provides strong evidence for the view that explicit and implicit memory for new associations are mediated by representational components -- pair and episodic representations, respectively -- that are established by different types of elaborative processing during the study trial.

TABLE 5. Completion and Cued Recall Test Performance as a
Function of Study Task and Test Context (from Graf and
Schacter, 1986, Experiment 1)

Completion Test Performance:

Study Task	Type of Test Item	
	Same Context	Different Context
Theme Sort	.43	.24
Length Sort	.39	.26
Baseline	.10	

Cued Recall Test Performance:

Study Task	Type of Test Item	
	Same Context	Different Context
Theme Sort	.83	.42
Length Sort	.60	.26

PRIMING FOR NEW AND OLD ITEMS

At the beginning of this chapter, a number of questions
were raised about the nature of the processes that mediate
explicit and implicit memory for new associations, about how
these processes are related to those that mediate implicit
memory for old items that have pre-existing representations
in long-term memory, and about the sparing of these
processes in amnesic patients and in elderly individuals.
The proposal that implicit and explicit memory for new
associations are mediated by different representational
components (pair and episodic representations, respecitvely)
that are newly established as a result of different types of
elaboration during the study trial offers only a partial
answer to these questions. An attempt to provide a more
complete answer is outlined in the final section of this
chapter.

This section addresses the following findings: First,
and most important, that priming for new items (new items is
used as a short-hand label for new associations) occurs only
with study tasks that require some form of elaborative
processing during the study trial, whereas priming for old
items occurs independently of the type or degree of
elaborative processing (see Graf and Mandler, 1984; Graf and

Schacter, 1985; Jacoby and Dallas, 1981; Schacter and Graf, 1986); second, that priming for both new and old items is independent of the type or degree of elaborative processing that is engaged by different study tasks (Graf and Schacter, 1986; Schacter and Graf, 1986); third, that both types of priming occur normally in elderly individuals and in amnesic patients (e.g., Graf and Schacter, 1985; Graf, Squire, and Mandler, 1984). This combination of findings can be readily accommodated by a modified version of an activation view of priming.

Activation views for priming of old items that have pre-existing representations in long-term memory have been proposed by several authors (cf. Graf and Mandler, 1984; Mandler, 1980; Morton, 1979; Rozin, 1976; Wickelgren, 1979). One view has highlighted the role of two memory organizing processes: integration and elaboration (Graf and Mandler, 1984; Graf et al., 1982; Mandler, 1980), the effects of which can be envisaged in terms of a distributed feature set (cf. Hinton and Anderson, 1981; Knapp and Anderson, 1984). Consider a set of features that represents all possible -- that is, all previously relevant -- aspects of an item. Integration refers to the coherence among these features and is related to the probability that when some features are activated, they will preferentially activate other features in the set. Elaboration refers to the richness and complexity of an item's representation which is defined by the nature and number of its features and by its associations with other mental contents.

According to this view, priming for an old item occurs as a result of an increase in the integration of its representation; a representation increases its level of integration when a subset of its features is simultaneously activated (McClelland and Rumelhart, 1985; Rumelhart and McClelland, 1982). As a consequence, when part of a recently studied item, such as its stem, is re-presented on a completion test, the whole item can become reactivated more easily or quickly because of the increased integration of its representation. Previously, several authors have used the word redintegration to describe this process of re-activation (Hollingworth, 1928; Horowitz and Prytulak, 1969). Rozin (1976) has suggested an analogy with the vacuum tubes in a radio; a vacuum tube takes an appreciable amount of time to become functional, but once heated up, it can become functional more quickly for some time afterwards.

In its present form, this activation view cannot accommodate priming for new items. However, it can readily be modified for this purpose. By a modified activation view, priming for old items is different from priming for new items because for old items, but not for new items, redintegrative processing occurs also during the study trial. That is, because there is a pre-existing representation in long-term memory for an old item, its processing can be accomplished by the redintegration of this representation. It has been assumed that the new memory representation for an item that is established during the study trial is a record of how the item was processed (e.g., Kolers, 1973, 1979). On this assumption, it follows that for an old item, such as the pair of strongly related words TABLE – CHAIR, the content of the pair representation that is established during the study trial is determined primarily by its pre-existing representation. Thus, because processing depends on redintegration, it is likely that similar pair representations would be constructed across different study tasks, even if they involve different levels of processing (e.g., Graf and Mandler, 1984; Graf et al., 1982; Jacoby and Dallas, 1981; Schacter, 1985). In contrast, for two unrelated words, there is no pre-existing representation whose redintegration can guide processing during the study trial and, consequently, a pair representation is constructed only if the study task requires relating paired words to each other in a meaningful manner. As a result, priming for new items depends on the nature of processing that is engaged to meet the study task requirements. However, despite this difference in how pair representations are established for old versus new items, this modified activation view of priming assumes that at the time of testing, priming for both items is mediated by the same process -- redintegration of a recently established representation.

Two major questions remain to be considered: First, why is implicit memory for new associations constant across study tasks that involve different types of degrees of elaborative processing, and second, why is implicit memory preserved in elderly individuals and in amnesic patients? The first finding suggests that similar pair representations were established across different elaborative study tasks. It is possible that this outcome was an accident due to the selection of the study tasks that were used in the experiments conducted this far. An alternative and more

interesting possibility, however, is that pair
representations remained constant across study tasks because
the content of these representations is determined primarily
by basic properties of the two words that form each pair.
That is, pair representations may be established as a result
of processing that is suggested, guided, or afforded by
properties of each pair of words and, thus, may be invariant
across a range of study task that have different performance
requirements. This view also suggests an account for the
results obtained with elderly individuals and amnesic
patients: It is possible that these individuals can show
normal priming for new associations because the elaborative
processing that is required for the construction of pair
representations is constrained or guided by properties of
the specific words in each pair. Such a view has been
proposed recently by Craik (1983) who drew a distinction
between environmentally guided processing and subject
initiated processing. By Craik's view, the latter type of
processing, which is involved in the construction of
episodic representations, is impaired in amnesic patients
and in elderly individuals because it depends more on the
availability of attentional resources and conscious
awareness than does the former type of processing.

Preparation of this manuscript was supported by Grant No.
U0299 from the Natural Sciences and Engineering Research
Council of Canada. I thank Kelly Nakamura for help in
preparing the manuscript.

REFERENCES

Barnes JM, Underwood BJ (1959). "Fate" of first-list
    associations in transfer theory. J Exp Psychol 58:97-105.
Cermak LS (1982). "Human Memory and Amnesia." Hillsdale,
    NJ: Erlbaum.
Cermak LS, Craik FIM (1979). "Levels of Processing in
    Human Memory." Hillsdale, NJ: Erlbaum.
Cohen NJ, Squire LR (1980). Preserved learning and
    retention of pattern-analyzing skill in amnesia:
    Dissociation of "knowing how" and "knowing that." Science
    210:207-209.
Craik FIM (1977). Age differences in human memory. In
    Birren JE and Schaie KW (eds), "Handbook of the Psychology
    of Aging." New York: van Nostrand Reinhold.

Craik FIM (1983). On the transfer of information from temporary to permanent memory. Phil Trans Royal Society London B302:341-359.

Diamond R, Rozin P (1984). Activation of existing memories in the amnesic syndrome. J Abnorm Psychol 93:98-105.

Eysenck MW (1979). Depth, elaboration and distinctiveness. In Cermak LS, Craik FIM (eds): "Levels of Processing in Human Memory," Hillsdale, NJ: Erlbaum.

Graf P (1982). The generation effect and a related memory phenomenon: An interpretative framework. J Verb Learn Verb Behav 21:539-548.

Graf P, Mandler G (1984). Activation makes words more accessible but not necessarily more retrievable. J Verb Learn Verb Behav 23:553-568.

Graf P, Mandler G, Haden M (1982). Simulating amnesic symptoms in normal subjects. Science 218:1243-1244.

Graf P, Schacter DL (1986). Effects of organization and concreteness on implicit and explicit memory. Paper presented at the meeting of the Psychonomic Society, New Orleans, Louisiana.

Graf P, Schacter DL (1985). Implicit and explicit memory for new associations in normal and amnesic patients. J Exp Psychol: Learning, Memory and Cognition 11:501-518.

Graf P, Schacter DL (in press). Selective effects of interference on implicit and explicit memory for new associations. J Exp Psychol: Learning, Memory and Cognition.

Graf P, Squire LR, Mandler G (1984). The information that amnesic patients do not forget. J Exp Psychol: Learning, Memory and Cognition 10:164-178.

Hinton GE, Anderson JA (1981). "Parallel Models of Associative Memory." Hillsdale, NJ: Erlbaum.

Hollingworth HL (1928). General laws of redintegration. J Gen Psychol 1:79-90.

Humphreys MS (1978). Item and relational information: A case for context independent retrieval. J Verb Learn Verb Behav 17:175-188.

Horowitz LM, Prytulak LS (1969). Redintegrative memory. Psychol Rev 84:519-531.

Jacoby LL, Craik FIM (1979). Effects of elaboration of processing at encoding and retrieval: Trace distinctiveness and recovery of initial context. In Cermak LS, Craik FIM (eds): "Levels of Processing in Human Memory," Hillsdale, NJ: Erlbaum.

Jacoby LL, Dallas M (1981). On the relationship between

autobiographical memory and perceptual learning. J Exp Psychol: General 110:306-340.

Kolers PA (1973). Remembering operations. Memory and Cognition 1:347-355.

Kolers PA (1979). A pattern-analyzing basis of recognition. In Cermak LS, Craik FIM (eds): "Levels of Processing in Human Memory," Hillsdale, NJ: Erlbaum.

Knapp A, Anderson JA (1984). A signal averaging model for concept formation. J Exp Psychol: Learning, Memory and Cognition 10:616-637.

Light LL, Anderson PA (1983). Memory for scripts in young and older adults. Memory and Cognition 11:435-444.

Mandler G (1980). Recognizing: The judgment of previous occurrence. Psychol Rev 87:252-271.

McClelland JL, Rumelhart DE (1985). Distributed memory and the representation of general and specific information. J Exp Psychol: General 114:159-188.

McGovern JB (1964). Extinction of associations in four transfer paradigms. Psychol Monogr 78 (16, Whole No. 593).

McKoon G, Ratcliff R (1979). Priming in episodic and semantic memory. J Verb Learn Verb Behav 18:463-480.

Morton J (1979). Facilitation in word recognition: Experiments causing change in the logogen model. In Kolers PA, Wrolstad ME, Bouma H (eds): "Processing of Visible Language," New York: Plenum.

Moscovitch M (1984). The sufficient conditions for demonstrating preserved memory in amnesia: A task analysis. In Squire LR, Butters N (eds): "Neuropsychology of Memory," New York: Guilford Press.

Postman L, Stark K (1969). Role of response availability in transfer and interference. J Exp Psychol 79:168-177.

Rabinowitz JC (1986). Priming in episodic memory. J Gerontol 41:204-213.

Rozin P (1976). The psychobiological approach to human memory. In Rosenzweig MR, Bennett EL (eds): "Neural Mechanisms of Learning and Memory," Cambridge, MA: M.I.T. Press.

Rumelhart DE, McClelland JL (1982). An interactive activation model of context effects in letter perception: Part 2. The contextual enhancement effect and some tests and extensions of the model. Psychol Rev 89:60-94.

Salasoo A, Shiffrin RM, Feustel TC (1985). Building permanent memory codes: Codification and repetition effects in word identification. J Exp Psychol: General 114:50-77.

Schacter DL (1985). Priming of old and new knowledge in
  amnesic patients and normal subjects. Annals New York
  Acad Sciences 444:41-53.
Schacter DL, Graf P (1986). Effects of elaborative
  processing on implicit and explicit memory for new
  associations. J Exp Psychol: Learning, Memory and
  Cognition 12:432-444.
Schacter DL, Harbluk JL, McLachlan DR (1984). Retrieval
  without recollection: An experimental analysis of source
  amnesia. J Verb Learn Verb Behav 23:593-611.
Squire LR, Shimamura AP, Graf P (1985). Independence of
  recognition memory and priming effects: A
  neuropsychological analysis. J Exp Psychol: Learning,
  Memory and Cognition 11:37-44.
Talland GA (1968). "Human Aging and Behavior," New York:
  Academic Press.
Tulving E, Schacter DL, Stark HA (1982). Priming effects in
  word-fragment completion are independent of recognition
  memory. J Exp Psychol: Learning, Memory and Cognition
  8:336-342.
Warrington EK, Weiskrantz L (1968). New method of testing
  long-term retention with special reference to amnesic
  patients. Nature 217:972-974.
Warrington EK, Weiskrantz L (1970). Amnesia: Consolidation
  or retrieval? Nature 228:628-630.
Warrington EK, Weiskrantz L (1982). Amnesia: A
  disconnection syndrome? Neuropsychologia 20:233-248.
Wechsler D (1917). A study of retention in Korsakoff
  psychosis. Psychiatric Bulletin, N.Y. State Hospital
  2:403-451.
Wickelgren WA (1979). Chunking and consolidation: A
  theoretical synthesis of semantic networks, configuring
  in conditioning, S-R versus cognitive learning, normal
  forgetting, the amnesic syndrome, and the hippocampal
  arousal system. Psychol Rev 86:44-60.

Neuroplasticity, Learning, and Memory, pages 301-325
© 1987 Alan R. Liss, Inc.

SITE FRAGILITY THEORY OF CHUNKING AND CONSOLIDATION IN A
DISTRIBUTED ASSOCIATIVE MEMORY

Wayne A. Wickelgren

Department of Psychology
University of Oregon
Eugene, OR 97403

George Miller (1956) and those who further developed
the idea of chunking as a learning process have produced a
powerful new type of associative learning that goes
substantially beyond the classical notions of associations
of ideas, extant since Aristotle. In classical associative
learning, two ideas activated contiguously in time had the
connection between them strengthened, intuitively a
horizontal association. In chunking, two ideas activated
simultaneously in the mind recruit a new internal
representative (node or nodes) to represent them and
associations are strengthened from the constituent ideas
to the new chunk idea and in the reverse direction.

Intuitively, chunking is a learned vertical
association, with hierarchical structure similar to that
found in the more genetically specified peripheral sensory
and motor systems. Chunking is an important new type of
learning for at least two reasons. First, chunking greatly
reduces associative interference, by permitting associations
to a chunk that are distinct from the associations to its
constituents. Second, chunking permits high level
representation of a complex idea that is as simple as the
representation of the more elementary constituent ideas at
their level.

In terrestrial biological minds, the mutations that
produced learning by chunking appear to be those that
produced the capacity for cognitive, as opposed to stimulus-
response, thinking. Chunking permits the minds of birds
and mammals to have mental maps or models of the world,

with mental entities representing objects and actions, not just stimuli and responses. Chunking permits us to have expectations of what our actions will accomplish, not just a strong urge to perform some response in a stimulus situation; the latter being, I believe, a fair description of the mind of a fish. I am basing these claims in part on the ideas and findings of Thorndike (1898), Tolman (1948), Bitterman (1969, 1975), and Razran (1971), but probably none of them would endorse all that I have just said concerning the difference between the minds of higher and lower vertebrates. One of my primary intellectual goals is to provide mathematical formulations of minds with and without chunking, to determine and compare the capacities of such minds more precisely.

Many of the ideas in this paper are incomplete and imprecise. Furthermore, my primary interest at present is theoretical cognitive science, not theoretical cognitive or physiological psychology. I hope some of these theoretical ideas will apply to real biological brains and the minds they make possible, and I will include a number of statements about the human mind and brain. However, my principal goal is to develop theories of possible minds, whether or not they correspond to any existing minds, though I will use what I have learned about real minds as the main stimulus for my thinking. One final warning: I will shift back and forth between statements about possible minds and statements about real minds and brains. This is ideal for theoretical exposition, so long as you remember that no careful attempt is being made in this paper to evaluate empirically any statements about real minds and brains.

CHUNKS

George Miller (1956) invented the chunk, in the context of processing and short-term memory, as a unit of coding in the mind. Although Miller noted that a great deal of learning had gone into the formation of chunks, he did not attempt to explain the learning process that formed the internal representative of a chunk, which is my focus. Miller defined a processing strategy of "recoding", which is the use of an already learned chunk to represent a sequence (order set) of smaller chunks. Although we clearly have the ability to learn ordered sets, the manner

in which orderings are represented in an associative memory
is beyond the scope of this paper. Briefly, I think that
downward (implies) associations from chunks prime the
unordered set of constituents, with the ordering of the
constituents given by horizontal (lateral) associations
among (context-sensitive) constituents (Wickelgren, 1969b,
1979b). In any case, here I am only concerned with the
unordered set of constituents of a chunk.

ASSOCIATIVE NETWORKS AND LINK TYPES

   Throughout this paper I will work within a
connectionist or network theoretical framework for
describing a mind. Specifically, a mind is a digraph
(directed graph), consisting of a set of nodes connected
by directed links (that is, the link from A to B is distinct
from the link in the reverse direction, from B to A). You
should think of the mind discussed in this paper as an
abstract model of the "association areas" of the human
cerebral cortex with some of the nodes receiving specific
sensory input (relayed through lower levels of the mind
not modelled here) and all of the nodes receiving
nonspecific arousal input from two arousal systems, the
learning arousal system and the retrieval arousal system.
Some of the nodes would output to lower levels of the mind
as well, but I am not concerned with this, and you should
assume that we can directly measure the activation output
of each node in this mind.

   Nodes in this mind are all of one type (excluding the
arousal systems, which are considered external to this
mind). In particular, there are no inhibitory nodes
analogous to inhibitory neurons. Inhibitory functions will
be modelled by inhibitory links between nodes. However,
there are several types of links. Links are classified on
four dimensions: conditionable or not, excitatory vs.
inhibitory, specific vs. nonspecific, and implies vs.
coimplies. Not all of the 16 possible link types exist,
and I will concentrate on just two types in this paper:
(a) conditionable excitatory specific implies links and
(b) conditionable excitatory specific coimplies links.
Hereafter, I will just refer to these as implies or
coimplies links, with the other adjectives understood.

   I will also make some use of two other link types,

unconditionable specific inhibitory links (referred to as inhibitory) and unconditionable nonspecific excitatory links (referred to as nonspecific), with the implies vs. coimplies dimension being irrelevant for these link types. The nonspecific links connect each node in the mind to the learning arousal system, not to each other. At a few points in the paper I will refer to another type of nonspecific link that might connect each node to the retrieval arousal system, but the properties of this system and its links to the mind are not discussed very much.

Previously, I assumed not two but three types of conditionable specific excitatory links -- up, down, and lateral (Wickelgren, 1979a). The correspondence is roughly as follows: Coimplies links will do the same job as the old up links, activating a node when the sum of the inputs from the link set that jointly coimplies the node exceeds an activation threshold. Coimplies links are for two-to-one or many-to-one associations. Implies links are for one-to-one associations and do the job of the old down links. At present, I assume that all excitatory lateral links are of the implies type, but some may be of the coimplies type.

Do not be misled by the word "implies" into assuming that if node A has an implies link to node B and A is strongly activated at time i that node B will necessarily be strongly activated at time i + 1. B will be activated above the threshold for possible inclusion in the next thought (consisting of all strongly activated nodes). However, a decision process (mediated by lateral inhibition) limits the next thought to the most strongly activated nodes within some limited attention span, and B may not make it. I am not prepared to provide a mathematical formulation of this decision process beyond this intuitive property, and indeed I will largely ignore all inhibitory links in this paper.

RANDOM CONNECTIONS AND BINARY CHUNKING

In discussing mechanisms of chunking it is helpful to deal with the concrete case of chunking two nodes A and B into a site on some chunk node, which I will here call node (AB). Such binary chunking is the simplest case, but repeated binary chunking is sufficient to chunk sets of larger size, albeit with some form of binary syntactic structure, such as ((AB)C), ((AB)(CD)), etc. There is also a strong probabilistic argument in favor of binary branching in (genetically) randomly connected associative networks where the total number of nodes is approximately the square of the average number of links per node. Throughout this paper, I will assume a concrete model with 10^8 nodes and 10^4 links per node. These exact numbers are not important, but it is important that the number of nodes in the mind is roughly the square of the number of links per node. Incidentally, the total number of neurons in the human cerebral cortex is roughly the square of the number of synapses per cortical neuron (Cragg, 1975; Pakkenberg, 1966).

Of course, we do not know that the chunking associative memory in humans is randomly connected. Part or all of it may be partitioned on the basis of the particular types of input or output connections to the more genetically specified sensory and motor modules of the mind. The transition from genetic to learned structuring of the connections of the mind may involve several steps or levels, even within chunking associative memory. Genetic guidance of chunking could easily result in the single-step chunking of sets of constituents larger than two. However, consideration of the case of binary chunking in genetically random associative networks will give us enough to chew on for the moment.

LINKS, SITES, NODES: ACTIVATION, STRENGTH, FRAGILITY

A node has a set of input sites, with each site containing a set of input links to that node. Sites will be classified into three types: (a) a single implies link, (b) two coimplies links, or (c) one specific (implies or coimplies) link and one nonspecific link to the learning arousal system. For reasons that will be discussed later, these three types are called <u>bound implies</u> sites, <u>bound coimplies</u> sites, and <u>free</u> sites, respectively. Links, sites, and nodes all have a positive real-valued <u>activation</u> property. Links also have a positive real-valued <u>strength</u> property, and sites have a positive real-valued <u>fragility</u> property, with site fragility being some monotonic increasing function of the strength of the nonspecific link to that site from the learning arousal system. Sites with no nonspecific link are really sites with a very weak nonspecific link (close to zero strength) and therefore close to zero fragility. For reasons that will be discussed later, fragility will serve as the theoretical measure of the degree of consolidation of a memory trace, with low-fragility representing high consolidation.

If node i has activation x_i and the link from node i to node j has strength z_{ij}, then link ij has activation $x_i z_{ij}$. Greater link activation produces greater site activation for the site at which the link terminates, and greater site activation produces greater node activation. I do not wish to commit myself to any particular functions summing link activation to get site activation and summing site activation to get node activation. Obviously, there are advantages to assuming as much linear combination as possible with at least one nonlinear threshold parameter at the site, node, or both.

However, in this paper, I wish to consider the possibility that the summation of two coimplies link activations in a single site produces greater node activation than if the same coimplies link activations occurred in different sites. If this nonlinear property holds and if chunking could somehow bring two coimplies links to the same site, then if links a & b were in one site and links c & d were in another site on the same node, the node would be more strongly activated by (a&b) or (c&d) than by (a&c), (a&d), (b&c) or (b&d). I call this set of assumptions the site grouping hypothesis. Site grouping permits a single node to function more like a logical conjunction unit than it could with only link strengthening as a learning mechanism. I am not convinced this is either desirable or true of the cerebral cortex, but it is worth considering.

CONTIGUITY CONDITIONING BY CROSS-CORRELATION

I make the standard assumption of contiguity conditioning of nodes (Hebb, 1949; Grossberg, 1967) that the strength of the link from node i to node j increases when the nodes are strongly activated at about the same time, more specifically when the activation of nodes i and j has a positive cross-correlation, typically with a temporal asymmetry (θ) to reflect link delay times in transmission of activation and perhaps other factors.

Grossberg (1967) expresses this very elegantly by the
equation:
$$z_{ij} = -uz_{ij} + \beta x_i (t - \theta)x_j(t),$$
where z_{ij} is the strength of the link from i to j, z_{ij} is
its time derivative (rate of change of strength, $-uz_{ij}$
represents forgetting via an exponential decay of link
strength (with which I disagree for long-term memory), and
$\beta x_i(t - \theta)x_j(t)$ represents learning due to cross-
correlation of the activation of node i at time $t - \theta$,
$x_i(t - \theta)$, and the activation of node j at time t, $x_j(t)$.

Elegant theoretical work, such as that of Grossberg,
demonstrates that there is much to be learned by careful
study of contiguity conditioning in the context of varying
assumptions about other aspects of network minds. Although
it has not been formulated mathematically, my previous
theory of chunking (Wickelgren, 1979a) describes a network
mind in which chunking, as well as conventional association
of ideas, can occur via the contiguity conditioning
learning mechanism. In the present theory, both implies
and coimplies links are assumed to be strengthened by some
cross-correlation type of contiguity conditioning.
However, as mentioned previously, changes in link strength
via contiguity conditioning may not be the only mechanism
mediating chunking. Chunking may also group two or more
coimplies links into a common site on the target node.

FREE AND BOUND SITES

Recall that I classified the sites of the mind into
three types: bound implies sites, bound coimplies sites,
and free sites. For the moment collapse the first two
types into one type. Thus, there is a partition of all of
the sites of the mind into two subsets: free and bound.
A free site has one specific link with low strength and
one nonspecific link with high strength. Activation of a
free site requires input activation of both the high
strength nonspecific link and the low strength specific
link. If a free site is consistently activated at about
the same time as its node is activated, activation of the
free site becomes a useful predictor of activation of the
entire node, and the strength of the specific link to that
free site is increased via the cross-correlation learning
mechanism. Although the nonspecific link to that site
contributed substantially to site activation, its

activation is random with respect to events to be
represented by the mind and nonspecific links are assumed
not to be strengthened by contiguity conditioning. Indeed,
when the specific link to a site is strengthened by learning,
this weakens the nonspecific link. Thus, learning is assumed
to strengthen the specific link at a site and weaken the
nonspecific link at the same site, converting it from a free
site to a bound site. Basically, the notion is that, at
birth, each node (whose links are not entirely specified
genetically) has a bunch of weak specific links to (free)
sites on other nodes. Some of these weak specific links
will prove to be predictive of activation of the nodes they
connect to, thus becoming strong specific links. The sites
with strong specific input links are said to be bound to
those links.

    The preceding paragraph only describes the process of
converting a free site to a bound site with a single
specific link, that is a 1-1 association. How do we get
the 2-1 association necessary for chunking? We get them
from having two sites activated in temporal contiguity with
activation of the target node. By the process described in
the preceding paragraph, this converts both free sites to
bound sites. Then the site grouping mechanism takes over
and collapses the two sites into a single bound site, or
perhaps the specific links of each newly bound site send
collateral links to the other newly bound site. In the two
cases, one gets either one or two bound coimplies sites.
Note that it is not necessary to assume that the specific
links of free sites are of two types, implies and coimplies.
There need be only one type of specific link to free sites.
A bound implies site results from a learning event that was
1-1. A bound coimplies site results from a learning event
that was 2-1 and the site grouping process that follows
such a learning event.

CHUNKING AND THE REVERSE LINK HYPOTHESIS

    There is undoubtedly a considerable degree of genetic
constraint on the randomness of neural connections in
animals, even in the cerebral cortex, and strong cases can
doubtless be made for many different types of nonrandomness
in the connections of minds, from a cognitive science
standpoint. However, in this paper, I will assume a mind
in which each node has specific links to a random sample of

other nodes, with one exception. The exception is the
reverse link hypothesis, that whenever node i connects to
node j, node j connects to node i. The link from i to j
may have different strength than the link from j to i, but
there is always a structural link from j to i, whenever
there is a link from i to j.

If nodes i and j connect to node k, but nodes i and j
do not connect to each other (the latter being the typical
case for the sort of mind envisioned in this paper), then
chunking i and j by binding them to node k will also
strengthen 1-1 (implies) associations from node k to node i
and from node k to node j. Thus, chunking not only
strengthens two coimplies links from the constituent nodes
to the chunk node, it also strengthens two implies links
from the chunk node to the constituent nodes. Logically,
nodes i and j together coimply node k, while node k implies
both nodes i and j. The sense of this is that node k
represents the conjunction of nodes i and j, so the
conjunction implies its constituents.

NONSPECIFIC LINKS AND THE LEARNING AROUSAL SYSTEM

There are some relatively obvious questions concerning
the mechanisms by which chunking could be accomplished in
a network mind such as the nervous system. The first
question is how do we know there is any node that receives
specific links from both A and B nodes in a genetically
random network? In my first theory of chunking (Wickelgren,
1969a), I assumed that some electrochemical gradient created
by the simultaneous activation of nodes A and B caused them
to grow links toward each other until they met, whereupon
they would link to the nearest node. Such a long distance
growth process would be difficult to engineer and is
generally deemed unlikely to occur in the adult nervous
system as a mechanism of learning.

A selectional theory of learning is far more plausible
for the human mind and more practical to engineer in an
artificial mind. One could also develop a model of
chunking in which one or more interneurons were enslaved by
the chunking process purely for the purpose of getting some
node that indirectly (via a chain of interneurons) received
input links from both A and B nodes, but I have little
interest in doing this. Furthermore, as I have argued

before (Wickelgren, 1979a), the ratio of synapses to neurons
in the human cerebral cortex is such that, while it is very
unlikely that any set of three or more neurons synapse with
a common (possible chunk) neuron, it is highly likely that
any set of two neurons do synapse on some common neuron.
In an arbitrary random network there is no guarantee of this,
but, if the ratio of links to nodes is great enough, the
probability can be made as close to one as you wish.

For two contiguously activated nodes to be chunked,
they must have their links to the chunk node strengthened.
The only link strengthening process we have assumed is
contiguity conditioning. This requires the chunk node to
be strongly activated at about the same time as the
constituent nodes are strongly activated. Since, prior to
chunking, the constituent nodes have only weak links to the
chunk node, how does the chunk node get activated? I still
like the basic mechanism described in Wickelgren (1979a) in
which a (spontaneously active) learning arousal system
provides strong nonspecific input to combine with the
converging weak specific input to the (AB) chunk node from
the constituent A and B nodes. By providing each free site
with a strong nonspecific input link to compensate for the
weak specific link, one could probably design a network
(and the mammalian cerebral cortex may be one) in which
input from two weak specific links is enough to activate
the node strongly enough to trigger contiguity conditioning.
A precise mathematical model is really important here, but
the foregoing argument is intuitively persuasive.

Furthermore, we can postulate alternation of activation
of learning vs. retrieval arousal systems, so that during
the learning phase of mental functioning (occurring several
times a second like the alpha rhythm) only free sites can
be activated (Wickelgren, 1979a). Routtenberg (1968)
presented considerable evidence to support the existence of
two such arousal systems in the human brain, a limbic
(hippocampal) arousal system and the more familiar reticular
activating system. The former could serve as the learning
arousal system and the latter the retrieval arousal system.
I no longer think it is necessary to alternate learning and
retrieval phases to permit free sites to activate their
nodes in competition with existing strong links from
constituent nodes, but it might be.

Nonspecific input would also assist the weak implies

links from the (AB) chunk node in activating the relevant
sites on the constituent A and B nodes. A positive feedback
loop is thus created between the chunk node and its
constituents, which produces a relatively long period of
paired activation of the chunk node and its constituents.
This strengthens both upward coimplies and downward implies
connections to the relevant sites by the plausible
contiguity conditioning mechanism.

FRAGILITY, CONSOLIDATION, UNLEARNING, DECAY AND AMNESIA

Although the learning event of contiguous activation
can be accomplished in a second or less and I assume that
the consequent increase in the strength of the specific
link(s) occurs almost immediately thereafter, a long-
lasting period of consolidation of this learning follows
the learning event. The consolidation consists of the
reduction in the strength of the nonspecific link(s) to
the learning arousal system at the newly bound site(s).
The nonspecific link has served its purpose of permitting
a new site to be bound via the contiguity conditioning
mechanism. Now that the site has been bound, a strong
nonspecific link would only cause more rapid forgetting
of the newly strengthened specific link. It is for this
reason that the strength of the nonspecific link is also
called the fragility of the site or, equivalently, the
fragility of the newly strengthened specific link.

Once a free site has been bound, its association to
the learning arousal system (fragility) begins to decrease,
rapidly at first, then progressively more slowly over time.
As fragility decreases, the probability of activation of
the site by the learning arousal system and other random
weak input decreases. Thus, there is less chance that the
bound site will be activated without input from the specific
link(s) it was bound to. Such uncorrelated activation is
assumed to weaken the previously strengthened specific
associations. The reduction in site fragility is, thus, a
consolidation process which protects the memory traces
(strengthened associations) from disruption by one kind of
forgetting. This forgetting results from activation of the
site without activation of the proper specific input links.
This is a kind of (backward) unlearning, but, strangely
enough, it behaves like a pure time decay process, because
the events that drive the loss of trace strength are

unrelated to the events that produced the original learning.

Furthermore, as the trace consolidates, this decay slows down over time since learning, a prediction that has been overwhelmingly confirmed (Wickelgren, 1972, 1974). Finally, although several facts concerning human memory indicate that consolidation continues for years following learning, most of the consolidation occurs within the first few hours or days following learning.

Retrograde amnesia is loss of memory for events that occurred before some insult to the brain such as concussion, electroconvulsive shock, lesions of the hippocampus, etc. The same consolidation process can be used to explain the reduced susceptibility of older memories to retrograde amnesia. The theory also accounts for why subjects with retrograde amnesia show anterograde amnesia, a reduction in ability to learn new associations, the so-called amnesic syndrome (for an explanation, see Wickelgren, 1979a). Since the amnesic syndrome seems to apply precisely to learning that might be presumed to employ new chunking (Wickelgren, 1979a), the explanation of normal chunking, normal forgetting, and both retrograde and anterograde amnesia via a common mechanism is appealing. The evidence indicates that the long-term memories that are disrupted in the amnesic syndrome are located in the cerebral cortex, but that a neural circuit involving the cortex and the hippocampus (and perhaps other structures) is critically involved in the learning and consolidation processes.

CONSOLIDATION, SITE RECYCLING, AND DENDRITIC SPINES

Apparently, virtually all excitatory synapses on mammalian cortical neurons are on dendritic spines. Thus, to apply the current theory to the mammalian cerebral cortex, let us assume that a site is a single spine or a set of nearby spines receiving one or more (specific) synapses from another cortical neuron and one or more (nonspecific) synapses from the learning arousal system. Although the nonspecific synapses start out stronger than the specific synapses at free sites, there is a sense in which the specific synapses are the genetically preferred synapses, because once the specific synapses are strengthened, this causes the nonspecific synapses to weaken at the same site. This is not all implausible, and examples of just such a process were cited in Wickelgren (1979a). It is also possible that if the nonspecific synapses are on different spines from the specific synapses, then what consolidation does is somehow to protect the newly bound specific spine from the effects caused by input to nearby nonspecific spines. There are many ways this could be done.

If a specific link becomes sufficiently weakened by forgetting, the consolidation process might reverse itself, recycling the site to the free state once more. There is also the more pessimistic version of this theory in which no site recycling is possible, and we gradually use up all of our free sites as we learn.

LEARNING AND UNLEARNING VIA CROSS-CORRELATION

Both learning and unlearning can be obtained from the cross-correlation term of Grossberg's equation for contiguity conditioning provided we change the activation terms, x_i and x_j, from absolute levels of activation to deviations in activation from some intermediate point. This permits negative contributions to link strength (unlearning) from the cross-correlation term whenever x_i is high and x_j is low (forward unlearning) and whenever x_i is low and x_j is high (backward unlearning). The effects of consolidation would then have to be reflected in a reduction of the β cross-correlation parameter. This will reduce backward unlearning, but it will also reduce both forward unlearning and further learning at the same synapse.

The reduction in further strengthening of the same synapse is not in obvious conflict with the facts since learning is definitely subject to diminishing returns, and many theorists suspect that multiple-trial learning involves trace replication at different synapses more than trace strengthening at the same synapse. However, the reduction in forward unlearning does not appear to be in accord with the facts of human learning (Wickelgren, 1974). Furthermore, it is only the kind of neurally backward unlearning produced by nonspecific activation of the postsynaptic neuron that can be assumed to diminish with consolidation, since it is only that kind of unlearning that, behaviorally, appears to be a pure time decay process (and not an unlearning process). In human forgetting, consolidation reduces the time decay factor and apparently not the unlearning factor, whether forward or backward, though the invariance of unlearning with time since original learning is a result in need of much further replication before we can be sure of it (Wickelgren, 1974). It is probably better to account for the reduction in forgetting due to time since learning (consolidation) by altering Grossberg's exponential decay term to one more in accord with the facts of long-term forgetting (Wickelgren, 1974). This is also more in accord with everyone's intuition (including Grossberg's) concerning the separation of learning and forgetting processes.

Nevertheless, it is interesting and worth remembering that modification of link strengths by cross-correlation of activation can be used to produce both forward and backward unlearning as well as learning. While I would be the last to downgrade intuitive verbal theory formulation, I am also a great admirer of mathematical theory formulation, in part because it can serve as a basis for, previously unsuspected, grand unifications of apparently disparate phenomena, such as the possible unification of learning and unlearning via the cross-correlation mechanism. Even though this particular unification may well be wrong for the mammalian brain, it is a fascinating possibility that would never have occurred to me without Grossberg's mathematical formulation of associative learning.

SITE GROUPING AND LOCAL GROWTH

This section describes a speculative neural mechanism of site grouping following learning. You may have heard the old saying about how a little knowledge is a dangerous thing. You need to be warned that I have a little knowledge of the nervous system. Also, I do not think that old saying applies to me or to anyone else who is careful to encode the degree of support for an idea and something about the nature of that support. Of course if you are one of those people to whom the old saying does apply, please skip to the next section. For those of you coming along for the ride, it is time to fasten your seatbelt.

The first question that concerns me is whether there

is any plausible neural mechanism by which constituent links that coimply a chunk node could be grouped into a common site, nearby sites, or sites with some other kind of synergism that provided a superadditive combination of their input link strengths. The purpose of such site grouping is to make a chunk node represent something closer to a conjunction of its constituents, instead of an additive combination. Of course, it may be that chunks do respond additively to constituent input in the brain. Consideration of whether there is a plausible neural mechanism for conjunctive grouping is relevant to this issue and interesting in its own right.

One possibility is that the dendritic tree might grow and contract so as to keep all free sites on a connected subtree containing no bound sites. The bound subtree would also be connected and contain no free sites. The bound subtree might be proximal to the cell body and the free subtree distal, or the main dendritic trunk might divide near the cell body into a bound subtree and a free subtree. Either way, when free sites become bound, the entire portion of the free subtree between these newly bound sites and boundary with the bound subtree contracts so as to transfer the newly bound sites to the bound subtree. If two or more sites were bound at about the same time, both would be transferred to about the same place in the bound subtree and thus might have a conjunctive-like, superadditive combination in retrieval. Once the newly bound sites were pushed onto the bound subtree, the free subtree would grow back to approximately its previous size, perhaps observing some sort of constancy in the total number of free and bound sites or just the total number of free sites. When bound links decrease in strength to some low level, the terminals might either remain on the bound subtree or grow a very short distance to reconnect to a site on the free subtree, recycling the sites.

If all of this degeneration and regrowth of the dendritic tree seems implausible, consider the possibility of local presynaptic terminal growth. When two sites are bound at about the same time, they may set up some local electrochemical gradient in the intracellular space or within the portion of the dendritic tree that connects them. This gradient might direct the growth of an axonal branch from each terminal to the vicinity of the other terminal, where it might synapse with the postsynaptic neuron in a nearby site, on the same spine perhaps or on adjacent spines.

Doubtless there are other possibilities for learned synaptic grouping that are as plausible as these or more plausible. Some sort of axonal or dendritic growth is probably required to achieve conjunctive-like superadditive site grouping, unless the entire dendritic tree of a chunk neuron is devoted to computing a single conjunction of two, three, or more synaptic inputs, with the rest of the 40,000 synapses per cortical neuron (Cragg, 1975) being wasted. However, the neural growth is of an extremely local kind that seems plausible. What is probably most exciting about such theories of site grouping is that they permit a neuron the potential to bind all of its sites in one-to-one or two-to-one combinations as desired. Furthermore, the number of remaining possible groupings of two or more free sites on a neuron degrades gracefully and minimally with increased binding of sites according to either theory. Recycling of decayed or unlearned previously bound sites and their specific links seems possible with either theory. All of this is of some importance in the distributed associative memory to be discussed next.

DISTRIBUTED ASSOCIATIVE MEMORY

Previously, I have defined chunking in the context of the specific-node ("grandmother cell") theory of coding in associative memory, once defining a chunk idea to be a single node that represented a disjunction of conjunctions of constituent nodes (Wickelgren, 1969a) and once emphasizing only the "conjunctive" aspect by defining a chunk idea to be a single node representing an unordered set of constituents (Wickelgren, 1979a). The question of this section is, "What is the representative of an idea in the mind, whether a constituent idea or a chunk idea?" Network minds offer some interesting alternative answers to this question. I will briefly describe six different classes of idea coding systems. These six systems do not exhaust the possibilities for idea representation in network minds, nor are they even mutually exclusive. The human brain makes some use of at least two of these six.

The six classes of coding systems include two nonassociative systems: (a) <u>coding by temporal pattern</u> of

activation in any single node or small set of nodes and
(b) coding by spatial pattern of activation in a small set
of nodes (like the pattern of Os and ls in a von Neuman
computer's memory registers). The human brain is known to
make some use of temporal pattern coding in the more
peripheral parts of the auditory nervous system, namely,
periodicity information in pitch perception and phase
information in localization. However, the brain converts
both of these temporal pattern codes into some kind of
"which set of neurons fire" code at higher levels, since
the temporal spiking pattern of neurons at higher levels
has no correlation with the auditory input in periodicity
and phase. Spatial and temporal pattern coding may be
used to some extent in motor control systems if there is
any truth to the coupled oscillator theory (see Gallistel,
1980, for an insightful review).

However, there is every reason to believe that higher
sensory, motor, and cognitive coding in the human mind uses
some version of one of the four following classes of
associative "which neuron fires" codes: (c) specific node
coding (the grandmother cell theory), in which activation
of a particular node represents thinking of an idea (your
grandmother, for example), (d) overlapping set coding, in
which thinking of an idea is represented by activation of
a set of nodes that will generally overlap with the
representation of different ideas (e) node activation
function coding, in which the representation of an idea is
a particular activation function defined over all of the
nodes in the mind, and (f) link activation function coding,
in which the representation of an idea is an activation
function defined over the links. Note that (e) can be
considered to be a generalization of (c) and (d), and (f)
can be considered to be a generalization of (c).

The extreme version of specific node coding in which
there is only one node for every idea is not very fault
tolerant, so one probably wants to have several similarly
linked nodes to represent each idea. As long as the set
of nodes representing one idea do not overlap with the set
of nodes representing another idea, I will classify this
as a version of specific node coding because the properties
appear to be quite similar.

Overlapping set coding is a discrete (all-or-none)
version of node activation function coding, and both can be

used to represent distributed associative memories. In
overlapping set coding, an idea is represented by a set of
nodes that generally overlaps the node sets representing
other ideas. The degree of distribution in the
representation of an idea can vary enormously within each
of these two classes. In the overlapping set coding system,
the maximum size set for representing an idea might vary
from two nodes to all of the nodes in the network. If one
defines a special "don't care" value for activation or
considers levels of activation that are close to zero to
be "don't care" values, then similar wide variability in
the degree of distribution of coding is possible in the
node activation function coding system. Distributed
memory versions of node and link activation function
coding pose fascinating conceptual problems about which I
need to think more. Overlapping set coding seemed more
tractable for my first step into the distributed
associative memory area, and so I will describe a theory
of chunking in terms of coding by overlapping sets of nodes.

I think it is of some interest that it was possible
to present most of the ideas about chunking that are in
this paper without explicit adoption of either this
distributed memory model or the specific node model.
Finally, I should note that I am not at all convinced
that human associative memory uses distributed as opposed
to specific node coding. Randomly connected associative
memories probably function better with distributed node
coding, but when there is some "genetic" guidance to
restrict the possible connections intelligently, specific
node coding may be functionally superior. I chose to
investigate chunking in a distributed memory context
mainly because I had not done so before and wanted to
become more familiar with the properties of distributed
associative memories.

DISTRIBUTED ASSOCIATIVE MEMORY VIA OVERLAPPING SET CODING

An idea is represented by a set of nodes, which I
currently imagine to vary in size from a few hundred for a
newly formed idea to around 10,000 for a highly familiar
idea. Different ideas are represented by different, but
overlapping, sets of nodes. Two constituent ideas
specify a new chunk idea when specific links from the two
sets of nodes representing the constituent ideas help

activate some free sites in a set of other nodes that will
become the set representing the chunk idea. Those links
ending on the chunk nodes are strengthened by contiguity
conditioning, binding the sites on the chunk node that they
end on. Because nodes are always connected in both
directions, the reverse, chunk to constituent, links also
get strengthened and bind their sites on the constituent
nodes. So an idea is represented by a set of nodes and
the various sites on a node represent many different ideas
that may have no conceptual relation to each other. A
node represents a random collection of ideas.

IDEA INTEGRATION IN LEARNING AND IDEA COMPLETION IN
RETRIEVAL

    Although a chunk node must receive inputs from two
weak specific links to be activated and bind its respective
input sites, nothing guarantees that these two links will
be one from one constituent idea set and one from the
other. Both may be from different nodes in the same
constituent idea set. Initially, I thought it was a
problem that the chunking mechanism of the theory would
chunk pairs of nodes that were members of the same idea
set (intrachunking) as well as chunking pairs of nodes that
were members of different idea sets (crosschunking). Then
I realized that intrachunking might serve a very useful
function, similar to Hebb's (1949) cell assemblies, that
of integrating the nodes of an idea set.

    Some definitions are useful for a precise explanation
of the role of idea integration in thinking:
(D1) A thought is a set of idea sets that are simultaneously
activated.
(D2) A initial subset is the subset of an idea set activated
by the last thought.
(D3) The completion subset is the subset of an idea set
generated asymptotically from the initial set by intraidea
links adding nodes to the activated subset of the idea set
until no further nodes can be added via intraidea links.
The completion of some initial subsets might be the entire
idea set, but the completion of other initial subsets might
be less than the entire idea set. The completion function
maps initial subsets to completion subsets.

    Of course, you should note that this is not a

completely precise model, as we need to deal with the
intra- vs. inter-idea retrieval problem, that each node will
have many strong interidea links besides those intraidea
links involved in idea integration. Indeed, these interidea
links are essential for activating the next thought, as in
Hebb's phase sequence. My current semiprecise working
hypothesis is that thinking consists of a cycle of phases
that repeats over and over. If we start the cycle with
the last thought's having activated an initial subset of
some current idea sets, then the cycle has three phases as
follows: initiation (inhibition of the last thought and
activation of the initial idea sets for the current thought),
completion (activation of the completion of some number of
these initial idea sets up to a limit set by the attention
span), and chunking (activation of new nodes, and link
strengthening to further integrate existing chunks and to
form new chunk ideas). Initiation and completion are two
phases of the retrieval process, while chunking is a
learning process.

IDEA DISCRIMINATION

Consider the following idea discrimination problem:
How big an initial subset of nodes in one idea set must be
activated (by the prior thought) to uniquely specify that
particular idea set? This form of the question demands
some further clarification. First of all, I am not
concerned with all of the complexities of the actual idea
retrieval process in this problem. For example, I am not
concerned with whether the completion of an initial set is
the entire idea set. Indeed, I am not concerned with any
aspect of the actual activation of nodes. I am asking
only about how big a subset of some particular idea set is
necessary in a logical sense to distinguish this idea set
from any other idea set encoded in the mind. That is to
say, you are to assume that there exists some number (N)
of idea sets in a particular mind, with all N idea sets
known completely by an omniscient observer. You give the
observer a subset of x nodes all of which are guaranteed
to be from one idea set, and the question is, "With what
probability (P) will the omniscient observer have enough
information to determine uniquely which set that is?"

P should be very close to unity for good idea
discrimination. That is, we want our initial set to

specify a unique idea with high probability, at least
logically, since otherwise there is no possible retrieval
mechanism that we could adjoin to this theory of idea
coding to make it work properly. Just because it seems
plenty high enough and works out conveniently, let's take
$P=.9999$ and see how big the size of the initial set X needs
to be to achieve this P for $n=10^8$ nodes in the mind, $d=10^4$
nodes/idea, and $N=10^8$ idea sets in the mind. The answer is
that $x=3$ gives $P=.9999$ that no other idea in this mind also
contains all 3 members of the initial set X! For $N=10^{12}$
ideas, x must be 4! For $N=10^{16}$, you need $x=5$. These are
very small numbers.

Since specific node (grandmother cell) coding can only
get a maximum of 10^8 ideas coded by 10^8 nodes (though $x=1$
for $P=1$), we are clearly able to realize an enormous
increase in idea coding capacity with overlapping set
encoding at a very modest cost in the logical
discriminability of ideas. Note also that the idea
discrimination capacity of overlapping set coding is so
great that there is no incentive on these grounds to use
more than two values (on or off) of node activation in
idea coding. Multiple or continuous values of node
activation may play some useful role in learning and
retrieval dynamics, but they are certainly unnecessary for
the coding of ideas in network minds.

REDUNDANCY, DIMINISHING RETURNS, AND SPACING EFFECTS IN
CHUNKING

With overlapping set coding, when constituents A and B
are chunked, sites on more than one chunk node are assumed
to have their input associations for A and B strengthened,
so that the AB idea is represented by a set of nodes.
Subsequent experience with the AB pair is presumed to
result in associating A and B to more chunk sites,
enriching the redundancy of representation of the AB idea.
However, while it doubtless makes sense to have more
frequently used ideas represented by larger sets, it is
probably not useful to add chunk sites in direct
proportion to the learning time or the number of learning
trials. Furthermore, we know that, by virtually any
commonly used measure of memory strength, the rate of
learning eventually slows down as a function of trials
or time--the law of diminishing returns in overlearning.

Indeed, although there is a variable period of time after
exposure to material before a person settles on an encoding
and gets that first huge learning increment, which I
presume to reflect the initial chunking, after that initial
chunking, the rate of further chunking appear to decrease
monotonically as strength increases. Of course, after some
time elapses, there is a reduction in the strength of
chunking due to forgetting, which permits a greater amount
of chunking to occur after a longer spacing interval between
learning trials (see Wickelgren, 1981, p.39-40 for a brief
review). This greater amount of learning (here presumed
to be chunking) after greater spacing between learning
trials usually more than compensates for the greater
amount of forgetting that also occurs, producing the
familiar benefits of spaced over massed practice.

By what mechanism might the rate of chunking be reduced
with increasing total strength of association from A and B
to AB chunk sites? Assume that the familiar lateral
inhibition mechanism constrains the total sum of
activation of all nodes, as in Milner (1957)--perhaps some
kind of conservation of activation law or in any case an
upper bound on total activation. Chunking might occur when
the active A and B nodes are less strongly associated to
each other via chunk nodes and thus not as strongly
activated as they would be if they were more strongly
chunked. When the A and B nodes are less strongly
activated and there are fewer AB chunk nodes activated,
there is less total activation, less lateral inhibition,
and thus more chance for new AB chunk sites and nodes to
become activated. As the number of AB chunk nodes
increases, this probability of activating and thereby
specifying, new AB chunk sites goes down, producing the
diminishing returns in chunking. Since recently chunked
AB sites are strongly linked to both A and B nodes and to
the learning arousal system, such recently chunked AB nodes
might be hyperactive, further reducing the probability of
new chunking. This provides an even greater benefit to
the spacing of learning trials in that spacing allows both
consolidation and forgetting to occur. Please note that
this is a quantitative argument that requires more than
verbal logic for adequate demonstration, and the present
argument is hardly more than superficial handwaving.
This is only the germ of an idea. Some of us are easily
infected by idea germs.

HIERARCHICAL LEARNING SUCH AS MATHEMATICS

In shallow learning, we chunk unrelated AB, CD, EF, etc. pairs. In deep learning, such as mathematics, we may chunk AB, then (AB)C, then ((AB)C)D, and so on sometimes to great depth. Though the AB chunk may have a strong trace immediately after initial learning, the hyperactivity of the recently chunked AB nodes may limit additional chunking, such as (AB)C, that uses AB as a constituent. The explanation is the same as for the spacing effect in further learning of AB. Although substantial forgetting of an AB chunk occurs from one session to the next, requiring time in review, such spacing may be optimal for new chunking that builds on the AB chunk. In addition, such review benefits the learning and retention of AB.

Of course, it is dangerous to prescribe educational practice from even a well-verified theory. Subject to that warning, the present theory suggests that there might be advantages in mathematics teaching to increasing the number of different topics covered in one session and restricting the depth of learning about each topic, reviewing each topic and adding another layer of learning in the next session. Since review takes time, this undoubtedly means that a smaller number of concepts and propositions could be covered in a term, but those that were presented might be vastly better learned and remembered in subsequent terms. Of course, this one-layer-at-a-time approach is more disorganized within a single session than presenting layer after layer of definitions, lemmas, and propositions, culminating in some beautiful theorem, in one continuous stretch of time. But the beautiful view from the top of the mountain is missed if one gets lost on the way up, and that happens all too frequently. Following the one-layer-at-a-time approach, it might take a few more days to get to the first beautiful view, but, except for the time lost to review, the number of beautiful views need not be drastically reduced, and the number of students getting the views might be increased.

The prediction that spacing between AB learning and (AB)C learning will be beneficial is novel, and, to my knowledge, there is no relevant experimental evidence. However, it agrees with my intuition that you cannot cram mathematics learning into as short a time as you can

shallower subjects. Spaced study may be even more
important to hierarchically deep learning than to shallow
learning, though students of any subject should be told to
to study at least a little every day, because crammed
knowledge is poorly learned and quickly forgotten. In
learning, it is wise to revere the turtle.

REFERENCES

Bitterman ME (1969). Thorndike and the problem of animal
   intelligence. Amer Psychol 24:444-453.
Bitterman ME (1975). The comparative analysis of learning.
   Science 188:699-709.
Cragg BG (1975). The density of synapses and neurons in
   normal, mentally defective, and aging human brains.
   Brain 98:81-90.
Gallistel CR (1980). "The Organization of Action: A New
   Synthesis." Hillsdale, NJ: Erlbaum, p 432.
Grossberg S (1967). Nonlinear difference-differential
   equations in prediction and learning theory. Proc Natl
   Acad Sci USA 58:1329-1334.
Hebb DO (1949). "The Organization of Behavior." New York:
   Wiley, p 335.
Miller GA (1956). The magical number seven, plus or minus
   two: some limits on our capacity for processing
   information. Psychol Rev 63:81-97.
Milner PM (1957). The cell assembly: Mark II. Psychol
   Rev 64:242-252.
Pakkenberg H (1966). The number of nerve cells in the
   cerebral cortex of man. J Comp Neurol 128:17-20.
Razran G (1971). "Mind in Evolution." Boston: Houghton
   Mifflin, p 430.
Routtenberg A (1968). The two-arousal hypothesis:
   Reticular formation and limbic system. Psychol Rev 75:
   51-80.
Thorndike EL (1898). Animal intelligence: An experimental
   study of the associative process in animals. Psychol Rev
   Monograph Supplements 2 (No. 8).
Tolman EC (1948). Cognitive maps in rats and men. Psychol
   Rev 55:189-208.
Wickelgren WA (1969a). Learned specification of concept
   neurons. Bull Math Biophysics 31:123-142.
Wickelgren WA (1969b). Context-sensitive coding,
   associative memory, and serial order in (speech)
   behavior. Psychol Rev 76:1-15.

Wickelgren WA (1972). Trace resistance and the decay of long-term memory. J Math Psychol 9:418-455.

Wickelgren WA (1974). Single-trace fragility theory of memory dynamics. Memory & Cognition 2:775-780.

Wickelgren WA (1976). Network strength theory of storage and retrieval dynamics. Psychol Rev 83:466-478.

Wickelgren WA (1979a). Chunking and consolidation: a theoretical synthesis of semantic networks, configuring in conditioning, S-R versus cognitive learning, normal forgetting, the amnesic syndrome, and the hippocampal arousal system. Psych Rev 86:44-60.

Wickelgren WA (1979b). "Cognitive Psychology." Englewood Cliffs, NJ: Prentice-Hall, p 436.

Wickelgren WA (1981). Human learning and memory. Annual Rev Psychol 32:21-52.

Index